DAVID P. LANE
CANCER RESEARCH CAMPAIGN
EUKARYOTIC MOLECULAR GENETICS GROUP
DEPARTMENT OF BIOCHEMISTRY
IMPERIAL COLLEGE OF SCIENCE & TECHNOLOGY
LONDON SW7 2AZ

DAVID P. LANE
CANCER RESEARCH CAMPAIGN
EUKARYOTIC MOLECULAR GENETICS GROUP
DEPARTMENT OF BIOCHEMISTRY
IMPERIAL COLLEGE OF SCIENCE & TECHNOLOGY
LONDON SW7 2AZ

ADVANCES IN VIRAL ONCOLOGY

Volume 3

Advances in Viral Oncology
Volume 3

DNA-Virus Oncogenes and Their Action

Editor

George Klein, M.D., D. Sc.
Department of Tumor Biology
Karolinska Institutet
Stockholm, Sweden

Raven Press ■ New York

Raven Press, 1140 Avenue of the Americas, New York, New York 10036

Library of Congress Cataloging in Publication Data
Main entry under title:

DNA-virus oncogenes and their action.

(Advances in viral oncology ; v. 3)
Includes bibliographical references and index.
1. Oncogenic viruses.   2. Viruses, DNA.   3. Cell
transformation.   I. Klein, George, 1925–
II. Series.   [DNLM: 1. DNA tumor viruses.   W1 AD888 v.3 /
QW 166 D629]
QR201.T84D58   1983   616.99′40194   83-9623
ISBN 0-89004-824-X

Made in the United States of America

The material contained in this volume was submitted as previously unpublished material, except in the instances in which credit has been given to the source from which some of the illustrative material was derived.

Great care has been taken to maintain the accuracy of the information contained in the volume. However, Raven Press cannot be held responsible for errors or for any consequences arising from the use of the information contained herein.

Preface

The first volume of this series dealt with the retrovirally transmitted oncogenes. Originally, these oncogenes were thought of as viral genes. Eventually, they became unveiled as cellular genes, acquired by the virus through a process of illegitimate recombination. For the virus, they represent an unnecessary burden, in the best case, but more usually result in a crippling replacement of an important viral gene, with defectivity as the result.

The present volume deals with the second oncoviral kingdom, the DNA tumor viruses. They represent the last citadel of the original viral oncogene concept. In all probability, they will remain in that position. Unlike the RNA viruses that are all members of the same closely related family, the DNA tumor viruses fall into three very different categories, ranging from the small papovaviruses, through the medium sized adeno- and to the large herpesviruses. As a further contrast against the retroviruses, their productive cycle is incompatible with cell growth and survival. Transformation can therefore only take place in non-productively infected cells. In spite of the great diversity among the oncogenic DNA viruses, they all appear to have one common property: latently infected, transformed cells all express a nuclear antigen that binds to DNA, whereas none of the retroviral transformants do so.

Due to the incompatibility between the productive viral cycle and cell survival, it is not surprising that all DNA tumor viruses show exclusive horizontal transmission, in contrast to the frequent vertical transmission among some of their retroviral counterparts. This has important consequences for their epidemiology and immunology. Some of the ubiquitous highly transforming DNA tumor virus systems provide the best examples of host immune surveillance against virally transformed cells.

The high selective impact of the long symbiosis between viruses like polyoma or EBV and their natural host is no doubt responsible for this.

This volume reviews some of the many advances in this vast area of research, without any claim of completeness. The small papovaviruses are examined in the first three chapters from the biochemical and structural points of view. The transforming action of the middle-sized adenoviruses is the subject of the fourth chapter. A major portion of this book is devoted to the large herpesviruses. These chapters reflect the rapid recent progress in this previously unexplored field. One of them, Epstein-Barr virus, and the "newcomer" of the last chapter, hepatitis B-virus, are the best candidates among the DNA-tumor viruses as causative or contributing agents in the origin of some human neoplasms.

This book is written for the specialist in cancer research and/or viral oncology who wishes to be informed about the recent developments in this area.

George Klein

Acknowledgments

I would like to express my thanks to all authors for their painstaking work.

George Klein

Contents

3   The Biochemical Basis of Transformation by Polyoma Virus
Alan E. Smith and Barry K. Ely

31   Structure and Function of the Simian Virus 40 Large T-Antigen
Peter W.J. Rigby and David P. Lane

59   Structure and Function of Papillomavirus Genomes
Olivier Danos and Moshe Yaniv

83   Molecular Biology of Adenovirus Transformation
Ulf Pettersson and Göran Akusjärvi

133   Epstein-Barr Virus Transformation and Replication
Elliott Kieff, Timothy Dambaugh, Mary Hummel, and Mark Heller

183   Epstein-Barr Virus Transformation: Biological and Functional
Aspects
Jesper Zeuthen

213   Esptein-Barr Virus-Induced Transformation: Immunological Aspects
A.B. Rickinson and D.J. Moss

239   Transcription Patterns in HSV Infections
Edward K. Wagner

271   Biochemical Aspects of Transformation by Herpes Simplex Viruses
Gary S. Hayward and Gregory R. Reyes

307   Oncogenic Transformation by *Herpesvirus saimiri*
Ronald C. Desrosiers and Bernhard Fleckenstein

325   Hepatitis B Virus and Primary Hepatocellular Carcinoma
W. Thomas London

343   *Subject Index*

Contributors

Göran Akusjärvi
Department of Medical Genetics
The Biomedical Center
S-751 23 Uppsala, Sweden

Timothy Dambaugh
Division of Biological Sciences
The University of Chicago
Chicago, Illinois 60637

Olivier Danos
Tumor Viruses Unit
Department of Molecular Biology
Institut Pasteur
25, rue du Dr. Roux
75724 Paris, Cedex 15, France

Ronald C. Desrosiers
New England Regional Primate
* Research Center*
Harvard Medical School
Southborough, Massachusetts 01772

Barry K. Ely
Biochemistry Division
National Institute for Medical Research
Mill Hill
London NW7 1AA, United Kingdom

Bernhard Fleckenstein
Institut für Klinische Virologie
University of Erlangen-Nürnberg
Loschgestrasse 7
D8520 Erlangen
Federal Republic of Germany

Gary S. Hayward
Department of Pharmacology and
* Experimental Therapeutics*
Johns Hopkins University School of
* Medicine*
Baltimore, Maryland 21205

Mark Heller
Division of Biological Sciences
The University of Chicago
Chicago, Illinois 60637

Mary Hummel
Division of Biological Sciences
The University of Chicago
Chicago, Illinois 60637

Elliott Kieff
Division of Biological Sciences
The University of Chicago
Chicago, Illinois 60637

David P. Lane
Cancer Research Campaign
Eukaryotic Molecular Genetics
* Research Group*
Department of Biochemistry
Imperial College of Science and
* Technology*
London SW7 2AZ, United Kingdom

W. Thomas London
Institute for Cancer Research
Philadelphia, Pennsylvania 19111

D. J. Moss
Queensland Institute of Medical
* Research*
Bramston Terrace
Herston, Queensland 4006, Australia

Ulf Pettersson
Department of Medical Genetics
The Biomedical Center
S-751 23 Uppsala, Sweden

Gregory R. Reyes
Department of Pharmacology and
* Experimental Therapeutics*
Johns Hopkins University School of
* Medicine*
Baltimore, Maryland 21205

A. B. Rickinson
Department of Pathology
The Medical School
University of Bristol
Bristol BS8 1TD United Kingdom

Peter W. J. Rigby
Cancer Research Campaign
Eukaryotic Molecular Genetics
Research Group
Department of Biochemistry
Imperial College of Science and
Technology
London SW7 2AZ, United Kingdom

Alan E. Smith
Biochemistry Division
National Institute for Medical
Research
Mill Hill
London NW7 1AA, United Kingdom

Edward K. Wagner
Department of Molecular Biology
and Biochemistry
University of California, Irvine
Irvine, California 92717

Moshe Yaniv
Tumor Viruses Unit
Department of Molecular Biology
Institut Pasteur
25, rue du Dr. Roux
75724 Paris, Cedex 15, France

Jesper Zeuthen
Institute of Human Genetics
The Bartholin Building
University of Aarhus
DK-8000 Aarhus C, Denmark

DNA-Virus Oncogenes
and Their Action

Advances in Viral Oncology, Volume 3, edited by
George Klein. Raven Press, New York © 1983.

The Biochemical Basis of Transformation by Polyoma Virus

Alan E. Smith and Barry K. Ely

*Biochemistry Division, National Institute for Medical Research,
Mill Hill, London NW7 1AA, United Kingdom*

Polyoma virus has two outstanding characteristics: It has a very small genome, and it causes tumors when injected into susceptible animals. The virus also has the ability to transform the growth properties of certain cells to a state of uncontrolled proliferation. Because the transformation of cells is probably analogous to some stages of tumor formation and is amenable to detailed analysis in the laboratory, polyoma virus has been studied intensively in the recent past. The simplicity of the virus means that a detailed description of the mechanism of viral transformation should be possible within the foreseeable future, and such an understanding should lead to new insights into tumorigenicity. Furthermore, because it is likely that in bringing about transformation the virus interacts with or mimics cellular regulatory elements, knowledge of this process may also lead to better understanding of normal cellular regulation.

The bulk of this review concentrates on the biochemical basis of transformation by polyoma virus. Work in this area addresses two broad questions: Which component of the virus has the ability to transform? What is the biochemical basis of its activity? Recent advances in our knowledge of the molecular biology of polyoma virus, and particularly use of the methods of recombinant DNA technology, have led to rapid progress in answering the first question. We now know that transformation by polyoma virus results from the integration and expression of viral DNA sequences and that the minimal sequences required to transform Rat-1 cells code for a single viral transforming protein called middle T antigen. By contrast, studies to establish the biochemical basis of the action of middle T antigen are less advanced, and so far we do not know how it functions.

The results presented here are highly selective, and they concentrate largely on middle T antigen as a transforming protein. For example, because the structures of polyoma virus DNA and mRNAs are not considered to be directly related to the biochemistry of transformation, these topics are largely omitted. Similarly, where recent experiments have proved unambiguous, we have ignored earlier data that proved difficult to interpret. We also omit a detailed description of the biology of polyoma virus transformation. For more extensive reviews of the molecular biology of polyoma virus and more comprehensive historical treatments of transformation, readers are referred to recent publications (21,29,45,60,99,104). A large amount of related work is also reported in the 1979 Cold Spring Harbor symposium on viral oncogenes.

GENOMIC ORGANIZATION OF POLYOMA VIRUS

The polyoma virus genome consists of a double-stranded circular molecule of DNA. The entire nucleotide sequence has been determined (16,94). The physical map of the viral DNA, the location of protein coding sequences, and other important features are shown schematically in Fig. 1. The site from which bidirectional DNA replication begins is called the origin (O_R) and is located near the junction of the *Hpa*II-3 and *Hpa*II-5 restriction enzyme fragments. The unique *Eco*RI restriction enzyme site is taken as map position zero, and the genome is divided clockwise into 100 map units (29,99).

The genome is most conveniently considered as two halves. The half extending clockwise from the origin is called the early region, because it is expressed early in the productive infection cycle, prior to the onset of viral DNA replication. The other half of the genome is called the late region, and this is transcribed after DNA replication.

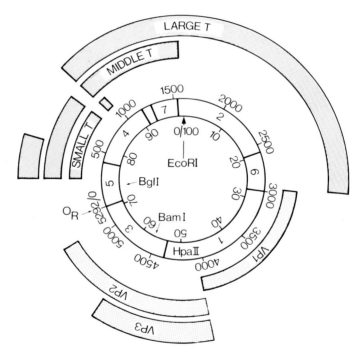

FIG. 1. Physical map of polyoma virus DNA. The figure shows the positions of cleavages by restriction enzymes *Hpa*II, *Eco*RI, *Bgl*I, and *Bam*I, the origin of DNA replication (O_R), and the locations of the sequences coding for the early *(heavy stippling)* and late *(light stippling)* proteins. The scales given are map units *(inner circle)* and nucleotide numbers *(outer circle)*.

mRNAs and Proteins

The late region of polyoma virus codes for the three structural proteins of the virus. The proteins themselves and the mRNAs that encode them have been characterized in detail (99), but because these are not involved in transformation, they will not be considered further.

The T antigens of the virus are defined as those proteins, present in transformed or tumor cells, that react with antiserum from animals bearing virus-transformed or tumor cells (anti-T serum). The tumor antigens were first detected by immunofluorescence and complement fixation. When they were analyzed by immunoprecipitation followed by SDS gel electrophoresis, three major species were detected (Fig. 2). These are referred to as large T, middle T, and small T, and they have

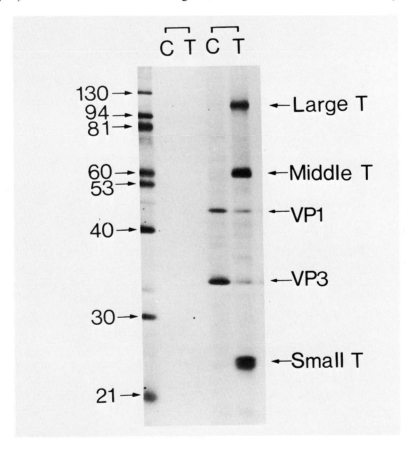

FIG. 2. Polyoma virus tumor antigens. ³⁵S-methionine-labeled extracts of uninfected **(left)** and infected 3T6 cells **(right)** were reacted with control (C) or rat anti-T serum (T). Immunocomplexes were collected by adsorption to protein-A-bearing bacteria, separated on a 15% polyacrylamide gel, and autoradiographed. Molecular weight markers are indicated (×10⁻³) in the left-hand track.

molecular weights of approximately 100,000, 55,000, and 22,000, respectively (42,47,79). The total molecular weight of the three proteins appeared to exceed the coding capacity of the early region of polyoma virus, and this suggested that they might be virus-induced cellular proteins rather than virus-coded. However, this interpretation was shown to be incorrect when it was established that the primary transcript of the early region of polyoma virus is spliced in three alternative ways. The detailed structures of the three major early mRNAs, including several alternative cap sites, the splice junctions, and the poly(A) addition site, have been established at the nucleotide level (99,101).

The structures of the three early proteins have also been shown to be consistent with the splicing model (Fig. 3). Thus, large T, middle T, and small T share a number of peptides that originate from the amino terminus; middle T and small T share additional peptides that are absent from large T; and middle T and large T have additional unique peptides from the carboxy-terminal ends of the two proteins (40,42,86). Perhaps the most striking feature of the arrangement of early genes is that the sequences between 86 and 99 map units are read in two alternative reading frames to give the unique carboxy-terminal half of middle T and a portion of large T.

Viral Mutants

A large number of polyoma virus early region mutants are now available. They can be classified in three broad groups, each of which maps to a different region of the genome (Fig. 3).

All the temperature-sensitive mutants of polyoma virus that affect early functions so far fall into one complementation group (called ts-a mutants) mapping in a restricted area of the sequences coding for the carboxy terminus of large T (20,26,28,29). Mutants of this class were mostly selected as being temperature-sensitive for replication. At the nonpermissive temperature, such mutants fail to synthesize viral DNA and overproduce early mRNAs and proteins (10,47).

Host-range-transformation (hr-t) mutants were originally isolated by using a screening procedure designed to identify transformation-defective mutants (4). Mutated viruses were screened for the ability to grow on virally transformed cells but not on untransformed cells. The various mutants isolated by this procedure belong to a single complementation group, and all are defective in replication in certain cells as well as in transformation. Marker rescue experiments and sequence analysis have shown that the lesion is usually, though not always, a small deletion and that it maps to a region of the early region between 78 and 84 map units (7,25,37,95). These sequences are shared by small T and middle T but are removed from the large T mRNA by splicing. The hr-t lesion sometimes affects the efficiency of splicing and results in synthesis of very small amounts of the mRNAs for small T and middle T. In other cases the proteins are produced, but in a truncated or an altered form (79,83). Because all hr-t mutants are competent to replicate in some cell lines, they provide evidence to show that middle T and small T are not essential for replicative growth of polyoma virus.

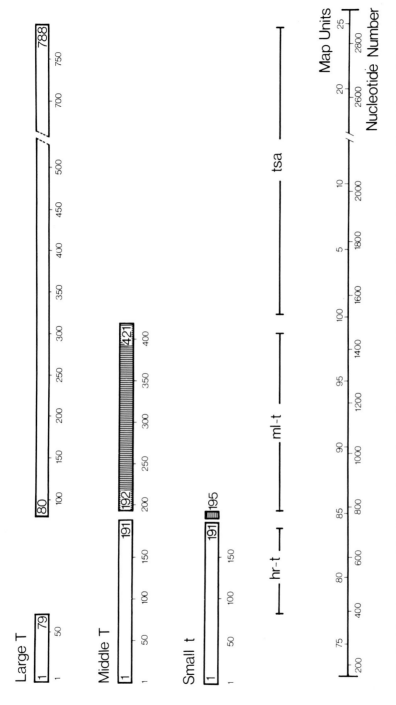

FIG. 3. The structures of the three polyoma virus early proteins and the locations of lesions defining hr-t, ml-t, and ts-a mutations. The approximate locations of the sequences coding for large T, middle T, and small T are shown relative to the scale given in map units and nucleotide numbers. The amino acid numbers are given, and the vertical hatching and horizontal hatching indicate sequences unique to middle T and small T, respectively.

Another broad group of mutants has been isolated that map to the region between 87 and 99 map units, the sequences shared between middle T and large T (3,34,59). Such mutants were largely constructed by manipulation of isolated viral DNA and were selected as being replication-competent. There is no single phenotype for mutants of this class, and we refer to them as ml-t mutants because they code for truncated versions of middle T and large T.

The methods of site-directed and site-specific mutagenesis are being used increasingly to generate precisely engineered mutant forms of the early proteins. Such mutants are referred to at the relevant places in the text.

Comparison with Simian Virus 40

The genetic organization of polyoma virus is very similar to that of simian virus 40 (SV40). If the circular map of each viral DNA is linearized at the origin, the positions of early and late functions and the relative positions of several classes of mutants coincide (29). Despite their similarities, however, there are significant differences between the two early regions. SV40 codes for only two proteins, large T and small T, and there is no SV40 counterpart to polyoma virus middle T (14,91). Thus, although there is significant homology between the predicted amino acid sequences of large T and small T, there is no SV40 equivalent to the sequences between 86 and 99 map units on the polyoma virus genome (30,93). This corresponds to the region encoding the unique carboxy-terminal region of middle T.

Recent analysis has also indicated that there are differences between cells transformed by polyoma virus and by SV40; in general, the polyoma-virus-transformed cells appear more transformed than their SV40 counterparts (68). It appears, therefore, that the resemblances between the genome organizations and replicative functions of polyoma virus and SV40 do not extend to their mechanisms of transformation.

PROPERTIES OF TRANSFORMED CELLS

Polyoma virus replicates in permissive mouse cells. The infection cycle consists of the early phase, when the viral early region is expressed, and the late phase, when the capsid proteins and progeny virions are produced. The transition between the two phases occurs following an increase in cellular DNA synthesis and the onset of viral DNA synthesis. In nonpermissive or semipermissive cells, such as rat or hamster, the virus does not replicate. In this case many of the infected cells go through some of the stages of early productive infection; for example, cellular DNA synthesis is stimulated, and changes in morphology occur. Such cells are said to be abortively infected or abortively transformed (96). The phenomenon is only transient, and most cells revert back to normal. A small proportion of nonpermissive cells become stably altered, and these are referred to as transformed.

Transformed cells are isolated by one of several methods. These select for cells that can grow under conditions where their untransformed parents fail to grow. For example, the ability to grow in low concentrations of serum, to grow as a focus of cells above a monolayer of normal cells, or to grow in semisolid medium are all used routinely. When a transformed cell is selected by one of these methods and subsequently examined using another of the selection techniques, it does not necessarily follow that it will behave as if transformed. For example, a cell selected as transformed by the ability to grow as a focus of cells over a monolayer may not have the ability to grow efficiently in soft agar (99).

In addition to the selection procedure, many other factors influence transformation. For example, the growth conditions of the cells undergoing transformation are crucial; the type of serum used and the degree of confluence can influence both the efficiency and the quality of transformation (6,61,73,85). Major differences in the transforming properties of polyoma virus are observed, depending on the cell types used (72,102). Thus, it cannot be assumed that results obtained with one cell line necessarily apply to a similar cell line of the same species. Presumably some cell lines produce constitutively some of the factors required for transformation, whereas others require the virus to code for or to stimulate the production of such factors. Any description of the process of transformation must therefore recognize the multiple alternative phenotypes of cells that fall into this category and accommodate the different results obtained using closely related cell lines.

These comments notwithstanding, transformed cells differ, in general, from their untransformed parents in a number of biological and biochemical properties (60,99). Rather than attempt to list all these properties, it is perhaps more useful to attempt to place them in different categories that may aid subsequent attempts to understand their biochemical bases.

Transformed cells differ from their parents in a number of properties that reflect the method used to select them and that provide the definition of transformation. They differ in terms of morphology, growth characteristics, and, most important, the ability to form tumors. Such cells tend to be more rounded, to grow in a more disordered array, and not to be subject to density regulation of growth in monolayers. They grow to high density before growth ceases, and their growth is not anchorage-dependent. Some reports have claimed that there is a hierarchy in some of these properties, and cells usually are not considered to be fully transformed unless they have the ability to grow in soft agar and to form tumors in animals (69).

In general, transformed cells differ from their untransformed parents in a number of other somewhat ill-defined characteristics that probably result from or reflect the changes mentioned earlier. Thus, their shape tends to be different, the cytoskeleton is more disordered and has fewer stress fibers (particularly actin cables), and elements of the extracellular matrix (for example, fibronectin) are sometimes disrupted. Transformed cells excrete plasminogen activator and transforming factors, they have a low threshold for growth and serum factors, and when grown in parallel with normal cells their proliferation rate is more rapid (99).

Many biochemical activities are also altered in polyoma-virus-transformed cells (60). In general, the rates of macromolecular synthesis are elevated. Reflecting this, the activity of a large number of enzymes is high. For example, the activity of enzymes that catalyze the synthesis of nucleotide precursors is enhanced, presumably to meet the increased demand for DNA synthesis. Similarly, a number of changes can be measured in membrane and transport properties; for example, the rates of entry of amino acids, sugars, and ions are all enhanced. Many of these biochemical changes can be considered to be related to and dependent on one another. They parallel the overall increase in the rate of cellular proliferation.

Many of the biological and biochemical changes described are not unique to transformed cells. They can occur, for instance, at certain stages during the normal cell cycle or following stimulation of cells with hormones or growth factors. Furthermore, it is quite possible that changes in one of the characteristics may inevitably lead to changes in others. For example, there is evidence that changing the shape of the cell (27) or disrupting the cytoskeleton will lead to an alteration in the rate of DNA synthesis (15). The major aim of much of the research on the cellular biology of transformation is to identify those altered properties of transformed cells that are central to the transformation process, those that are merely an inevitable consequence of the altered metabolic activity of the cell, and those that are virtually irrelevant. Research into the biochemistry of transformation seeks to describe in molecular terms the events that trigger the initial steps of the process and to define precisely the resulting cascade of biochemical and biological changes.

VIRAL GENES ASSOCIATED WITH POLYOMA VIRUS TRANSFORMATION

Experiments with the first ts-a mutants of polyoma virus showed that the initiation of transformation by the mutants was temperature-sensitive. Other early studies showed that polyoma virus DNA is stably associated with the chromosomal DNA of transformed cells. Furthermore, the tumor antigens were expressed in such cells, as well as early in the productive infection cycle, whereas the coat proteins were not expressed. Similarly, mRNA corresponding to transcripts of the early region could be detected. All these data supported the view that continued expression of at least part of the early region of polyoma virus was necessary to initiate and maintain the transformed state. This suggested a model predicting that the early proteins themselves brought about transformation. Subsequent experiments have established that this conclusion is correct and that the ability to transform is largely associated with middle T antigen.

Middle T Antigen is a Transforming Protein

When extracts of polyoma-virus-transformed cells are immunoprecipitated with anti-tumor-cell serum, middle T and small T are almost invariably detected. By contrast, full-size large T is seldom found (42,48). This result argues that the continued presence of full-size large T is unnecessary for maintenance of transformation. Analysis of the mRNA present in transformed cells had already shown that the early transcripts were less than full length, but the significance of this result was not appreciated at the time (50).

Consistent with the protein data, detailed analysis of the viral DNA integrated into the host cell chromosome showed that the early sequences were often truncated or interrupted within the sequences coding for the carboxy-terminal region of large T (5,17,52). At least one complete copy of the sequences coding for middle T was invariably found. These results imply that the integrated viral genome will be incapable of synthesizing full-size large T, but that middle T and small T can be made.

Transformation studies using mutants with lesions mapping at different positions in the early region support the view that middle T is associated with the maintenance of transformation. The ts-a mutants, which all map in the distal portion of the early region coding for the unique sequences of large T, are able to give rise to transformation at low temperature, but in the majority of cases the resulting transformants remain transformed on shift-up (28,73). The hr-t mutants, which map in the region shared by middle T and small T and mostly result in the synthesis of reduced amounts of truncated versions of the two proteins, are defective in transformation (4,83). Because these mutants are capable of synthesizing normal amounts of large T, the continued presence of this protein is insufficient to bring about transformation. Indeed, in other experiments a cell line containing integrated hr-t mutant DNA was isolated. This cell line (called 18.37) expresses normal large T, but does not have a transformed phenotype (53). Because the 18.37 cell line contains some free polyoma virus DNA, it was argued that the large T is functional, at least in excision, and yet unable to transform.

The more recently isolated ml-t mutants with deletions in the region shared by middle T and large T that code for shortened versions of the two proteins also have altered transformation properties. In some cases the mutants are less effective than wild-type virus, whereas in others they are more effective (3,34,49,59). Mutants of this class are all capable of synthesizing normal amounts of small T. Together, the results using the three classes of mutants indicate that large T and small T are incapable of transformation and imply that middle T has this activity.

Fragments purified from restriction enzyme digests of polyoma virus DNA, or from bacterial plasmids containing cloned viral DNA sequences, have been used to establish the minimal sequence requirement for transformation following transfection of the DNA into Rat-1 cells. These studies showed that fragments of early region DNA containing all the sequences necessary for expression of middle T and small T, but lacking sequences coding for the carboxy-terminal half of large T, are capable of transforming cells (36,66). Such fragments of DNA are also capable of causing tumors when injected into animals (64). These experiments not only demonstrate, like those described earlier, that the minimal requirement includes sequences coding for middle T and small T but also show that the requirement for full-size large T in the initiation of transformation can be bypassed when using DNA as the transforming agent.

All the experiments described here suffer from the complication that the sequences encoding middle T give rise not only to middle T itself but also, by the operation of alternative splices, to small T and part of large T. This makes it difficult to deduce unequivocally the properties of the different proteins. This problem was overcome by cloning a cDNA copy of the sequences spanning the different splices in the early transcripts and using this to construct DNA sequences coding individually for each of the early proteins without the need for splicing. When these were used to transfect cells, the DNA coding for middle T only was able to transform Rat-1 cells to a state that gave rise to colonies in soft agar and to tumors in animals (102). Surprisingly, the transcripts of the middle-T-only plasmid were able to function without the need for splicing elsewhere in the molecule. The major alternative splices to generate large T and small T are not possible because the relevant acceptor and/or donor sites are not present in the cloned sequences, and this result establishes unequivocally that the sequences coding for middle T alone have the ability to transform Rat-1 cells. It seems reasonable to conclude that middle T is a transforming protein.

Large T Antigen Plays a Role in the Initiation of Transformation by Virus and Induces a Measurable Phenotype

Experiments using ts-a mutants of polyoma virus have implied that large T has a role in the initiation of transformation by virus (28). Analysis of the integrated DNA present in polyoma-virus-transformed rodent cells has shown that the viral DNA is often arranged as at least a partial tandem head-to-tail repeat (5,17,52). This has been interpreted to mean that under normal circumstances viral DNA is partially replicated prior to integration. Because large T is required for DNA replication, this would explain the involvement of large T in initiation.

Large T is also required for the excision of integrated viral DNA from the chromosomes of transformed cells (2). Excision and subsequent DNA replication occur in cells that are semipermissive for viral replication. Because replication of the virus could be lethal, and because large T is required for this activity, the finding that transformed rodent cells seldom contain full-size large T may mean not only that the whole molecule is not required for maintenance but also that its presence is selected against (52,54). Indeed, it is striking that when the full-size large T that was detected in one transformed cell line was examined, it was found to be defective in DNA replication (38). Similarly, permissive cells may be transformed by polyoma virus mutants containing an intact early coding sequence but a defective origin of DNA replication. Presumably the so-called COP cells are transformed by middle T, but the defective origin prevents large T from excising and replicating the integrated DNA (105).

Large T controls the transcription of polyoma virus DNA and has the ability to regulate the synthesis of the early mRNAs (10). Presumably, therefore, large T or fragments thereof may modulate the levels of mRNA in transformed cells, and this might modulate transformation by a protein dosage effect.

Although large-T-mediated integration, excision, and control of transcription are all involved in transformation by polyoma virions, these activities may be considered peripheral, secondary activities. The processes are not essential for transformation of Rat-1 cells by polyoma virus middle T, because they can all be bypassed using plasmid DNAs. Indeed, such secondary effects probably contributed to the difficulties encountered in interpreting earlier experiments with different mutants.

Productive infection by polyoma virus induces a round of cellular DNA synthesis in the host cell. This may be required to prepare the cell for the large amount of subsequent viral DNA synthesis. This mitogenic effect of polyoma virus appears to be a property of large T, because cells abortively infected by hr-t mutants still undergo a round of DNA synthesis even though they do not become morphologically transformed (80). It has been claimed that this demonstrates that the mitogenic and transforming functions of polyoma virus can be separated. However, it could be argued that middle T, because it has the ability to induce cells to divide rapidly and repeatedly, might also be considered to be mitogenic. In any event, it is not clear whether or not the mitogenic effect of large T has an effect on viral transformation.

Under some circumstances it is possible to obtain Fischer Rat-3T3 cells that are transformed by polyoma virus ts-a mutants and that have a temperature-sensitive phenotype (73). This result implies that large T is able to modulate the extent of transformation in the so-called N-type transformed cells, and it has prompted further studies to establish which viral sequences are required to rescue the transformed phenotype at the nonpermissive temperature. The results have shown that the amino-terminal portion of large T coded by the sequences extending to the EcoRI site can rescue, and they have predicted that the presence of this part of the protein is necessary to achieve a fully transformed phenotype in Rat-3T3 cells (72,103).

This conclusion contrasts with the results obtained using the middle-T-only plasmid, which showed that large T was not required to transform Rat-1 cells (102). Subsequent examination of the middle-T-only-transformed Rat-1 cells revealed differences between these and cells transformed by the complete early region. The middle-T-only cells failed to grow in low concentrations of serum under conditions where so-called normal transformed cells grow readily (71). This result implies that although the amino-terminal half of large T is not essential for transformation of Rat-1 cells, it does alter the growth properties of the cells and induces a measurable phenotype. Further experiments have examined this in more detail.

Normally, cells taken directly from an animal into culture are referred to as primary cells, and they have a limited life-span. Only a small proportion of such cells survive the crisis that occurs after a certain number of passages in culture and go on to become established or immortalized as permanent cell lines. Experiments using the plasmid that codes for the amino-terminal fragment of large T have shown that these sequences have the ability to establish primary rat cells to give permanent cell lines. Presumably the fragment of large T provides a function that is lacking in primary cells but that is constitutive in established cells that have survived the selection that occurs at crisis.

Further experiments have shown that the middle-T-only plasmid is unable to transform primary rat cells. Together, these results imply that the transformation of primary cells requires the presence of middle T and part of large T to provide the transforming and immortalization functions, respectively, whereas the transformation of established cell lines requires only middle T. Even though large T is not required to transform established cell lines, cells containing large T have an altered phenotype, including a decreased requirement for serum factors. It is striking that the transforming region of adenovirus also appears to have two separable activities. The E1A region is required for immortalization of rat kidney cells, whereas E1B is required for full transformation (39).

The Role of Small T Antigen in Transformation

Relatively few direct studies on the role of polyoma virus small T have been possible, partly because it shares virtually all its amino acid sequence with middle T. However, similar experiments using mutants of SV40 (analogous to hr-t mutants) that synthesize reduced levels of truncated small T have shown that they are capable of transforming cells and forming tumors (58,61). Nonetheless, it is possible to measure defects in their transforming activity (6,85). Under some conditions the latent period for tumor production is longer than with wild-type virus, and the metastatic potential of the tumor cells is reduced (19,58). It has been argued that SV40 small T provides a growth-factor activity but that some cells provide this activity constitutively (60). Indeed, small T does share a number of sequences with small polypeptide hormones (30). However, because the mechanism of transformation by SV40 differs from that used by polyoma virus, the significance of these findings is unclear. It would be surprising, however, if the sequences coding for small T were present in the polyoma virus genome and were conserved at least in part in SV40 and human BK virus, to find that the protein has no role in replication or transformation.

BIOCHEMICAL PROPERTIES OF POLYOMA VIRUS MIDDLE T ANTIGEN

The evidence presented here supports the view that polyoma-virus-induced transformation of Rat-1 cells can be brought about by the action of a single viral transforming protein. A similar conclusion, namely that a single viral protein is sufficient to transform cells, has been reached for a number of other tumor viruses, and this raises the question of how transforming proteins function.

As outlined earlier, transformed cells differ from their untransformed parents in a vast number of properties. It is very unlikely that these all result from the direct action of a single protein. It is much more probable that transforming proteins, like mitogens or hormones, interact with or mimic key regulatory elements within the cell. This interaction probably triggers a number of secondary actions, and eventually, by the operation of a cascade, the multitude of changes results. Perhaps it is the continued presence of the transforming protein resulting in the permanent operation of a pathway normally subject to cellular regulation that gives rise to the uncontrolled malignant growth characteristic of transformed cells.

Studies to establish the mechanism of action of middle T are hampered by the very small amount of the protein present in productively infected or transformed cells. No other abundant source of the protein has been found or engineered, and there are no reports of extensive purification. Most of the work on the biochemistry of middle T has centered on a possible associated kinase activity and the finding that middle T is probably membrane-associated.

Protein Kinase Activity

The finding that polyoma virus middle T is nonnuclear and in all probability is associated with cellular membranes has influenced studies on the possible biochemical basis of its action. For example, it is very unlikely to transform cells by a direct effect on gene expression. One powerful mechanism whereby a single cytoplasmic protein may influence a wide spectrum of cellular events is the phosphorylation of regulatory enzymes to bring about a change in their activity or structure. Perhaps the best example of this is the modulation of glycogen metabolism in rabbit muscle cells by the enzyme phosphorylase kinase, which itself is controlled by hormones such as adrenalin acting via the cAMP-dependent protein kinase or by neuronal excitation via Ca^{2+} fluxes (11). Control by protein kinases and their complementary phosphatases is rapid and readily reversed. These considerations led to an investigation of the possible involvement of protein kinases in transformation and to the discovery that the transforming protein of Rous sarcoma virus, called pp60[src], has an associated protein kinase activity (12,56). This finding prompted a similar investigation using polyoma virus.

Middle-T-associated Protein Kinase

The most rapid and simple assay for a possible protein kinase associated with a protein that is present in only small amounts is an immune-complex assay. In this procedure the protein in question is reacted with a specific antibody, and the immune complex is collected using protein-A-bearing bacteria. After extensive washing, the bacteria are resuspended in a solution containing γ-^{32}P-ATP. If a protein kinase is present, it may phosphorylate any suitable substrate present in the immune complex. In the case of pp60[src], the heavy chain of IgG becomes phosphorylated (12).

When unlabeled extracts of polyoma-virus-infected cells are immunoprecipitated using anti-T serum and incubated with γ-^{32}P-ATP, proteins with a molecular weight of approximately 55,000 become labeled (22,76,89,90). When control serum or extracts of uninfected cells are used, no labeling is detected. By using a variety of different mutants with deletions or alterations at different positions in the early region, it is possible to establish that the products of the reaction are middle T and rat IgG heavy chain and that the presence of the kinase activity is strictly dependent on the presence of middle T (Table 1). Kinase activity is also detected in immunoprecipitates obtained using an antibody raised against the carboxy-terminal six amino acids of middle T (107) and using monoclonal antibodies against middle T (S. Dilworth, 1982, *personal communication*).

The kinase activity is detected in a wide range of polyoma-virus-transformed cells, including those transformed by middle T only, but not in cells transformed by SV40 or Rous sarcoma virus. There is also good correlation between the transforming activities of various different viral mutants and the levels of kinase they induce.

TABLE 1. *Kinase activity* in vitro *for polyoma virus mutants*

Mutant	Large T	Middle T	Small T	Kinase activity	Transforming activity
ts-a					
32°	+	+	+	+	+
39°	−	−	−	−	
32°→39°	↓	↑	↑	+ +	
hr-t					
NG-59	+	Altered	Altered	−	−
SD-15	+	Shortened	Shortened	−	−
NG-18	+	Absent	Absent	−	−
ml-t					
dl 8	Shortened	Shortened	+	+ +	+ +
dl 45	Shortened	Shortened	+	+	+
dl 23	Shortened	Shortened	+	−	−
dl 1013/14	Shortened	Shortened	+	+	+

Correlation between kinase activity *in vitro* for polyoma virus mutants, transforming activity, and presence of middle T. Kinase activity refers to the ability of middle T to accept phosphate *in vitro*. Arrows indicate that the amount of the protein is increasing (↑) or decreasing (↓). A plus sign indicates the presence of wild-type amounts of protein; two pluses indicate elevated amounts; a minus sign indicates absence of the protein or activity. Data from Smith et al. (89) and Schaffhausen and Benjamin (77).

Subcellular fractionation studies have shown that the kinase activity is associated with the plasma membrane fraction of cells (88,90). Although there is a clear association between the presence of middle T and the kinase activity, the experiments described earlier are not capable of distinguishing between a model that predicts that middle T has an intrinsic protein kinase activity and one predicting that it specifically associates with a cellular kinase.

Phosphotyrosine

When the amino acid to which the phosphate residue is attached during the middle T-associated kinase reaction was examined, it was found to separate from phosphoserine or phosphothreonine, which account for over 99% of the phosphate residues on total cellular proteins. Characterization of the modified amino acid showed it to be tyrosine (22). This was the first demonstration of a protein kinase with specificity for tyrosine, but subsequent analysis of other systems has shown that the kinases associated with pp60[src] and a number of other viral transforming proteins also phosphorylate tyrosine (41). Kinases associated with a cellular protein related to pp60[src] and with the epidermal growth factor (EGF) receptor also phosphorylate tyrosine residues (106). It appears, therefore, that there is a class of protein kinases present in cells with the ability to phosphorylate tyrosine. To date, these are all associated with regulatory systems and all associated with membrane proteins.

A large body of evidence has accumulated to show that the tyrosine kinase activity of pp60[src] is intimately associated with the protein; pp60[src] synthesized *in vitro* from purified viral RNA and the protein expressed in bacteria from cloned viral DNA both have kinase activity (23,33,62). Similarly, the kinase activity present in cells transformed by temperature-sensitive mutants is itself temperature-sensitive, and highly purified preparations of pp60[src] retain kinase activity (24,57,81).

Some of the corresponding experiments have been attempted using polyoma virus, but so far no convincing data to show that the kinase activity is a property of middle T have been reported. Thus, attempts to obtain middle T active in the kinase reaction either by translation of polyoma mRNA in cell-free systems or following expression in bacteria have been unsuccessful. Enriched preparations of middle T are not yet sufficiently pure to conclude that the protein itself has kinase activity, and no temperature-sensitive mutants of middle T have yet been reported.

Phosphotyrosine and Transformation

Irrespective of whether the polyoma virus protein kinase is a property of middle T itself or of an associated cellular enzyme, the unusual specificity of the reaction places it in an interesting class of protein kinases. It could play an important role in the transformation process. However, experiments to detect changes in phosphotyrosine metabolism in polyoma-virus-transformed cells have been inconclusive.

In the case of Rous-sarcoma-virus-transformed cells, there is a 10-fold increase in the abundance of phosphotyrosine following transformation (82). Furthermore, a number of possible substrates for the enzyme have been identified, including a 36,000-dalton protein that is specifically phosphorylated on tyrosine on transformation (70). Purified preparations of pp60[src] phosphorylate purified preparations of the 36,000-dalton protein (24).

By contrast, there is no increase in the level of phosphotyrosine in polyoma-virus-transformed cells (82). Similarly, attempts to detect phosphotyrosine-containing proteins that appear following transformation by polyoma virus have been unsuccessful (A. E. Smith, 1980, *unpublished results*). These data demonstrate that transformations by polyoma virus and by Rous sarcoma virus do not use an identical pathway that includes, for example, phosphorylation of the 36,000-dalton protein.

None of the experiments described here establish in themselves that pp60[src] has intrinsic phosphotyrosine kinase activity that is directly responsible for transformation, but the weight of evidence supports this view. This contrasts with the almost total lack of direct evidence to show that middle T has a kinase activity that is relevant to the transformation process. It could be argued that middle T associates with a cellular phosphotyrosine kinase during the extraction procedure and that this association is fortuitous and irrelevant. On the other hand, none of the data exclude the possibility that polyoma virus middle T or a protein with which it specifically interacts phosphorylates a regulatory enzyme that is not sufficiently abundant or soluble to be detected by the methods used and that this induces transformation without a gross change in phosphotyrosine level.

Membrane Association

Cell fractionation studies have shown that middle T is associated largely with the plasma membrane fraction of cells, with smaller amounts present in the endoplasmic reticulum fraction (44,46). However, no successful attempts to characterize the association have been reported. Procedures that should label the proteins present on the external surfaces of cells have not yielded labeled middle T, thus suggesting that the protein does not extend to the outer surface of the cell.

Characterization of the amino terminus of middle T shows that it is Ac-Met-Asp-Arg and that the methionine residue originates from initiator tRNA (40,63). This result excludes the possibility that middle T is directed to the plasma membrane by a transient N-terminal signal sequence similar to that used, for example, by the vesicular stomatitis virus G (VSV G) protein or HLA antigens (75). This, and the observation that large T and small T do not associate with membranes, suggests that the membrane targeting signal and the anchoring signal are both present in the carboxy-terminal unique sequences of middle T. It probably implies that the mRNA for middle T, like that for pp60^{src}, is translated on free polysomes and that the protein is transported to the membrane after synthesis (55). Taken together, all the data suggest that middle T is associated with the inner surface of the plasma membrane. However, a more detailed analysis of its orientation relative to the lipid bilayer and to the membrane itself is required.

The DNA sequence of polyoma virus predicts the presence of a hydrophobic segment of 20 amino acids very close to the carboxy-terminal end of middle T (Fig. 4). This sequence resembles the transmembrane segments of various proteins that span the lipid bilayer (75). Experiments to study the role of the predicted hydrophobic sequence have suggested that it is important. A cloned fragment of polyoma virus DNA containing sequences coding for middle T was used to transform cells, and the effect of removing sequences from the carboxy-terminal end of the protein was studied (67). This analysis showed that removing part of the sequence and replacing it with plasmid sequences drastically reduced the ability to transform. A more recent study used techniques of site-specific mutagenesis on similar cloned DNA to convert the triplet coding for glutamine 385 of middle T to a termination codon (8). This generates a truncated middle T molecule lacking 37 amino acids from the carboxy terminus, including the 20 hydrophobic residues. The truncated middle T is defective in transformation.

The truncated middle T is not associated with membranes, thus suggesting that the hydrophobic sequence is involved in the interaction. To demonstrate that the

----

FIG. 4. The amino acid sequence of polyoma virus middle T predicted from the DNA sequence (94) and known position of splice sites (101). The N-terminal 79 amino acids are shared by all three early proteins, the amino acids between residues 80 and 91 *(light stippling)* are shared by middle T and small T, and the remainder are unique to middle T. The boxed amino acids appear to be essential for transformation, and the *heavily stippled* sequence is the hydrophobic putative membrane binding segment. Note that the DNA sequence determined by Deininger et al. (16) predicts that glycine 328 is glutamic acid.

MET ASP ARG VAL LEU SER ARG ARG ALA ASP LYS 10 GLU ARG LEU LEU GLU LEU LEU LYS LEU PRO 20

ARG GLN LEU TRP GLY ASP PHE GLY ARG MET 30 GLN GLN ALA TYR LYS GLN GLN SER LEU LEU 40

LEU HIS PRO ASP LYS GLY SER HIS ALA 50 LEU MET GLN GLU LEU ASN SER LEU TRP GLY 60

THR PHE LYS THR GLU VAL TYR ASN LEU ARG 70 MET ASN LEU GLY GLY THR GLY PHE GLN VAL 80

ARG ARG LEU HIS ALA ASP GLY TRP ASN LEU 90 SER THR LYS ASP THR PHE GLY ASP ARG TYR 100

TYR GLN ARG PHE CYS ARG MET PRO LEU THR 110 CYS LEU VAL ASN VAL LYS TYR SER SER CYS 120

SER CYS ILE LEU CYS LEU ARG LYS GLN 130 HIS ARG GLU LYS ASP LYS CYS ASP ALA 140

ARG CYS LEU VAL LEU GLY GLU CYS PHE CYS 150 LEU GLU CYS TRY MET GLN TRP PHE GLY THR 160

PRO THR ARG ASP VAL LEU ASN LEU TYR ALA 170 ASP PHE ILE ALA SER MET PRO ILE ASP TRP 180

LEU ASP ASP VAL HIS SER VAL TYR ASN PRO 190 LYS ARG ARG SER GLU GLU LEU ARG ARG 200

ALA ALA THR VAL HIS TYR MET THR THR THR 210 GLY HIS SER ALA MET GLU ALA SER THR SER 220

GLN GLY ASN GLY MET ILE SER SER GLU SER 230 GLY THR PRO ALA THR SER ARG ARG LEU ARG 240

LEU PRO SER LEU SER ASN PRO THR TYR 250 SER VAL MET ARG SER HIS SER TYR PRO PRO 260

THR ARG VAL LEU GLN GLN ILE HIS PRO HIS 270 ILE LEU LEU GLU GLU ASP GLU ILE LEU VAL 280

LEU LEU SER PRO MET THR ALA TYR PRO ARG 290 THR PRO PRO LEU TYR PRO GLU SER VAL 300

ASP GLN ASP GLN LEU GLU LEU GLU GLU GLU 310 GLU GLU GLU TYR MET PRO MET GLU ASP 320

LEU TYR LEU ASP ILE LEU PRO GLY GLY GLN 330 VAL PRO GLN LEU ILE LEU PRO PRO ILE ILE 340

PRO ARG ALA GLY LEU SER PRO TRP GLU GLY 350 LEU ILE LEU ARG ASP LEU GLN ARG ALA HIS 360

PHE ASP PRO ILE LEU ASP ALA SER GLN ARG 370 MET ARG ALA THR HIS ARG ALA ALA LEU ARG 380

ALA HIS SER MET GLN ARG ARG LEU ARG ARG 390 LEU GLY ARG THR LEU LEU LEU VAL THR PHE 400

LEU ALA ALA LEU LEU GLY ILE CYS LEU MET 410 LEU PHE ILE LEU ILE LYS ARG SER ARG HIS 420

PHE. 421

involvement is direct, rather than mediated by a conformational change elsewhere in the molecule, requires cross-linking experiments, but these have not yet been reported. It was also found that the truncated middle T coded by the chain-termination mutant lacks kinase activity. A similar shortened form of middle T can be generated by treating membrane preparations from normal cells with proteases, but in the latter case the preparation retains kinase activity. Taken together, these data suggest that middle T must interact with membranes in order to transform and that this interaction requires the carboxy-terminal amino acids of middle T. The interaction with the membrane either activates an intrinsic phosphotyrosine kinase or allows association with a cellular kinase (8).

It is striking that the transforming protein of Rous sarcoma virus is also associated with the plasma membrane of transformed cells. There is no evidence that the protein spans the membrane, and some results suggest that it is concentrated on the inner surface in regions of cell–cell and cell–substratum contact (43). Other data suggest that pp60[src] lacks kinase activity until it associates with two cellular proteins and is deposited in the membrane (13). The predicted amino acid sequence does not include a hydrophobic segment, but the membrane binding domain has been mapped to the amino-terminal half of the molecule (55).

Mapping Functions of Polyoma Virus Middle T

Experiments described here indicate that at least some of the sequences involved in the interaction between middle T and membranes map to the carboxy-terminal region of the molecule. Further attempts to map functional domains on middle T have tentatively identified a phosphorylation site and a sequence that appears to be essential for transformation.

Phosphotyrosine in Middle T

To identify the phosphotyrosine residue labeled during the *in vitro* kinase reaction, middle T has been subjected to partial proteolysis, and the fragments have been separated on polyacrylamide gels. By comparing materials labeled with γ-^{32}P-ATP, with ^{35}S-methionine or -cysteine, or with ^{35}S-methionine from initiator tRNA it was shown that the phosphate is attached to the carboxy-terminal portion of the molecule. The analysis was extended by similar experiments using mutant forms of middle T with deletions that remove each of the tyrosine residues in turn. Assuming that the phosphorylation site and the proteolytic cleavage sites remain constant in all of the different forms of middle T, the results show that the phosphate residue is attached to tyrosine 315 (Fig. 4). This residue follows a tract of six glutamic acids (77,88; A. E. Smith, 1980, *unpublished results*).

The sequence of the phosphorylated peptide has not been confirmed unequivocally by direct sequencing methods. However, the synthetic peptide Ac-Leu-Glu-Glu-Glu-Glu-Glu-Glu-Tyr-Met-Pro-Met-Lys inhibits the kinase activity *in vitro*, supporting the idea that this is the phosphate acceptor site (Harvey, Belsham, and A. E. Smith, 1981, *unpublished results*). On the other hand, it should be emphasized that the amount of phosphate attached to middle T isolated from cells is extremely low, and we are not aware of any evidence showing that tyrosine 315 is phosphorylated *in vivo*.

The sequence preceding tyrosine 315 bears some resemblance to the tyrosine phosphorylation site in pp60[src] (Fig. 5). Perhaps an acidic sequence preceding a tyrosine residue is a common feature of the recognition site for tyrosine kinases (87). The sequence in middle T has an even more striking homology with a sequence in gastrin (1). In this case, a sequence of five glutamic acids lies adjacent to a tyrosine residue that in about 50% of gastrin molecules is sulfated. It is not clear if this remarkable structural similarity implies a corresponding common function that is associated with the two proteins.

Essential Amino Acid Sequences

In addition to their use to identify properties of the different polyoma virus proteins, the early region mutants may also be used for more detailed mapping of the transforming activity of middle T. Most of the hr-t mutants are defective in transformation because they contain deletions that alter the efficiency of the different splices and result in the synthesis of very small amounts of truncated versions of middle T and small T (37,83). A few of the hr-t mutants do appear able to splice normally and produce approximately normal amounts of truncated versions of middle T and small T. One of these mutants, NG-59, is striking in that it codes for an inactive middle T species that differs from the wild type only by the replacement of aspartic acid 179 by isoleucine-asparagine (Table 2). Another mutant (SD-15) codes for an inactive truncated middle T (7). Presumably the lesions in NG-59 and SD-15 induce conformational changes in middle T that affect its activity.

A large number of ml-t mutants have been isolated that remove sequences from the carboxy-terminal half of middle T (3,34,59,65). Two of these are interesting in that although both remove long tracts of middle T sequences, one of the mutants (dl 23) is transformation-defective, whereas the other (dl 8) appears to transform

Leu. Glu. Glu. Glu. Glu. Glu. Glu. Tyr. Met.   middle-T

311   P

Ile. Glu. Asp. Asn. Glu. Tyr.Thr.   pp60[src]

415   P

Leu. Glu. Glu. Glu. Glu. Glu. Ala. Tyr. Gly.   gastrin

25   S

FIG. 5. Amino acid sequences around the sites of tyrosine modification in middle T, pp60[src], and gastrin.

TABLE 2. *Transforming activity of polyoma virus middle T mutants*

Mutant	Middle T	Transformation	Amino acid sequences deleted	Comments	Ref.
hr-t					
SD-15	Shortened	−	83–129	Other point mutations	7
B-2	Absent	−	105–421	Out of phase	37
NG-18	Absent	−	114–421	Out of phase	37,95
NG-59	Altered	−	179	Insert Ile-Ile-Asn; residue 151 is Phe	7
ml-t					
dl 8	Shortened	+ +	253–282		92
dl 45	Shortened	+	281–302		3
dl 2210	Shortened	+	294–310		65
dl 2208	Shortened	−	298–316		65
dl 23	Shortened	−	301–335		92
dl 1020	Shortened	+	319–332		65
dl 1015	Shortened	+	338–347		59
Termination					
MOP 1033	Truncated	−	261–421		97
1387-T	Truncated	−	384–421		8

more effectively than wild-type virus (34,49). It is striking that the phosphate acceptor activities associated with the two truncated middle Ts parallel their transforming ability: dl 23 is defective, whereas dl 8 is an exceptionally active acceptor (90). Furthermore, dl 23 lacks sequences including the glutamic-acid-rich region (92).

Subsequent analyses of the transforming activities of a large number of other ml-t deletion mutants have refined the map of sequences required for transformation (65). The results (Table 2) show that surprisingly long tracts of middle T from approximately residue 253 to 347 can be removed in one or another of the deletion mutants without apparent effect on transformation, with one very striking exception: All mutants lacking the sequence Glu-Glu-Glu-Glu-Tyr-Met-Pro-Met are transformation-defective (Fig. 4).

Although not all the mutants have been examined directly, middle T coded by any mutant lacking this sequence would not be expected to be phosphorylated *in vitro* because it lacks the phosphate acceptor site. It is not yet known if all such mutants also lack the kinase activity that phosphorylates rat IgG. Thus, it is not yet clear whether the sequence defined earlier is essential for transformation (a) because phosphorylation of tyrosine 315 is necessary, (b) because the region is an essential part of the active site of an intrinsic kinase activity or part of the binding site of a cellular kinase, or (c) because of some other unrelated activity. It would certainly be unwise to conclude at this stage that the apparent requirement for sequences surrounding tyrosine 315 means that phosphorylation of this residue or a phosphotyrosine kinase activity is essential for polyoma virus transformation.

Minor Forms of Middle T

Immunoprecipitates containing polyoma virus early proteins include a variety of minor protein components. Some of these are present in the immunoprecipitates, because they specifically interact with the early proteins and are coprecipitated with them. For example, large T interacts with a cellular phosphoprotein called NVT or p53 (51), and small T binds to two other host cell proteins (74). In addition to these cellular proteins, minor components with molecular weights of approximately 63,000 and 37,000 have been detected in several laboratories (42,79,83,84). Fingerprint analysis of these proteins has shown that they are related to the other polyoma virus early proteins. Other studies have shown that they are lacking in cells infected with hr-t mutants (83).

The minor early proteins have received little attention, partly because no viral mRNA species containing alternative splices and present in the same relative abundance have been detected. If such mRNAs do not exist, then presumably the minor proteins arise by posttranslational modification or by proteolytic cleavage of other early proteins. The results with hr-t mutants would indicate that the minor proteins are related to middle T or small T. Clearly, these minor proteins and any possible very minor mRNAs coding for them require further study. If other splices are possible at a low level in early region transcripts, their presence could complicate the experiments using the plasmids presently believed to code for only one early protein.

Analysis of the middle T species labeled *in vitro* during the kinase reaction has revealed approximately equal amounts of two labeled species of middle T (77). Closer examination of ^{35}S-labeled middle T isolated from cells has shown that two species of corresponding mobility were present, but in this case the slower-migrating species was approximately 10-fold less abundant than the other species. This was interpreted to mean that the minor species is much more active in the kinase reaction. Presumably the modification that results in the altered mobility is responsible for the difference in kinase activity; however, the nature of the modification is unknown.

Sucrose density-gradient fractionation of extracts of polyoma-virus-infected or -transformed cells has shown that the species active in the kinase reaction sediments as a broad peak at about 6S (78). This could mean that the kinase activity is associated with an oligomeric form of middle T or that middle T sediments rapidly because it is associated with a cellular protein.

The presence of minor forms of middle T has also been predicted by experiments using monoclonal antibodies against middle T (18). Some of the antibodies are able to recognize virtually all of the middle T present in cell extracts, whereas others interact with only a small fraction. This may mean that such antibodies recognize a determinant present on only a minor population of middle T molecules, but the nature of such a determinant is presently unknown.

BIOCHEMICAL BASIS OF ACTION OF LARGE T AND SMALL T

Neither large T nor small T is essential to bring about transformation of Rat-1 cells by the polyoma virus early region. Nevertheless, large T is able to induce a measurable phenotype in transformed Rat-1 cells (71). Furthermore, the amino-terminal half of large T is required to transform primary rat cells, and it has the ability to establish or immortalize such cells. It is not yet known whether these three properties of large T are different manifestations of the same activity or represent three separate functions. For convenience we refer to these properties collectively as the immortalization function.

Virtually nothing is known about the biochemistry of small T. The presence of the protein may be required to bring about changes in the cytoskeleton and cellular membranes, because in the case of SV40 small T it is necessary to disrupt the actin cable network and to stimulate the release of plasminogen activator (100). Polyoma virus small T interacts with two cellular proteins, but their functions and cellular locations are unknown (74).

Polyoma virus large T is a multifunctional protein. It has the ability to bind specifically to the origin region of polyoma virus DNA (32), it has an associated ATPase activity (31), and it interacts with NVT (51). The binding of large T to the origin region almost certainly controls transcription and replication of the viral DNA during the productive infection cycle (98). These properties could also influence transformation by modulating the amount of mRNA synthesized and by controlling replication prior to integration and excision. However, these are secondary effects in the transformation process. It is not obvious what biochemical property of large T catalyzes the immortalization function.

There is some evidence to show that polyoma virus large T stimulates a round of cellular DNA synthesis (80). This activity is probably required in the productive infection cycle to prepare the cell for the burst of viral DNA synthesis. The continued expression of this function in primary cells might be the basis of the immortalization effect. Because only a limited amount of the large T sequence is required for immortalization, the property involved must map in the amino-terminal half of the molecule. No functions of polyoma large T have yet been mapped, but in the case of SV40 it is known that truncated versions of the protein retain the ability to bind to DNA but not to interact with NVT (9). Sequences homologous to those present in the truncated SV40 molecules are present in the minimal polyoma-virus-truncated large T that retains the immortalization function.

SUMMARY AND FUTURE PROSPECTS

From the data presented here it seems reasonable to conclude that middle T is responsible for the bulk of the transforming activity of polyoma virus. It is very likely that the protein interacts with membranes, probably with the inner side of the plasma membrane. Possibly, therefore, transformation results because middle T somehow modifies components of the membrane.

Although the modification to the membrane could be mediated by the action of a tyrosine-specific protein kinase, all the evidence to support this view is very circumstantial. We emphasize that we do not know if tyrosine 315 is phosphorylated *in vivo*; we do not know if middle T has an intrinsic kinase activity capable of phosphorylating both itself and/or other proteins or if middle T interacts with a cellular tyrosine kinase; we do not know if the putative interaction with a cellular kinase is physiologically meaningful, and we do not know any of the substrates for the putative kinase. On the other hand, we are not aware of any experiments that exclude the possibility that the mechanism of action of middle T involves a kinase activity.

It is to be expected that work in the immediate future will concentrate on attempts to unravel the biochemistry of middle T, particularly to establish the role of the putative kinase. The use of plasmid DNAs coding for middle T only will probably play a major part in these studies, as will the construction of specific mutant forms of the protein. An abundant source of middle T and a simple purification scheme would also be invaluable.

Irrespective of how middle T might bring about a modification to the plasma membrane, there are several possible consequences of such a modification. For example, middle T might alter cellular architecture. This would result in changes in cell shape, and this in itself might be sufficient to catalyze an increase in cellular proliferation. An alternative possibility is that middle T alters transmembrane traffic, alters the sensitivity of cells to growth factors, transforming factors, or growth-promoting agents, or alters the release of these factors into the extracellular fluid. Future studies are likely to concentrate on properties of the plasma membrane of polyoma-virus-transformed cells, particularly any biochemical alterations that can be detected, and on the virus-induced transforming factors.

Another area where much remains to be learned concerns the function of the amino-terminal half of large T. Its role in transformation, immortalization, and inducing the altered phenotype is now established, but virtually nothing is known of the biochemistry associated with these properties. Further studies are also likely to attempt to find a role for small T. Again, the use of plasmid DNAs capable of coding separately for these proteins is likely to prove fruitful.

Ultimately, studies on virus-induced transformation seek to describe in molecular terms the events occurring in the cell following exposure to virus. Any such description necessarily requires that we have a clear definition of the end result, that is, of transformation itself. From the preceding discussion it is obvious that we do not yet have such a definition. Transformed cells display a wide array of different phenotypes, and they differ in many properties from their untransformed parents. It is unclear which of the altered properties are central to the transformation process, which are secondary, and which are largely irrelevant. The inability to define precisely what is meant by transformation remains a major hurdle in further attempts to describe the biochemical events that catalyze the process. Any future advances in our knowledge of the biochemistry of transforming proteins must be accompanied by a clearer understanding of the cellular biology of normal and transformed cells.

ACKNOWLEDGMENTS

We thank our colleagues at Mill Hill for helpful comments on the manuscript, Drs. R. Kamen, G. Magnusson, and S. Dilworth for permission to quote unpublished results, and Mrs. Lydia Pearson for typing the manuscript.

REFERENCES

1. Baldwin, G. S. (1982): Gastrin and the transforming protein of polyoma virus have evolved from a common ancestor. *F.E.B.S. Lett.*, 137:1–5.
2. Basilico, C., Gattoni, S., Zouzias, D., and Della Valle, G. (1979): Loss of integrated viral DNA sequences in polyoma virus transformed cells is associated with an active viral A function. *Cell*, 17:645–659.
3. Bendig, M., Thomas, T., and Folk, W. (1980): Viable deletion mutant in the medium and large-T antigen coding sequences of the polyoma virus genome. *J. Virol.*, 33:1215–1220.
4. Benjamin, T. L. (1970): Host range mutants of polyoma virus. *Proc. Natl. Acad. Sci. USA*, 67:394–399.
5. Birg, F., Dulbecco, R., Fried, M., and Kamen, R. (1979): State and organisation of polyoma virus DNA in transformed rat cell lines. *J. Virol.*, 29:633–648.
6. Bouck, N., Beales, N., Shenk, T., Berg, P., and di Mayorca, G. (1978): New region of the simian virus 40 genome required for efficient viral transformation. *Proc. Natl. Acad. Sci. USA*, 75:2473–2477.
7. Carmichael, G. G., and Benjamin, T. L. (1980): Identification of DNA sequence changes leading to loss of transforming ability in polyoma virus. *J. Biol. Chem.*, 255:230–235.
8. Carmichael, G. G., Schaffhausen, B. S., Dorsky, D. I., Oliver, D. B., and Benjamin, T. L. (1982): The carboxy terminus of polyoma middle-T antigen is required for attachment to membranes, associated protein kinase activities, and cell transformation. *Proc. Natl. Acad. Sci. USA*, 79:3579–3583.
9. Chaudry, F., Harvey, R., and Smith, A. E. (1982): Structure and function of four SV40 truncated large-T antigens. *J. Virol.*, 44:54–66.
10. Cogen, B. (1978): Virus specific early RNA in 3T6 cells infected by a mutant of polyoma virus. *Virology*, 85:222–230.
11. Cohen, P. (1978): The role of cAMP-dependent protein kinase in the regulation of glycogen metabolism in mammalian skeletal muscle. *Curr. Top. Cell Regul.*, 14:117–126.
12. Collett, M. S., and Erikson, R. L. (1978): Protein kinase activity associated with the avian sarcoma virus *src* gene product. *Proc. Natl. Acad. Sci. USA*, 75:2021–2024.
13. Courtneidge, S. A., and Bishop, J. M. (1982): The transit of pp60[src] to the plasma membrane. *Proc. Natl. Acad. Sci. USA*, *(in press)*.
14. Crawford, L. V., Cole, C. N., Smith, A. E., Paucha, E., Tegtmeyer, P., Rundell, K., and Berg, P. (1978): Organization and expression of early genes of simian virus 40. *Proc. Natl. Acad. Sci. USA*, 75:117–121.
15. Crossin, K., and Carney, D. (1981): Evidence that microtubule depolymerisation early in the cell cycle is sufficient to initiate DNA synthesis. *Cell*, 23:61–71.
16. Deininger, P., Esty, A., LaPorte, P., Hsu, H., and Friedman, T. (1980): The nucleotide sequence and restriction enzyme sites of the polyoma genome. *Nucleic Acids Res.*, 8:856–860.
17. Della Valle, G., Fenton, R., and Basilico, C. (1981): Polyoma large-T antigen regulates the integration of viral DNA sequences into the genome of transformed cells. *Cell*, 23:347–355.
18. Dilworth, S., and Griffin, B. G. (1982): Monoclonal antibodies against polyoma virus T-antigens. *Proc. Natl. Acad. Sci. USA*, 79:1059–1063.
19. Dixon, K., Ryder, B., and Burch-Jaffe, E. (1982): Enhanced metastasis of tumours induced by a SV40 small-t deletion mutant. *Nature*, 296:672–675.
20. Eckhart, W. (1977): Complementation between temperature-sensitive (ts) and host range non-transforming (ht-t) mutants of polyoma virus. *Virology*, 77:589–597.
21. Eckhart, W. (1981): Polyoma T-antigens. *Adv. Cancer Res.*, 35:1–25.
22. Eckhart, W., Hutchinson, M. A., and Hunter, T. (1979): An activity phosphorylating tyrosine in polyoma T-antigen immunoprecipitates. *Cell*, 18:925–933.
23. Erikson E., Collett, M., and Erikson, R. L. (1978): *In vitro* synthesis of a functional ASV transforming gene product. *Nature*, 274:919–921.
24. Erikson, E., and Erikson, R. L. (1980): Identification of a cellular protein substrate phosphorylated by the ASV transforming gene product. *Cell*, 21:829–836.
25. Feunteun, J., Sompayrac, L., Fluck, M., and Benjamin, T. L. (1976): Localization of gene functions in polyoma virus DNA. *Proc. Natl. Acad. Sci. USA*, 73:4169–4173.
26. Fluck, M. M., and Benjamin, T. L. (1979): Comparisons of two early gene functions essential for transformation in polyoma virus and SV40. *Virology*, 96:205–228.

27. Folkman, J., and Moscona, A. (1978): Role of cell shape in growth control. *Nature*, 273:345–349.
28. Fried, M. (1965): Cell transformation ability of a temperature-sensitive mutant of polyoma virus. *Proc. Natl. Acad. Sci. USA*, 53:486–491.
29. Fried, M., and Griffin, B. E. (1977): Organization of the genomes of polyoma virus and SV40. *Adv. Cancer Res.*, 24:67–113.
30. Friedman, T., Esty, A., LaPorte, P., and Deininger, P. (1979): The nucleotide sequence and genome organization of the polyoma early region: Extensive nucleotide and amino acid homology with SV40. *Cell*, 17:715–724.
31. Gaudrey, P., Clertant, P., and Cuzin, F. (1980): ATP phosphohydrolase activity of polyoma virus T-antigen. *Eur. J. Biochem.*, 109:553–560.
32. Gaudrey, P., Tyndall, C., Kamen, R., and Cuzin, F. (1981): The high affinity binding site on polyoma virus DNA for the viral large-T antigen. *Nucleic Acids Res.*, 9:5697–5710.
33. Gilmer, T., and Erikson, R. L. (1981): The Rous sarcoma virus transforming protein pp60[src] expressed in *E. coli* functions as a protein kinase. *Nature*, 294:771–773.
34. Griffin, B. E., and Maddock, C. (1979): New classes of viable deletion mutants in the early region of polyoma virus. *J. Virol.*, 31:645–656.
35. Hand, R. (1981): Functions of T-antigens of SV40 and polyoma virus. *Biochim. Biophys. Acta*, 651:1–24.
36. Hassell, J. A., Topp, W. C., Rifkin, D. B., and Moreau, P. E. (1980): Transformation of rat embryo fibroblasts by cloned polyoma virus DNA fragments containing only part of the early region. *Proc. Natl. Acad. Sci. USA*, 77:3978–3982.
37. Hattori, J., Carmichael, G. G., and Benjamin, T. L. (1979): DNA sequence alterations in hr-t deletion mutants of polyoma virus. *Cell*, 16:505–513.
38. Hayday, A., Ruley, H. E., and Fried, M. (1982): Structural and biological analysis of integrated polyoma virus DNA and its adjacent host sequences cloned from transformed rat cells. *J. Virol.*, 44:*(in press)*.
39. Houweling, A., Van den Elsen, P. J., and Van der Eb, A. (1980): Partial transformation of primary rat cells by the leftmost 4.5% fragment of adenovirus 5 DNA. *Virology*, 105:537–550.
40. Hunter, T., Hutchinson, M. A., Eckhart, W., Friedman, T., Esty, A., LaPorte, P., and Deininger, P. (1979): Regions of the polyoma genome coding for T-antigens. *Nucleic Acids Res.*, 7:2275–2288.
41. Hunter, T., and Sefton, B. (1980): Transforming gene product of Rous sarcoma virus phosphorylates tyrosine. *Proc. Natl. Acad. Sci. USA*, 77:1311–1315.
42. Hutchinson, M. A., Hunter, T., and Eckhart, W. (1978): Characterization of T antigens in polyoma-infected and transformed cells. *Cell*, 15:65–77.
43. Hynes, R. O. (1980): Cellular location of viral transforming proteins. *Cell*, 21:601–602.
44. Ito, Y. (1979): Polyoma virus-specific 55K protein isolated from the plasma membrane of productively infected mouse cells is virus-coded and important for cell transformation. *Virology*, 98:261–266.
45. Ito, Y. (1980): Organization and expression of the genome of polyoma virus. In: *Viral Oncology*, edited by G. Klein, pp. 447–473. Raven Press, New York.
46. Ito, Y., Brocklehurst, J. R., and Dulbecco, R. (1977): Virus-specific proteins in the plasma membrane of cells lytically infected or transformed by polyoma virus. *Proc. Natl. Acad. Sci. USA*, 74:4666–4670.
47. Ito, Y., Spurr, N., and Dulbecco, R. (1977): Characterization of polyoma virus T antigen. *Proc. Natl. Acad. Sci. USA*, 74:1259–1263.
48. Ito, Y., and Spurr, N. (1980): Polyoma virus T antigens expressed in transformed cells: Significant of middle T antigen in transformation. *Cold Spring Harbor Symp. Quant. Biol.*, 44:149–157.
49. Ito, Y., Spurr, N., and Griffin, B. (1980): Middle T antigen as a primary inducer of full expression of the phenotype of transformation by polyoma virus. *J. Virol.*, 35:219–232.
50. Kamen, R., Lindstrom, D. M., Shure, H., and Old, R. W. (1974): Virus-specific RNA in cells productively infected or transformed by polyoma virus. *Cold Spring Harbor Symp. Quant. Biol.*, 39:187–198.
51. Lane, D. P., and Crawford, L. V. (1979): Large-T antigen is bound to a host cell protein in SV40 transformed cells. *Nature*, 278:261–263.
52. Lania, L., Gandini-Attardi, D., Griffiths, M., Cooke, B., DeCicco, D., and Fried, M. (1980):

The polyoma virus 100K large T antigen is not required for transformation. *Virology*, 101:217–232.

53. Lania, L., Griffiths, M., Cooke, B., Ito, Y., and Fried, M. (1979): Untransformed rat cells containing free and integrated DNA of a polyoma non-transforming (HR-T) mutant. *Cell*, 18:793–802.

54. Lania, L., Hayday, A., and Fried, M. (1981): Loss of functional large-T and free viral genomes from cells transformed *in vitro* by polyoma virus after passage *in vivo* as tumor cells. *J. Virol.*, 39:422–431.

55. Levinson, A., Courtneidge, S. A., and Bishop, J. M. (1981): Structural and functional domains of RSV transforming protein pp60^{src}. *Proc. Natl. Acad. Sci. USA*, 78:1624–1628.

56. Levinson, A., Oppermann, H., Levintow, L., Varmus, H. G., and Bishop, J. M. (1978): Evidence that the transforming gene of ASV encodes a protein kinase associated with a phosphoprotein. *Cell*, 15:561–572.

57. Levinson, A. D., Oppermann, H., Varmus, H. E., and Bishop, J. M. (1980): The purified product of the transforming gene of ASV phosphorylates tyrosine. *J. Biol. Chem.*, 255:11973–11980.

58. Lewis, A. M., and Martin, R. G. (1979): Oncogenicity of simian virus 40 deletion mutants that induce altered 17-kilodalton t-proteins. *Proc. Natl. Acad. Sci. USA*, 76:4299–4302.

59. Magnusson, G., Nilsson, M.-G., Dilworth, S. M., and Smolar, N. (1981): Characterisation of polyoma virus mutants with altered middle and large T-antigens. *J. Virol.*, 39:673–683.

60. Martin, R. G. (1981): The transformation of cell growth and transmogrification of DNA synthesis by SV40. *Adv. Cancer Res.*, 34:1–68.

61. Martin, R. G., Petit Setlow, V., Edwards, C. A. F., and Vembu, D. (1979): The roles of the simian virus 40 tumour antigens in transformation of Chinese hamster lung cells. *Cell*, 17:635–643.

62. McGrath, J. P., and Levinson, A. D. (1982): Bacterial expression of an enzymatically active protein encoded by RSV src gene. *Nature*, 295:423–426.

63. Mellor, A. J. (1979): The translation of papovavirus mRNAs. Ph.D. Thesis. University of London.

64. Moore, J. L., Chowdhury, K., Martin, M. A., and Israel, M. A. (1980): Polyoma large tumour antigen is not required for tumorigenesis mediated by viral DNA. *Proc. Natl. Acad. Sci. USA*, 77:1336–1340.

65. Nilsson, S., Tyndall, C., and Magnusson, G. (1982): A small segment of polyoma middle T-antigen important for transformation defined by deletion mutants. *J. Virol.*, *(in press)*.

66. Novak, U., Dilworth, S. M., and Griffin, B. E. (1980): Coding capacity of a 35% fragment of the polyoma virus genome is sufficient to initiate and maintain cellular transformation. *Proc. Natl. Acad. Sci. USA*, 7:3278–3282.

67. Novak, U., and Griffin, B. E. (1981): Requirement for the C-terminal region of middle T-antigen in cellular transformation by polyoma virus. *Nucleic Acids Res.*, 9:2055–2073.

68. Perbal, B., and Rassoulzadegan, M. (1980): Distinct transformation phenotypes induced by polyoma virus and SV40 in rat fibroblasts and their control by an early viral gene function. *J. Virol.*, 33:697–707.

69. Pollack, R., Risser, R., Conlon, S., Freedman, V., and Rifkin, D. (1975): Production of plasminogen activator and colonial growth in semi solid medium are *in vitro* correlates of tumourigenicity. *Cold Spring Harbor Conf. Cell Proliferation*, 2:885–891.

70. Radke, K., Gilmore, T., and Martin, G. S. (1980): Transformation by Rous sarcoma virus: A cellular substrate for transformation-specific protein phosphorylation contains phosphotyrosine. *Cell*, 21:821–828.

71. Rassoulzadegan, M., Cowie, A., Carr, A., Glaichenhaus, N., Treisman, R., Favaloro, J., Cuzin, F., and Kamen, R. (1982): Separate but complementary roles for polyoma virus early proteins in the alteration of cell growth requirements leading to transformation. In: *Perspectives on Genes and the Molecular Biology of Cancer*. Raven Press, New York *(in press)*.

72. Rassoulzadegan, M., Gaudray, P., Canning, M., Trejo-Avila, L., and Cuzin, F. (1981): Two polyoma virus gene functions involved in the expression of the transformed phenotype in FR 3T3 rat cells. I. Localization of a transformation maintenance function in the proximal half of the large T coding region. *Virology*, 114:489–500.

73. Rassoulzadegan, M., Seif, R., and Cuzin, F. (1978): Conditions leading to the establishment of the N (a gene dependent) and A (a gene independent) transformed states after polyoma virus infection of rat fibroblasts. *J. Virol.*, 28:421–426.

74. Rundell, K., Major, E. O., and Lampert, M. (1981): Association of cellular 56,000 and 32,000 molecular weight proteins with BK and polyoma virus small-t antigens. *J. Virol.*, 37:1090–1093.
75. Sabatini, D., Kreibich, G., Morimoto, T., and Adesnik, M. (1982): Mechanisms for the incorporation of proteins in membranes and organelles. *J. Cell Biol.*, 92:1–22.
76. Schaffhausen, B. S., and Benjamin, T. L. (1979): Phosphorylation of polyoma T antigens. *Cell*, 18:935–946.
77. Schaffhausen, B. S., and Benjamin, T. L. (1981): Comparison of phosphorylation of two polyoma virus middle T antigens *in vivo* and *in vitro*. *J. Virol.*, 40:184–196.
78. Schaffhausen, B. S., and Benjamin, T. L. (1981): Protein kinase activity associated with polyoma virus middle T antigen. *Cold Spring Harbor Conf. Cell Proliferation*, 8:1281–1298.
79. Schaffhausen, B. S., Silver, J. E., and Benjamin, T. L. (1978): Tumour antigen(s) in cells productively infected by wild-type polyoma virus and mutant NG-18. *Proc. Natl. Acad. Sci. USA*, 75:79–83.
80. Schlegel, R., and Benjamin, T. (1978): Cellular alterations dependent upon the polyoma virus Hr-t function: Separation of mitogenic from transforming capacities. *Cell*, 14:587–599.
81. Sefton, B., Hunter, T., and Beemon, K. (1979): Temperature sensitive transformation by Rous sarcoma virus and temperature sensitive kinase activity. *J. Virol.*, 33:220–229.
82. Sefton, B., Hunter, T., Beemon, K., and Eckhart, W. (1980): Evidence that the phosphorylation of tyrosine is essential for cellular transformation by Rous sarcoma virus. *Cell*, 20:807–816.
83. Silver, J., Schaffhausen, B., and Benjamin, T. L. (1978): Tumour antigens induced by nontransforming mutants of polyoma virus. *Cell*, 15:485–496.
84. Simmons, D. T., Chang, C., and Martin, M. A. (1979): Multiple forms of polyoma virus tumor antigens from infected and transformed cells. *J. Virol.*, 29:881–887.
85. Sleigh, M. J., Topp, W. C., Hanich, R., and Sambrook, J. F. (1978): Mutants of SV40 with an altered small t protein are reduced in their ability to transform cells. *Cell*, 14:79–88.
86. Smart, J. E., and Ito, Y. (1978): Three species of polyoma virus tumor antigens share common peptides probably near the amino-terminal of the proteins. *Cell*, 15:1427–1437.
87. Smart, J. E., Oppermann, H., Czernilofsky, A. P., Purchio, A. F., Erikson, R. L., and Bishop, J. M. (1981): Characterisation of sites for tyrosine phosphorylation in the transforming protein of Rous sarcoma virus and its cellular homologue. *Proc. Natl. Acad. Sci. USA*, 78:6013–6017.
88. Smith, A. E. (1980): Role of protein kinases in replication and transformation by polyoma virus. In: *Protein Phosphorylation and Bio Regulation*, edited by G. Thomas, E. Podesta, and J. Gordon, pp. 219–228. Karger, Basel.
89. Smith, A. E., Fried, M., Ito, Y., Spurr, N., and Smith, R. (1979): Is middle-T of polyoma virus protein kinase? *Cold Spring Harbor Symp. Quant. Biol.*, 44:141–147.
90. Smith, A. E., Smith, R., Griffin, B., and Fried, M. (1979): Protein kinase activity associated with polyoma virus middle T antigen *in vitro*. *Cell*, 18:915–924.
91. Smith, A. E., Smith, R., and Paucha, E. (1979): Characterisation of tumour antigens present in SV40 transformed cells. *Cell*, 18:335–346.
92. Smolar, N., and Griffin, B. E. (1981): DNA sequences of polyoma virus early detection mutants. *J. Virol.*, 38:958–967.
93. Soeda, E., Arrand, J. R., and Griffin, B. E. (1979): Polyoma virus: The early region and its T-antigens. *Nucleic Acids Res.*, 7:839–857.
94. Soeda, E., Arrand, J. R., Smolar, N., Walsh, J. E., and Griffin, B. E. (1980): Coding potential and regulatory signals of the polyoma virus genome. *Nature*, 283:445–453.
95. Soeda, E., and Griffin, B. E. (1978): Sequences from the genome of a non-transforming mutant of polyoma virus. *Nature*, 276:294–298.
96. Stoker, M. (1965): Abortive transformation by polyoma virus. *Nature*, 218:234–238.
97. Templeton, D., and Eckhart, W. (1982): Mutation causing premature termination of the polyoma virus middle-T antigen blocks cell transformation. *J. Virol.*, 41:1014–1024.
98. Tjian, R. (1981): The regulation of viral transcription and DNA replication by SV40 large-T antigen. *Curr. Top. Microbiol. Immunol.*, 93:5–24.
99. Tooze, J. (1980): *DNA Tumour Viruses, Part 2*, ed. 2. Cold Spring Harbor Laboratory, Cold Spring Harbor, New York.
100. Topp, W. C., and Rifkin, D. B. (1980): The small-t protein of SV40 is required for loss of actin cable networks and plasminogen activator synthesis in transformed rat cells. *Virology*, 106:282–291.

101. Treisman, R. H., Cowie, A., Favaloro, J. M , Jat, P., and Kamen, R. (1981): The structures of the spliced mRNAs encoding polyoma virus early region proteins. *J. Mol. Appl. Gen.*, 1:83–92.
102. Treisman, R. H., Novak, U., Favaloro, J., and Kamen, R. (1981): Transformation of rat cells by an altered polyoma virus genome expressing only the middle T protein. *Nature*, 292:959–600.
103. Trejo-Avila, L., Gaudray, P., and Cuzin, F. (1981): Two polyoma virus gene functions involved in the expression of the transformed phenotype in FR 3T3 rat cells. II. The presence of the 56K middle-T protein in the cell membrane is not sufficient for maintenance. *Virology*, 114:501–506.
104. Turler, H. (1980): The tumor antigens and the early functions of polyoma virus. *Mol. Cell. Biochem.*, 32:63–93.
105. Tyndall, C., Lupton, S., Jat, P. J., Favaloro, J., and Kamen, R. (1982): Isolation and characterisation of mouse cells transformed by origin defective polyoma virus. *J. Virol. (in press)*.
106. Ushiro, H., and Cohen, S. (1980): Identification of phosphotyrosine as a product of EGF-activated protein kinase in A-431 cell membranes. *J. Biol. Chem.*, 255:8363–8365.
107. Walter, G., Hutchinson, M. A., Hunter, T., and Eckhart, W. (1981): Antibodies specific for the polyoma virus middle tumor antigen. *Proc. Natl. Acad. Sci. USA*, 78:4882–4886.

Advances in Viral Oncology, Volume 3, edited by
George Klein. Raven Press, New York © 1983.

Structure and Function of Simian Virus 40 Large T-Antigen

Peter W. J. Rigby and David P. Lane

*Cancer Research Campaign, Eukaryotic Molecular Genetics Research Group,
Department of Biochemistry, Imperial College of Science and Technology,
London SW7 2AZ, United Kingdom*

The initiation of transformation by simian virus 40 (SV40) requires the expression of only the early region of the viral genome, which encodes two proteins: the large T antigen (apparent molecular weight 94,000) and the small t antigen (apparent molecular weight 17,000). Studies with deletion mutants that cannot synthesize small t antigen have shown that this protein is required neither for transformation *in vitro* nor for tumor induction *in vivo* (54,62,115). These data and experiments with *tsA* mutants, temperature-sensitive mutants affecting only large T antigen, have shown clearly that large T antigen is the protein required for the initiation of transformation and have suggested very strongly that the continued expression of functional large T antigen is necessary for maintenance of the transformed phenotype. Although small t antigen is clearly not essential for transformation, the activities of this protein can affect the quality of the transformation event (34,114). However, in a formal genetic sense, the gene coding for large T antigen is the oncogene of SV40, and we shall therefore confine our attention to this genetic element and its protein product.

The roles played by large T antigen in both the productive infection of permissive cells and the transformation of nonpermissive cells have recently been authoritatively and comprehensively reviewed in Tooze (113), and Martin (60) has quite superbly discussed the roles of the SV40 tumor antigens in transformation. We shall not presume to duplicate those reviews, to which the reader is referred for background information relevant to the points we shall consider and for discussion of the many aspects of large T antigen that we shall not cover. We shall concentrate our attention on recently published work relevant to selected aspects of the structure and function of large T antigen. We shall attempt to define what seem to us to be the critical issues facing the student of large T antigen and to consider the experimental approaches that are likely to further our understanding of this extraordinary protein.

Large T antigen is capable of catalyzing a large number of biochemical reactions (Table 1). In some cases it is easy to see how these activities relate to each other. For example, the binding of large T antigen to the SV40 origin is required for the initiation of viral DNA replication, and the promoter for the SV40 early transcription

TABLE 1. *Biochemical reactions in which SV40 large T antigen has been implicated*

Function	Region of T antigen involved in function[a]	Ref.
1. Sequence specific binding to viral DNA	4600–4000	3,21,68,71,72,73,80, 81,90,94,104,105, 110
2. Initiation of viral DNA replication	Unknown, but by implication same as 1	11,12,63,71,72,76a, 102,103
3. Autoregulation of viral early transcription	Unknown, but by implication same as 1	37,71,86,113
4. Induction of viral late transcription	Unknown	113
5. ATPase	Unknown	3,10,10a,112
6. Protein kinase	Unknown	3,112,113
7. Adenovirus helper function	3200–2700	77,113
8. Induction of immunity to SV40 tumor cells	3200–2700 sufficient	1,5,6,18,19,33,42, 45,47,55,89,100, 107
9. Target for cytotoxic T cells	N-terminal half sufficient	83
10. Binding to cellular DNA	4100–3800	8,60,74,80,81
11. Initiation of cellular DNA replication	4300–4000	9,25,59,60,61,69, 97a,111
12. Binding to p53	Unknown	4,8,13,16,22,35,40, 50,66,85,89
13. Activation of rDNA transcription	3800–3500	25,97,97a,98
14. Induction of cellular enzyme synthesis	Unknown	60,78,113
15. Activation of RNA polymerase II transcription of cellular genes	Unknown	91,92
16. Initiation and maintenance of oncogenic transformation	Unknown but N-terminal half has limited capability	13,16,60,62

[a]As functions have generally been mapped against the DNA sequence rather than the amino acid sequence, functions are located according to nucleotide numbers using the numbering system of Buchman, Burnett and Berg (113). These locations should be regarded as highly tentative and interpreted with due regard to the reservations expressed in the text.

unit is known to overlap the origin. It is thus not difficult to see how large T antigen can autoregulate its own synthesis. It is much less easy to relate this DNA binding activity to the fact that a small proportion of the large T antigen in a cell is displayed on the surface, where it provides the antigen recognized during the immunological rejection of SV40-induced tumors. These widely disparate activities suggest that large T antigen is a multidomain protein, with each domain being responsible for a particular biochemical activity, and a major emphasis of current research is to map the protein's activities against both its primary sequence and its tertiary and quaternary structures.

We shall confine our attention to some particular aspects of the biochemistry and biology of large T antigen: (a) the biochemical and biological properties of cell-surface large T antigen; (b) the binding of large T antigen to SV40 DNA, the relationship of this binding to the initiation of DNA replication and the autoregulation of early transcription, and attempts to locate regions of the protein involved in DNA binding; (c) the existence of biochemically and functionally distinct subsets of large T antigen; (d) the unusual T antigens synthesized in SV40-transformed cells and their relationship to the interaction of the protein with the host cell genome; (e) the binding of large T antigen to cellular DNA and the possible role of such interactions in the alterations in cellular DNA replication and cellular transcription that characterize transformed cells.

We cannot, in the space of this chapter, deal comprehensively with any of these issues. We do hope to provide a critical review of the work that has been done and to point out what, in our view, will be profitable areas for future research.

SV40 LARGE T ANTIGEN ON THE CELL SURFACE

SV40-induced tumors can be rejected by immunologically competent animals. This rejection shows specificity, because animals that have rejected SV40-induced tumors are still susceptible to tumors induced by other agents but are able to reject more rapidly or at a higher dose other independently induced SV40 tumors.

In the most closely studied model system, BALB/c mice can be protected against the growth of a fixed dose of the SV40-transformed tumor cell line mKSA. In addition to protection by prior injection of irradiated tumor cells, prior injection of live virus or of partially or very highly purified SV40 large T antigen is protective (1,6,24,107). The effector mechanisms that are induced by large T antigen or virus immunization and that account for tumor protection are not precisely established, but the available evidence strongly implies that specific cytotoxic T cells are a major component of the antitumor response (31,106,116). It has been demonstrated clearly that specific H-2-restricted (32,76,107) cytotoxic T cells are primed *in vivo* by the injection of virus, tumor cells, or large T antigen. These cytotoxic T cells can be boosted *in vitro* and then used to kill chromium-labeled SV40-transformed target cells in a standard *in vitro* cytotoxicity test. The *in vitro* system shows acute target specificity, as only SV40-transformed H-2-compatible targets are killed.

The precise biochemical nature of the target antigen recognized by cytotoxic T cells is not understood in any system. In the SV40 system there is good evidence that a species antigenically related to SV40 large T antigen is at least a component of the target structure. This evidence is of two sorts; the first concerns the requirement for induction of immunity to SV40-induced tumors, and the second concerns the requirement for the target cell to be recognized by cytotoxic T cells.

Purified large T antigen, even large T antigen isolated as a single band from SDS polyacrylamide gels, is able to protect mice against mKSA tumors (6,24,107).

The entire large T antigen molecule is not required for the induction of tumor immunity, because both $Ad2^+ND_2$ and $Ad2^+ND_1$ viruses can, albeit at low efficiency, induce specific immunity (45,47,55). These experiments are often misinterpreted; they do indicate that the C-terminal region of large T antigen encoded by these hybrid viruses is protective, but they certainly do not exclude the possibility that other areas of the molecule have similar activity or that multiple areas are required for maximal protection. The availability of new deletion and point mutations affecting the gene for large T antigen (76a,77) and the production of small t antigen in bacteria (87,108) should allow more precise definition of the regions of large T antigen that can function to induce tumor immunity.

Recent studies by Tevethia's group have used a new approach to determine the nature of the target antigen recognized *in vitro* by *in-vivo*-primed cytotoxic T cells. They have transfected tk⁻ mouse L cells with hybrid tk⁺ plasmids encoding deleted large T antigen molecules. This approach has yielded some positive results; expression of the N-terminal region of large T antigen is sufficient to produce a target cell susceptible to kill by primed cytotoxic T cells (83). The simplest interpretation of these results is that large T antigen is present on the surfaces of SV40-transformed cells, where it "associates" with H-2 antigen to form a target structure susceptible to cytotoxic T cell recognition. An alternative hypothesis is that SV40 transformation induces the synthesis and display at the cell surface of a specific host structure that is the actual target species. This seems innately less likely, given the great specificity of the cytotoxic T cells for SV40-transformed cells, recently confirmed using cloned lines of SV40-specific cytotoxic T cells (3a). Definitive proof that large T antigen is the target structure requires specific blocking of the cloned cytotoxic T cells with antibody against large T antigen or incorporation of the target structures into liposomes. However, all reasonable current criteria for the identification of T cell targets suggest that structures antigenically related to SV40 large T antigen are involved and must therefore be present on the surface. The SV40 system is exceptional in that purified protein will induce cytotoxic T cells. Because the T cells are H-2-restricted and, furthermore, restricted by Class 1 antigens (32), the injected large T antigen must somehow be processed so that it is presented to cytotoxic T cell precursors in the context of Class 1 antigens. There is no other well-documented case of the induction of cytotoxic T cells by soluble antigen. This unusual property may relate to the affinity of large T antigen for the surfaces of normal and transformed cells (53). Because of the ease with which the early region of SV40 can now be manipulated, the SV40 tumor-specific transplantation antigen (TSTA) is likely to become an extremely fruitful system for structural studies on the nature of cytotoxic T cell target antigens.

The realization from tumor-protection experiments that a structure related to large T antigen is present on the cell surface has led to efforts to demonstrate surface large T antigen using biochemical and serological techniques. Two things need to be borne in mind when analyzing these studies: First, the number of molecules that need to be displayed at the cell surface to act as a target for cytotoxic T cells can be very small and below the theoretical limits of detection of immunofluorescent staining. Second, all SV40-transformed cells contain high concentrations of large T antigen in the nucleus, the bulk of which is readily extracted under physiological conditions. The investigator who wishes to prove that large-T-antigen-related proteins synthesized by a given cell are processed by that same cell into a surface form must therefore overcome the potential objections that the surface antigen detected is either cytoplasmic or nuclear contamination of plasma membrane preparations, or that it is acquired passively from lysed cells present in the culture. Although the means by which large T antigen is present at the surface is not of crucial importance to the tumor immunologist, it is of considerable importance to the virologist, because the surface form, if it is an actively produced subset of large T antigen, may have a specific function in both transformation and replication, as well as its more passive role as a target antigen.

Two recent studies offer fairly convincing proof for an active processing of large T antigen into a special surface form. Gooding et al. (33) used a wide range of anti-T monoclonal antibodies to stain the surface of an SV40-transformed mouse cell line using an indirect immunofluorescence technique. They were able to show quite convincing surface staining with some, but not all, of the antibodies, although all the antibodies had a very high titer against nuclear large T antigen when used in the same type of test. This study confirms earlier results from Butel's laboratory (52) and from Deppert and Henning's group (18,42). In these cases, antitumor sera, sera made against gel-purified large T antigen, or sera made against a small synthetic peptide corresponding to the extreme C-terminal region of large T antigen (118) were used. Deppert has claimed that the anti-gel-purified-T sera are relatively more potent against the surface form than the nuclear form when compared with antitumor sera. He has also shown (19a), using the antipeptide sera, that the extreme C terminus is exposed, and this would fit in general terms with the results of Gooding et al. (33), because it was predominantly monoclonals directed against the central area of large T antigen that failed to score in the surface assay. Deppert has also shown that the $Ad2^+ND_2$- and $Ad2^+ND_1$-encoded large-T-antigen-related proteins are expressed at the cell surface (19). The controls employed in these experiments were first to stain non-SV40-transformed cells and second to lyse cells in the culture deliberately and show that the lysate would not render non-SV40-transformed cells surface-T-positive. Finally, Gooding et al. showed loss of surface staining following mild trypsin treatment; surface large T antigen did not reappear in the absence of protein synthesis (33). Deppert performed an excellent control in plating a mixture of SV40-transformed and control cells, allowing them to grow together and then staining the mix; he was able to distinguish positive from negative cells. Gooding et al. stained cells in suspension (prepared using EDTA), and Deppert used monolayer cultures. The results are still open to some doubts, because in all cases the reactions were very weak, and a number of different cell line and serum combinations gave negative results.

Direct biochemical studies have also demonstrated the presence of surface large T antigen. Either metabolically labeled cells were fractionated into nuclear, cytoplasmic, and membrane fractions and then immunoprecipitated and analyzed by

SDS polyacrylamide gel electrophoresis or the surface proteins were iodinated using a lactoperoxidase technique and analyzed following solubilization by immunoprecipitation and gel electrophoresis. A number of groups have detected "surface T" by these methods (19,57,99,100). Many of the fractionation studies are unconvincing, because the purity of the plasma membrane fractions and the degree of contamination with cytoplasmic or nuclear membrane materials were not adequately assessed. Similarly, the lactoperoxidase results are open to the criticism that the labeled "external" T could have come from lysed cells. In all cases the essential problem is that the form of large T antigen detected on the surface is identical with that present in the nucleus and cytoplasm. If surface T were characterized by a specific modification, the problem would be much more easily resolved. Indeed, Klockmann and Deppert have demonstrated that the membrane form of large T antigen is acylated (47a). Santos and Butel (89), in a recent and very closely controlled study, have provided the most convincing biochemical evidence so far for surface large T antigen. They used a novel approach in that following lactoperoxidase iodination they incubated the cell monolayer with anti-T antibody before cell lysis. On solubilization they were thus able to selectively precipitate the T antigens available on the exterior surface of the cell monolayer without further addition of antibody. The results clearly demonstrated that they were selectively labeling a very small subset of the total large T antigen molecules present in the culture and that all of the labeled molecules were exposed to the exterior. To control for the possibility that large T antigen shed from dying cells was attaching itself to the surfaces of live cells, mixing experiments were performed using vast excesses of labeled, sonicated cell extracts, incubating them with the live monolayer, and then taking this through the external immunoprecipitation procedure. No significant contamination by the lysate was seen. This is in contrast to the results obtained by Lange-Mutschler and Henning (53), who have reported a specific association of large T antigen extracted from cell lysates with the surfaces of cells, although in this latter case the amounts of lysate applied were huge. An important conclusion from the data of Santos and Butel is that the "surface T" is still associated with the host p53 protein that is found in a complex with nuclear large T antigen. Furthermore, both the surface large T antigen and surface p53 are phosphorylated and available to external antibody.

If we accept the bulk of evidence in favor of a surface form of large T antigen, then it is legitimate to ask what role this species performs. Clearly it is a strong candidate for the viral tumor-specific transplantation antigen, TSTA, but this seems unlikely to be its sole purpose. A more active role may be imagined, perhaps involvement in active transport, because one of the properties of SV40-transformed cells is the ability to grow in restricted media. Alternatively, the plasma membrane form of large T antigen may be a passive consequence of a need to associate with internal membranes for function. In either case, the failure to select cells in tumors that have a nuclear-T-positive surface-T-negative phenotype strongly implies that these two properties and/or the property of transformation are not readily separated by mutation, particularly in view of the fact that Mora's group has shown that injection into mice of cells "doubly" transformed by SV40 and another agent allows the selection of T-negative variants *in vivo* (5). The application of modern *in vitro* mutagenic techniques should allow detailed analysis of the relationship between the ability of large T antigen to be displayed on the cell surface and the protein's other functions.

INTERACTION BETWEEN SV40 LARGE T ANTIGEN AND THE DNA SEQUENCES SURROUNDING THE VIRAL ORIGIN OF DNA REPLICATION

Tegtmeyer (103) observed many years ago that in cells infected with *tsA* mutants at the nonpermissive temperature the initiation of viral DNA replication is severely inhibited, but elongation is unaffected, suggesting that large T antigen, the product of the *A* gene, interacts in some way with the viral origin of DNA replication. That such an interaction does occur was demonstrated by electron microscopy and by nitrocellulose-filter binding experiments (46,84), but such analyses could not lead to a detailed description of exactly how large T antigen binds to a specific region of the viral genome. During the past few years, several groups have expended considerable effort in attempting to define exactly which regions of large T antigen are required for DNA binding and which nucleotides in the region surrounding the viral origin of DNA replication are involved in this interaction. In order to pursue such studies, it was necessary to obtain fairly large amounts of purified large T antigen protein and to develop techniques to identify those DNA sequences bound by it.

The SV40-transformed human cell line SV80 synthesizes high levels of large T antigen and was therefore used as a convenient source of the protein in many early studies. However, we now know that the SV80 large T antigen is a member of an interesting class of mutants, found quite frequently in transformed cells *(vide infra)*, in which the transformation function(s) of the protein is intact but the DNA replication function(s) is inactivated. All experiments that use this protein are thus severely compromised. An extremely attractive alternative to the purification of large T antigen from SV40-infected or -transformed cells was afforded by the isolation of the adenovirus-2-SV40 hybrid virus Ad2$^+$D2 (41). HeLa cells infected by this virus synthesize a protein, called D2T, that contains all of the SV40 sequences unique to large T antigen but none of the sequences shared by the large T and small t antigens (Fig. 1). The N-terminal segment of this protein derives from an adenovirus structural protein. Because D2T is synthesized under the control of the adenovirus major late promoter, relatively large amounts of the protein accumulate in infected HeLa cells, which can be grown in bulk in suspension culture. Tjian exploited these observations to purify D2T to near homogeneity (110), and both his group and that of Livingston have performed an extensive series of experiments to characterize the interactions of this protein with the SV40 genome (72,105,110). The standard experimental design has been to bind D2T, at various protein concentrations, to SV40 DNA, or to cloned fragments thereof, and then to analyze the

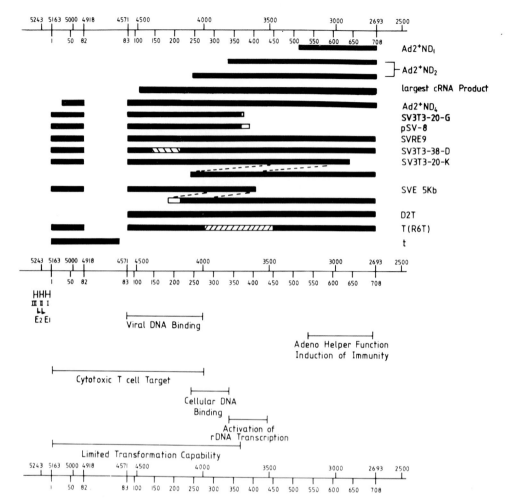

FIG. 1. A functional map of SV40 large T antigen. Map coordinates are given in nucleotide numbers, according to the system of Buchman, Burnett, and Berg (113), above the lines and in amino acid numbers below the lines. The upper panel shows the structures of the various large-T-antigen-related proteins discussed in the text. The data were taken from the following references: (a) Ad2+ND1, Ad2+ND2, and AD2+ND4 (80); only the largest Ad2+ND4 encoded protein is shown. (b) The largest cRNA translation product (81). (c) SV3T3-20-G (13); the open segment at the C terminus indicates amino acids encoded by the flanking cellular DNA. (d) pSV-8 (16); the open segment at the C terminus indicates that this region of the T antigen(s) encoded by pSV-8 is of uncertain structure. (e) SVRE9 (102); the discontinuity indicates the position of the single base substitution. (f) SV3T3-38-D (11); the cross-hatched region indicates the position of the deletion. (g) SV3T3-20-K (56); indicated is the extent of the perfect tandem duplication. (h) SVE 5Kb (63); indicated is the extent of the duplication; the open region indicates amino acids encoded by an inverted segment of SV40 DNA. (i) D2T (41). (j) T and t (113); the cross-hatched segment in T indicates the region in which most ts-a mutations map. (k) R6T (109). Immediately below the central line of map coordinates are shown the three binding sites for D2T and R6T (71,72,86,110) and the two starting points for viral early transcription (27,37). The lower panel shows the mapping of the functions of large T antigen. The relevant references are given in Table 1.

DNA sequences protected using either the DNase I footprinting procedure of Galas and Schmitz (26) or the specific chemical modifications developed for the Maxam and Gilbert DNA sequencing methods (28) or protection from digestion by exonuclease III (93).

The results of Tjian's group have led to the view that T-antigen-origin binding is closely analogous to the interactions between the λ repressor and operators. The protein binds, probably as tetramers (73), to three adjacent sites. Site I is on the early side of the origin, site II is coincident with the genetically defined minimal origin (20), and site III is located on the late side of the origin. Titration experiments in which increasing amounts of D2T are bound to a fixed amount of SV40 DNA have shown that site I is occupied first. As the D2T concentration is increased, sites II and III become occupied, and Livingston's group has also observed an additional site, called I', on the early side of site I, that becomes occupied at the same D2T concentrations as site II. These data suggest that the binding of D2T to site I may facilitate subsequent binding to sites II and III, i.e., that the interaction is cooperative. Such cooperativity could occur by one of two mechanisms. One could argue that sequence-specific binding occurs only to site I and that the subsequent occupation of sites II and III results from processive polymerization of the D2T onto the DNA via protein-protein interactions. This proposition seems somewhat unlikely in view of the fact that both sites II and III are on the same side of site I, and extensive invasion of early region sequences has not been observed. The alternative explanation is that the binding of D2T to site I alters the conformation of the DNA in such a way as to facilitate subsequent binding to sites II and III.

These possibilities have been tested by analyzing the binding of D2T to a series of deletion and substitution mutations generated within the origin region. As expected, deletion of site I greatly reduces the ability of D2T to bind to the DNA. Mutants in which site II is deleted, or substituted by foreign sequences, do not bind T antigen efficiently to the "Site-II-equivalent" sequences (71). Such data indicate that there are sequence requirements for binding to site II and that the occupation of this site is not the result of processive polymerization of the protein.

The relationships between the *in vitro* binding of D2T to the SV40 origin region and the role of large T antigen in the regulation of viral DNA replication and viral early transcription have also been studied. Myers and Tjian (72) correlated the ability of D2T to bind to the DNA of deletion mutants with the ability of these same mutant DNAs to replicate in permissive monkey cells. The DNA replication assay depends on the availability of COS cells (29). These are permissive CV-1 monkey kidney cells transformed by a cloned segment of SV40 DNA containing the entire early transcription unit, but in which the viral origin of DNA replication has been inactivated by a deletion. The resident viral genome can thus neither replicate nor be rescued, but the cells contain functional large T antigen and the cellular factors required for viral DNA replication. If such cells are transfected with plasmid vector DNA that cannot replicate, the DNA is rapidly degraded. However, if the plasmid has cloned into it a functional SV40 origin, it can replicate, and the transfected DNA thus not only persists but also increases in abundance. Replication is normally detected by analyzing the low-molecular-weight DNA present in transfected cells by agarose gel electrophoresis and Southern blotting. In accordance with previous data, site III is not required for efficient replication. A small deletion at the *Bgl*I site in site II abolishes DNA replication *in vivo*, although this mutant DNA is bound by D2T as efficiently as wild-type DNA. Conversely, a mutant lacking most of site I is only slightly impaired in its DNA replication ability, although its binding to D2T is considerably reduced. Deletion of all of site I and sequences between sites I and II abolishes replication and further reduces binding to D2T. These data thus do not provide a clear correlation between DNA replication *in vivo* under the influence of wild-type large T antigen and D2T binding. Although mutations in site I do show some correlation, it must be noted that the mutant deleted in site II does not replicate, although it binds normally in the *in vitro* assay.

Large T antigen regulates the transcription of its own mRNA in infected permissive cells. The relationship between this transcriptional regulation and D2T binding has not yet been tested by studying the *in vivo* transcription of mutant templates, but it has been intensively studied using the *in vitro* transcription system of Manley et al. (58). Rio et al. (86) showed that this *in vitro* transcription system accurately initiates at both SV40 promoters, early and late, and that transcription from the early promoter is specifically inhibited by D2T, which has no effect on late transcription or on transcription from the major late promoter of adenovirus 2. Moreover, the transcription of mutant DNAs lacking T antigen binding sites I and II is not repressed by D2T.

Hansen et al. (37) have performed similar experiments and have also addressed the question of the shift in the 5′ termini of the early mRNAs that occurs late during the productive infection of permissive cells. Early in infection the predominant 5′ termini are located close to the origin of DNA replication, within D2T binding site II; late in infection the majority of 5′ termini shift some 40 to 50 nucleotides upstream (27) to sites close to the early region proximal border of site III. Both of these early transcriptional initiation sites are utilized in the *in vitro* system, and again all early transcription is repressed by sufficiently high concentrations of D2T. However, more detailed mapping of the RNAs synthesized in the *in vitro* system by nuclease digestion of DNA/RNA hybrids shows that the "early" early 5′ termini are repressed at lower D2T concentrations than the "late" early 5′ termini. Measurements of the binding of D2T using the footprinting technique show that repression of the "early" early 5′ termini corresponds to the binding of D2T to site I, whereas repression of the "late" early 5′ termini appears to require binding to sites I and II. In agreement with these *in vitro* data, DiMaio and Nathans [cited by Hansen et al. (37)] have shown that mutants with deletions in site I overproduce early mRNA and large T antigen fivefold, i.e., they show decreased susceptibility to large-T-antigen-mediated autoregulation of early transcription. Moreover, Ghosh and Lebowitz (27) have shown by analyzing the early RNA at late times during infection by *tsA* mutants that functional large T antigen is required to maintain the upstream shift of 5′ termini. However, it is not clear that the shift of 5′ termini is mediated simply by the binding of large T antigen to site I and thus the repression of initiation at the "early" early start site. A mutant virus containing a deletion of site I undergoes a normal shift [Hansen and Sharp, cited by Hansen et al. (37)], and thus this process may also depend on interactions at site II.

A possible objection to much of the work discussed earlier is that it depends on the use of D2T, which may not be functionally identical with the wild-type large T antigen produced in productively infected or transformed cells. In order to obviate this objection, Thummel et al. (109) have constructed novel adenovirus-SV40 hybrid viruses that express the whole of the large T antigen coding sequence under adenovirus late control. The protein isolated from HeLa cells infected by the hybrid virus Ad-SVR6, which we shall call R6T, thus has exactly the same amino acid sequence as wild-type large T antigen, and thus one cannot object, as in the case of D2T, that the absence of some SV40 sequences and the presence of adenovirus sequences alters the interactions of the protein with SV40 DNA. The binding of R6T to SV40 DNA is qualitatively similar to that of D2T, site I being occupied at low protein concentrations, whereas sites II and III become occupied at higher concentrations (71). However, higher protein:DNA ratios are required for binding to sites II and III when D2T is used instead of R6T, suggesting that D2T may be somewhat impaired in its ability to bind to DNA. Like D2T, R6T does not bind efficiently to site II in mutants from which site I has been deleted. R6T also represses transcription from the SV40 early promoter *in vitro*, but is twofold to threefold more efficient than D2T, again suggesting that this latter protein is not fully functional (71).

Large T antigen could repress early transcription either by blocking the binding of RNA polymerase II to the SV40 early promoter or by preventing the elongation of preinitiated polymerase molecules. Myers et al. (71) have tested this latter possibility by constructing hybrid plasmids in which the three T antigen binding sites are positioned, in either orientation, downstream of the adenovirus 2 major late promoter. Transcription from the adenovirus promoter is not repressed by R6T, indicating that the presence of bound T antigen does not prevent the passage of preinitiated RNA polymerase. R6T does not repress the transcription of mutant templates from which site I has been deleted, in agreement with the results obtained with D2T. However, binding to site I alone is not sufficient to cause repression, which must depend on interactions between T antigen and, at least, sites I and II, as was also suggested by the work of Hansen et al. (37).

Although R6T clearly represents an improvement over D2T, there are still objections to its use. R6T may contain the entire amino acid sequence of SV40 large T antigen, but the protein is synthesized in the environment of a human cell late in adenovirus infection rather than in a monkey cell during SV40 infection or in an SV40-transformed cell. It is clear that wild-type large T antigen is extensively modified posttranslationally. There are considerable numbers of phosphorylation sites on the protein (117), and it has also been reported that some large T antigen is poly-ADP-ribosylated (30). Moreover, present evidence does not eliminate other forms of modification, for example, glycosylation. The large T antigen present in SV40-infected or -transformed cells exists in a variety of oligomeric structures, some involving the host-coded p53 protein, which may have distinct biochemical functions *(vide infra)*. It is not presently clear whether or not R6T is properly modified and/or oligomerized in Ad-SVR6-infected cells. It has also been argued that infected cells contain antigenically and biochemically distinct subsets of large T antigen *(vide infra)*. Although these data are open to objection, further experimentation on this point is clearly required, and until the precise form of large T antigen that binds to the origin in a productively infected permissive cell has been clearly identified, results obtained with proteins such as R6T must be interpreted with caution.

In addition to defining the regions of the viral genome bound by large T antigen, it is also of importance to identify the sequences within the protein that constitute the DNA binding site. In addition to binding with high affinity to the viral origin of DNA replication, large T antigen also binds with lower affinity to cellular DNA (74). This latter interaction could simply be a reflection of a general property of DNA binding proteins, namely that they interact with all DNA but with a significantly higher affinity for their specific recognition sequence, or it could indicate that there are two DNA binding sites on large T antigen. It is likely that the interaction of large T antigen with cellular DNA is not an *in vitro* artifact, because the protein can induce a round of cellular DNA replication in quiescent cells, and SV40-transformed cells exhibit a pattern of cellular DNA replication distinct from that of their untransformed parents *(vide infra)*.

The principal approach used to attempt to locate regions of large T antigen important for both types of DNA binding has been to analyze the DNA binding properties of a variety of T antigen derivatives produced by (a) *in vitro* translation of SV40 cRNA (81), (b) the nondefective adenovirus-2-SV40 hybrid viruses (80), and (c) SV40-transformed cells (8). SV40 cRNA is a colinear transcript of the entire early region and thus retains the intron normally removed from large T antigen mRNA by splicing. Translation of large-T-antigen-related proteins from this template can thus initiate only at AUG codons located after the splice acceptor sequence. *In vitro* translation of cRNA yields a family of large T-antigen-related proteins that derive from translational initiation at AUG codons within the large T antigen coding sequence. Only the largest *in vitro* translation product binds to SV40 DNA, suggesting that the segment of large T antigen encoded between nucleotides 4,600 and 4,400 approximately is required for origin binding (81). The adenovirus-SV40 hybrid viruses encode a series of large-T-antigen-related proteins that have the same C terminus as authentic large T antigen and extend for varying distances toward the N terminus of the protein. The DNA binding properties of these proteins implicate the same region of large T antigen in origin binding, if it is assumed that sequences shared by small t and large T antigens play no role in this process. The data also suggest that the segment of large T antigen encoded between nucleotides 4,100 and 3,800 approximately is required for binding to cellular DNA (80). Many SV40-transformed cells synthesize large-T-antigen-related proteins with an apparent molecular weight of less than 94,000 *(vide infra)*. Several of these truncated T antigens have been analyzed with respect to their ability to bind to cellular DNA, with the conclusion that a protein extending from the normal N terminus up to a region encoded around nucleotide 4,000 has the ability to bind, whereas shorter proteins do not (8).

Although these three types of experiment have been interpreted to provide more or less consistent data, they are open to severe criticism. They treat large T antigen as if it functions as a linear array of amino acids. Because the ability of a protein to bind to DNA is abolished by the deletion of certain amino acids, one cannot conclude that those amino acids are directly involved in DNA binding. It is intrinsically just as likely that those amino acids contribute to a tertiary or quaternary structure that is required either directly for DNA binding or, perhaps, because it allows some posttranslational modification that modulates the protein's affinity for DNA. Only positive results can thus be of any significance. However, just because a particular large T antigen derivative binds to either viral or cellular DNA, it cannot be concluded that the protein contains a fully functional DNA binding site. In none of the work published to date has the affinity of the protein for the DNA been measured, nor have footprinting or methylation protection experiments been performed to ensure that the protein binds in the same way as authentic large T antigen.

Proper identification of sequences that contribute to the DNA binding activity of large T antigen will require much more extensive genetic analysis. The power of this type of approach is exemplified by the elegant studies of Nathans and his colleagues. They used *in vitro* mutagenic techniques to generate a series of mutations in the viral origin of DNA replication that impair the ability of that template to be replicated by wild-type large T antigen (95). They then selected revertants (94) and found that some of the reversion mutations mapped in the gene for large T antigen, between nucleotides 4,376 and 4,002. Given that fully functional wild-type large T antigen cannot efficiently initiate replication at the mutant origins, whereas it can from wild-type origins, and that the revertant large T antigens can effectively initiate at the mutant origins, it is much more likely that these mutations will define regions of large T antigen intimately involved in DNA binding, although indirect effects cannot be eliminated *a priori*.

The development of techniques for site-directed mutagenesis can confidently be expected to lead to a renaissance in SV40 genetics, and already the first in what will surely be a very large series of new mutations within the *A* gene have been isolated and partially characterized (D. Nathans, K. Peden, J. Pipas, and A. E. Smith, *personal communications*). These mutants will surely be invaluable in dissecting the regions of large T antigen required for the protein's many biochemical activities, but they have also already shown clearly the problems inherent in all previous attempts to map the DNA binding site of large T antigen. It has been an article of faith in the field that only the sequences unique to large T antigen are involved in DNA binding; without such a belief, none of the work with D2T would have received credence. Yet a small deletion in the small t/large T common region severely affects the ability of large T antigen to bind to SV40 DNA (10a). It seems highly likely that in this case the defect in DNA binding is mediated via structural effects, but if this mutant had been discovered several years ago, the experiments discussed earlier might well have been interpreted in quite a different way. It will not be surprising if the DNA binding ability of large T antigen is inactivated by mutations located throughout the coding sequence. The mechanisms by which these mutations exert their effects will be revealed only by more direct biochemical analyses.

Of prime importance is the measurement of the affinities with which mutant large T antigens bind to DNA. A mutant with a 10-fold decrease in affinity for the SV40 origin may well bind to the origin, as judged by the McKay immunoprecipitation assay (68), but such a decrease in affinity would clearly be significant biologically. The immunoprecipitation assay is also prone to artifact, because different monoclonal antibodies bind to large T antigen with different affinities, a problem that severely compromises the recent report that there are functionally distinct subsets of large T antigen *(vide infra)*. If the extreme power of the modern genetic techniques is to be realized, it is necessary that the mutant large T antigens be analyzed by rigorous biochemical techniques. It will also be necessary to resort to some of the classical techniques of protein chemistry. In this regard, the pioneering work of Tjian with D2T, whatever the defects of this particular protein, clearly defines the route to be followed. It is necessary to purify large amounts of wild-type large T antigen from SV40-infected cells and, perhaps, to further fractionate this protein into preparations of defined oligomerization or posttranslational modification state. The interactions of such pure protein preparations with DNA can then be properly assessed. For example, there has been some controversy in the literature as to the relative DNA binding abilities of the monomeric, dimeric, tetrameric, and higher oligomeric forms of large T antigen, although the current consensus appears to be that dimers are the active species *(vide infra)*. However, these experiments simply ask about the activities of protein species that were of a particular oligomeric status when the gradient was run; they do not address the question of the oligomeric status of the protein when it binds to the DNA. If sufficient amounts of pure large T antigen were available, it would be possible to utilize protein–protein and protein–nucleic-acid cross-linking reagents to define precisely the form of the protein that binds to the origin. It should also be noted that *in vivo* large T antigen binds not to naked DNA but to the viral minichromosome in which the genome is complexed with histones and, probably, other host proteins that could dramatically modulate T-antigen–DNA interactions.

SUBSETS AND FORMS OF SV40 LARGE T ANTIGEN

When large T antigen extracted from transformed or infected cells is analyzed by gel filtration or zonal sedimentation, a variety of forms of different molecular weights can be detected (3,23,40,49,66,75,79). More recently, discrete large T antigen species have also been described based on specific binding to host proteins, reaction with monoclonal antibodies, posttranslational modifications, and enzymatic activities.

Zonal sedimentation of SV40-infected cell extracts in sucrose and glycerol gradients resolves a minimum of two forms of large T antigen, one sedimenting at 5S to 6S, the other at 15S to 16S. When extracts of transformed cells or infected cells are analyzed using broader gradients, a third form sedimenting at around 23S is apparent. This third species is specifically associated with the host p53 protein (23,40,66) and will be discussed in more detail later.

The peak at 5S to 6S has been analyzed for DNA binding activity, both specific and nonspecific, for ATPase and protein kinase activities (3), and for phosphorylation state (23,40,66). Pulse-chase experiments indicate that newly synthesized large T antigen first enters the "light" form and then "matures" into the heavier species (4,23). The results obtained by different groups on the properties of the light form are not entirely consistent, and this may be explained partly by technical differences, but also by the recent observation of Bradley et al. (3) that the peak at 5S to 6S can be resolved into two separate species, one of 5.5S and the other of 7S. This group has equated the 5.5S species with the monomer and the 7S species with the dimer and has found that only the dimeric form possesses ATPase and DNA binding activity, whereas both the monomer and dimer possess protein kinase activity. Whether this kinase activity is intrinsic to large T antigen or represents an exogenously bound protein is still in dispute (112), but it is clear that the activity cosediments with even the lightest forms of large T antigen. The 7S dimer is a quantitatively comparatively minor species and often would not be detected antigenically except as a very slight shoulder on the leading edge of the 5S peak. All groups seem to agree that these light (monomer/dimer) forms are underphosphorylated relative to the 16S forms and that they show specific binding to the SV40 origin of DNA replication.

The 16S form also has protein kinase, ATPase, and specific DNA binding activities associated with it. The 16S form showed a greater salt resistance for both its nonspecific and specific DNA binding (21), reaching an optimum at 150 to 200-mM NaCl rather than at 60 to 80 mM as for the lighter species. The 22S to 23S forms associated with the host p53 protein (23,40,66) also show specific DNA binding activity (21); because this activity can be immunoprecipitated with anti-p53 monoclonal antibodies, it is clear that the complex retains this potential (85).

Pulse-chase experiments have demonstrated that large T antigen takes a considerable time following synthesis to enter into the complex with the p53 host protein (4). The stabilities of the different species of large T antigen have not been closely investigated. In the experiments of Bradley et al. (3) the high-molecular-weight (16S and 23S) complexes were stable in 1-M NaCl, and no *in vitro* assembly of the low-molecular-weight species could be seen. Dilution of the 16S form in a medium of higher ionic strength (3) or purification on phosphocellulose (21) will lead to partial conversion to the 5S to 6S form. Recently, Montenarh and Henning (68a,68b) have demonstrated that the higher-molecular-weight species are stabilized by divalent cations, because following treatment with 20-mM EDTA they obtained conversion of the 16S form to lighter species. Furthermore, they were able to recover the 16S form by incubation in the presence of 22-mM Mg^{2+}.

The large T antigens encoded by *tsA* mutants have been shown by a number of groups to fail to assemble into the higher-molecular-weight forms at the nonpermissive temperature (23,35,48,49), although complexes formed at the permissive temperature are sometimes stable on shift up to the higher temperature (23). The formation of the T–p53 complex is also affected by the *tsA* lesion, but is, in addition, strikingly dependent on the host species from which the p53 is derived; human and monkey p53s bind to large T antigen with a much lower affinity than the rat and mouse forms of the protein (22,50; D. P. Lane, *unpublished data*). Disappointingly, none of these investigators has pinpointed a clearly significant difference in the properties of the different-molecular-weight forms of large T antigen or indeed any special property of the T–p53 complex not possessed by free large T antigen. Perhaps the most significant result is that of Bradley et al., that the monomer is inactive in DNA binding and ATPase activity (3). However, to prove that the monomer species is not in some way irreversibly denatured, it is necessary to show recovery of activity on dimerization *in vitro*. It is possible that Henning's discovery will make these *in vitro* reassembly experiments feasible.

The recent production of a large number of monoclonal antibodies to large T antigen (10,36,39) has provided a new tool for the potential definition of subsets. This approach faces two central problems: First, different monoclonal antibodies differ greatly in their affinity for large T antigen, which can be deceptive; second, subsets defined by the display of a given antigenic determinant will not necessarily reflect subsets of biological significance. The latter point is well illustrated by the variable sensitivity of different antigenic sites to loss by denaturation; for example, some epitopes are resistant to boiling in 2% (w/v) SDS (36,39,51). The former difficulty is well illustrated by a critical analysis of two recent papers. Gurney et al. (36) showed by sequential immunoprecipitation that they were unable to completely deplete a cell extract of large T antigen using the clone 7 antibody (PAb100), and Scheller et al. (90) showed that this antibody preferentially precipitated the large T antigen that bound specifically to SV40 DNA. The important implication of these results is that only a small and antigenically discrete subset of large T antigen is capable of specifically binding to the SV40 origin. However, as Gurney et al. pointed out in their original description of PAb100, the antibody appears to have a very low affinity for large T antigen, repeated cycles of immunoprecipitation bringing down small but detectable amounts of the antigen (36). Indeed, they showed that as much large T antigen was brought down in the fourth round of precipitation as in the second round. An antibody with low affinity for large T antigen will preferentially precipitate oligomeric forms of the antigen, as multiple interactions will occur between *Staphylococcus aureus* cells, the antibody, and the oligomeric antigen. So the results of Scheller et al. can be reinterpreted very differently as showing that large T antigen is oligomerized when it is bound to DNA. This would fit well with electron microscopic observations (73), and it emphasizes the potential problems of interpretation when using monoclonal antibodies. Another problem is the realization that protein molecules are not rigidly fixed in space, so that combination with an antibody can easily change the shape of the molecule, enhancing or reducing the binding of another antibody to the same antigen. This phenomenon has been well documented in the case of H-2 antigens. The functional importance of the different subsets of large T antigen is still unclear, but the ability to change the aggregation state by altering the divalent cation concentration *in vitro* may make more meaningful studies possible. New mutations in the large T antigen gene may also improve our ability to associate form with function.

NOVEL LARGE T ANTIGEN DERIVATIVES SYNTHESIZED IN SV40-TRANSFORMED CELLS

It has been known for several years that SV40-transformed cells often contain T antigens distinct from the small t and large T antigens that are the only known products of the early region during the productive infection of permissive cells (7,48,65,96,101). Peptide mapping studies have revealed that these proteins are structurally related to large T antigen (7,48,64,65,96,101). They have been divided into two classes: super T antigens, which are larger than wild-type large T antigen, and truncated T antigens, which are smaller. The application of recombinant DNA techniques to the analysis of the structure of the integrated viral DNA in SV40-transformed cells has led to the isolation of the templates for some of these novel T antigens. By sequencing the DNA templates it has been possible to precisely define the structures of the proteins, and by transfecting the cloned DNAs into both permissive and nonpermissive cells the biological properties of the proteins have been assessed.

Super T antigens are encoded by segments of integrated viral DNA that contain duplications of viral sequences. In one case, that of the super T antigen from the SV3T3 C120 line of transformed BALB/c 3T3 cells, the duplication is a perfect tandem that is in phase with the reading frame for large T antigen (56). This template directs the synthesis of a protein of apparent molecular weight 145,000. In the other case, that of the super T antigen of apparent molecular weight 115,000 synthesized by a subcloned line of transformed rat cells, the duplication is not a perfect tandem, and the template contains sequences of unknown origin (63). Transfection of these super T antigen templates into nonpermissive cells shows that both proteins retain the ability to transform, but transfection into permissive monkey cells reveals that the plasmids do not replicate, whereas analogous plasmids carrying the wild-type large T antigen coding region do replicate (12,63,63a). Cotransfection with plasmids encoding the wild-type protein allows replication, thus localizing the defect to the super T antigen rather than to the origin. Super T antigens are thus mutants that separate the replication and transformation functions of large T antigen.

Such mutant large T antigens are surprisingly common in transformed cells. Stringer (102) has shown that the integrated viral genome carried in the transformed rat cell line SVRE9 contains a point mutation, an A to G change at nucleotide 4,178, that converts a lysine to a glutamic acid. This large T antigen is also transformation-competent but replication-incompetent (102), as is the protein encoded by the integrated viral DNA segment SV3T3-38-D, isolated from the transformed BALB/c 3T3 cell line SV3T3 C138. This segment contains a deletion of 219 nucleotides, between nucleotides 4,396/4,392 and 4,177/4,173, that is in phase with the reading frame for large T antigen (11). It is interesting to note that both these mutations map in the region that has been suggested to encode the DNA binding site of large T antigen, but direct analyses of the interactions of these proteins with the viral origin of DNA replication have not been reported. The final case is that of SV80, the transformed human cell line from which large T antigen was purified for several early studies of the interaction of the protein with DNA. The integrated viral early region carried by SV80 contains a number of point mutations, one of which inactivates the viral DNA replication function [W. Gish and M. Botchan, cited by Clark et al. (10)]. Moreover, it should be noted that whereas super T antigens and deleted large T antigens of the type encoded by SV3T3-38-D are obviously distinct from wild-type large T antigen when analyzed by SDS polyacrylamide gel electrophoresis, the SVRE9 and SV80 large T antigens appear to be wild-type by this criterion. It may therefore be that many other trans-formed-cell large T antigens are also mutants, a possibility that can be tested only by the cloning of more integrated viral early transcription units.

However, it is clear from the examples quoted earlier that such novel T antigens are not a rarity. Indeed, Clayton and Rigby (14) found that of the seventeen viral early transcription units that they cloned from three lines of transformed BALB/c 3T3 cells only two encode wild-type large T antigen. Is there a selection against the presence of fully functional large T antigen? The way that the investigator grows the cells requires that the transformation function is retained; so it appears that the selection is against the DNA replication function. It seems likely that this selection operates because the DNA replication function of large T antigen, or some function intimately associated with it, is capable of catalyzing rearrangements of the cellular genome that are selectively disadvantageous. It is now well established that the integration patterns of SV40-transformed cells are not stable (2,43,44,88; M. Lovett, C. E. Clayton, and P. W. J. Rigby, *in preparation*). Considerable rearrangements of both the integrated viral sequences and the flanking cellular DNA continue to occur for many years after the cells were originally transformed. Moreover, am-plification of integrated viral sequences occurs when *tsA*-transformed mouse cells are subjected to selection for anchorage-independent growth (43), and extensive nucleotide sequencing studies on the segments of integrated viral DNA isolated by Clayton and Rigby (14) have revealed that both viral sequences and the flanking cellular DNA are amplified in wild-type-virus-transformed cells (D. Murphy and P. W. J. Rigby, *in preparation*). For SV40 there is no direct evidence that these rearrangements and amplifications are catalyzed by large T antigen. However, Basilico's group has shown clearly that the amplification of integrated polyoma virus DNA depends on the presence of functional large T antigen (15). More recent data from this group have shown that the frequency of sister chromatid exchanges is increased in polyoma *tsA*-transformed cells grown at the permissive temperature. More strikingly, methotrexate-resistant colonies occur more frequently at the per-missive temperature, suggesting that amplification of the cellular dihydrofolate reductase gene can be catalyzed by functional polyoma large T antigen (C. Basilico, *personal communication*). This latter result would be of particular importance because it implies that polyoma large T antigen is capable of amplifying replicons that do not contain a viral origin. Further evidence for the notion that expression of a replication-competent large T antigen is deleterious to the cell derives from studies in which the SV40 genome is cotransfected into nonpermissive cells with a dominant selectable marker gene, *Ecogpt*. In cells selected for the expression of this marker gene, SV40 small t antigen is synthesized, but intact large T antigen is not produced (70; T. Roberts and D. Livingston, *personal communication*).

Rather less is known about the truncated T antigens that are also commonly found in transformed cells. However, Clayton et al. (13) have shown that a segment of integrated viral DNA cloned from the transformed BALB/c 3T3 line SV3T3 C120 encodes a truncated T antigen of apparent molecular weight 48,000, the C-terminal amino acids of which are specified by the flanking cellular DNA, and Chaudry et al. (8) have studied the DNA binding properties of this protein. A most surprising result is that the template for this truncated T antigen, SV3T3-20-G, is capable of morphologically transforming Rat-1 cells, although the frequency is only 1% of that obtained with intact SV40 DNA, and the foci induced are quite distinct from those induced in parallel experiments by plasmids carrying the entire viral early transcription unit (13). Colby and Shenk (16) have constructed mutants of SV40 with almost exactly the same coding capacity as SV3T3-20-G, although the C-terminal segment in this case is viral in origin, and they have shown that such genomes can immortalize rat embryo cells and that some of the cell lines thus established have a transformed phenotype. These data suggest that the N-terminal half of large T antigen has some transforming ability, and they are particularly provocative in view of the recent results of Rassoulzadegan et al. (82), who have shown unequivocally that although polyoma virus middle T antigen is sufficient to transform established cell lines, an activity of the N-terminal half of large T antigen is required for the transformation of primary cells and that this segment of large T antigen alone is capable of alleviating the serum dependence of established cell lines. Further studies on the biological properties of SV40-truncated T antigens are thus clearly required in order to ascertain the precise capabilities of this segment of the protein.

EFFECTS OF SV40 LARGE T ANTIGEN ON CELLULAR DNA REPLICATION AND CELLULAR TRANSCRIPTION

Following the infection of both permissive and nonpermissive cells by SV40, the earliest detectable effects of large T antigen are the induction of a variety of cellular enzymes and the induction of a round of cellular DNA replication, even in quiescent cells. Although there is presently no direct evidence that these effects are mediated by direct interactions between large T antigen and cellular DNA sequences that control DNA replication or transcription, there is some circumstantial evidence to suggest that this is the case, and much current research effort is directed toward an analysis of this proposition. Such work is likely to be crucial to our understanding of the role of large T antigen during transformation. It seems highly unlikely that a single protein, even a protein with so many functions as large T antigen, can directly cause all of the biochemical and biological changes that distinguish a transformed cell from its untransformed parent. Rather, the protein must in some way reprogram the cell's metabolism and/or gene expression.

Microinjection of purified D2T into the nuclei of quiescent cells has shown that this protein is capable of inducing a round of cellular DNA replication (111). Martin and Oppenheim (61) showed by fiber autoradiography that the frequency of cellular origins is increased, and the origin-to-origin distance is decreased, in transformed cells relative to normal cells, and Marchionni and Roufa (59) have presented evidence that large T antigen affects the precise period during the S phase at which integrated viral sequences are replicated. Two questions thus arise: (a) Is there a specialized function on large T antigen for the induction of cellular DNA replication, or is this phenomenon a secondary manifestation of the viral DNA replication function(s)? (b) Are there sequences within the cellular genome that are recognized by large T antigen and used by it as replication origins?

Two approaches have been used to attempt to answer the first question. The classic approach has been analysis of deletion mutants of SV40, which suggests that the cellular induction function is separable from the viral DNA replication function (76a,97a), an answer not unexpected in view of the long-standing observation of Chou and Martin (9) that in certain *tsA* mutants inactivation of the cellular induction function requires a higher temperature than does inactivation of the viral replication function. The alternative approach, pioneered by Graessmann and his collaborators, has been to microinject fragments of the SV40 genome into the nuclei of quiescent cells. Mueller et al. (69) used this technique to show that the C-terminal one-third of large T antigen is not required for the induction of cellular DNA replication, although it is required for viral DNA synthesis. Galanti et al. (25) have performed similar experiments using both cloned and uncloned restriction fragments and the cloned DNAs of deletion mutants. Their data indicate that the segment of large T antigen required for the induction of cellular DNA synthesis is encoded between nucleotides 4,400 and 4,000 approximately. However, these experiments would be more convincing if it had also been shown that the microinjected cells synthesize only the predicted truncated T antigens.

The existence within the cellular genome of sequences that could be used as an origin by large T antigen has been assessed by screening libraries of genomic DNA with the origin fragment of SV40 DNA in the hope that segments of cellular DNA having sequence homology might also have functional homology. Conrad and Botchan (17) have isolated a human sequence with homology to the viral origin, and Singer's group has isolated similar sequences from the African green monkey genome (67). Although the cloned human segment carries an enhancer function similar to that possessed by the 72-base-pair repeats located on the late side of the SV40 origin (17), the monkey segments do not. Neither type of segment can initiate large-T-antigen-dependent replication (17; M. Singer, *personal communication*). If it is indeed the case, as suggested by Harland and Laskey (38), that the initiation of eukaryotic DNA replication is not a sequence-specific event, then there may be no special cellular "origins" with which large T antigen interacts. However, it is equally possible that the protein can interact with cellular sequences devoid of homology to the viral origin, and it will most certainly be of interest to try to clone directly cellular DNA capable of binding to large T antigen, although it must be borne in mind that the interactions responsible for the induction of cellular DNA replication may require other proteins, an obvious candidate being p53.

Infection by SV40 induces the synthesis of several cellular enzymes involved in nucleotide and nucleic acid metabolism, and, at least in the case of thymidine kinase, this induction depends on the presence of functional large T antigen (78). However, in such cases it has not been directly shown that the induction occurs at the level of transcription. There is one case in which a direct effect of large T antigen on cellular transcription has been clearly documented. In some human–mouse somatic cell hybrids only the human rDNA complement is normally expressed. The introduction of large T antigen into such hybrid cells by viral infection or DNA transfection leads to transcriptional activation of the previously quiescent mouse rDNA complement (97). The types of experiments discussed earlier with respect to the induction of cellular DNA replication have also been applied to try to locate the function responsible for the induction of rDNA transcription. It has been concluded that the two functions are separable, with the transcriptional induction function being encoded between nucleotides 3,800 and 3,500 (25,97a,98). These experiments are, however, open to the reservations discussed in the section on cellular DNA replication. Surprisingly, there is no evidence for a large T antigen binding site within or adjacent to the mouse or human rRNA transcription unit (53a). However, addition of purified D2T stimulates the transcription of human rDNA by RNA polymerase I in an *in vitro* system, raising the intriguing possibility that large T antigen may be able to interact directly with the transcriptional machinery (53a).

It is, however, clear that the ability of large T antigen to activate rDNA transcription is unlikely to be relevant to the mechanism of transformation. Alterations in cellular physiology will depend on changes in the expression of protein coding genes that are transcribed by RNA polymerase II. There are no clear examples of changes in gene expression in transformed cells that can be identified by alterations in the level of a particular protein. Thus, in order to identify genes that may be regulated by large T antigen, it is necessary to use differential transcription as the screening procedure. Two groups have now succeeded in using cDNA cloning techniques to identify and isolate cellular genes that are transcribed at higher levels in SV40-transformed cells than in the parental normal cells (91,92). In both cases, analyses of the transcription of these genes in *tsA*-transformed cells suggest a fairly direct regulation by large T antigen. More detailed analyses of these genes are likely to be of considerable importance for our understanding of the mechanism of transformation, and they should certainly provide appropriate experimental systems for detailed analysis of the effect of large T antigen on cellular transcription.

ACKNOWLEDGMENTS

We are grateful to Dan Nathans, Janet Butel, Bob Carroll, Wolfgang Deppert, Ellen Fanning, Linda Gooding, Tucker Gurney, Roland Henning, Bob Kamen, Arnie Levine, David Livingston, Evelyne and Pierre May, Jim Pipas, Tom Shenk, Maxine Singer, Alan Smith, Peter Tegtmeyer, Satvir Tevethia, and Bob Tjian for providing us with unpublished information and to Sue Hayman for her expert preparation of this manuscript.

P. W. J. R. holds a Career Development Award from the Cancer Research Campaign, which also paid for work from the authors' laboratories.

REFERENCES

1. Anderson, J. L., Martin, R. G., Chang, C., Mora, P. T., and Livingston, D. M. (1977): Nuclear preparations of SV40-transformed cells contain tumor-specific transplantation antigen activity. *Virology*, 76:420–425.
2. Bender, M. A., and Brockman, W. W. (1981): Rearrangement of integrated viral DNA sequences in mouse cells transformed by simian virus 40. *J. Virol.*, 38:872–879.
3. Bradley, M. K., Griffin, J. D., and Livingston, D. M. (1982): Relationship of oligomerization to enzymatic and DNA-binding properties of the SV40 large T antigen. *Cell*, 28:125–134.
3a. Campbell, A. E., Foley, F. L., and Teverthia, S. S. (1983): Demonstration of multiple antigenic sites of the SV40 transplantation rejection antigen by using cytotoxic T lymphocyte clones. *J. Immunol.*, 130:490–492.
4. Carroll, R. B., and Gurney, E. G. (1982): Time-dependent maturation of the Simian virus 40 large T p53 complex studied by using monoclonal antibodies. *J. Virol.*, 44:565–573.
5. Chang, C., Chang, R., Mora, P. T., and Hu, C.-P. (1982): Generation of cytotoxic lymphocytes by SV40-induced antigens. *J. Immunol.*, 128:2160–2163.
6. Chang, C., Martin, R. G., Livingston, D. M., Luborsky, S. W., Hu, C.-P., and Mora, P. T. (1979): Relationship between T-antigen and tumor-specific transplantation antigen in simian virus 40-transformed cells. *J. Virol.*, 29:69–75.
7. Chang, C., Simmons, D. T., Martin, M. A., and Mora, P. T. (1979): Identification and partial characterization of new antigens from simian virus 40-transformed mouse cells. *J. Virol.*, 31:463–471.
8. Chaudry, F., Harvey, R., and Smith, A. E. (1982): Structure and biochemical functions of four Simian virus 40 truncated large T-antigens. *J. Virol.*, 44:54–66.
9. Chou, J. Y., and Martin, R. G. (1975): DNA infectivity and the induction of host DNA synthesis with temperature-sensitive mutants of simian virus 40. *J. Virol.*, 15:145–150.
10. Clark, R., Lane, D. P., and Tjian, R. (1981): Use of monoclonal antibodies as probes of simian virus 40 T antigen ATPase activity. *J. Biol. Chem.*, 256:11854–11858.
10a. Clark, R., Peden, K., Pipas, J. M., Nathans, D., and Tjian, R. (1983): Biochemical activities of T-antigen proteins encoded by Simian virus 40 deletion mutants. *Mol. Cell. Biol.*, 3:220–228.
11. Clayton, C. E., Lovett, M., Murphy, D., Thomas, P. G., and Rigby, P. W. J. (1983): A deletion in viral DNA isolated from transformed cells separates the transformation and viral DNA replication functions of simian virus 40 large T-antigen. *J. Virol.*, *(submitted)*.
12. Clayton, C. E., Lovett, M., and Rigby, P. W. J. (1982): Functional analysis of a simian virus 40 super T-antigen. *J. Virol.*, 44:974–982.
13. Clayton, C. E., Murphy, D., Lovett, M., and Rigby, P. W. J. (1982): A fragment of the SV40 large T-antigen gene transforms. *Nature*, 299:59–61.
14. Clayton, C. E., and Rigby, P. W. J. (1981): Cloning and characterization of the integrated viral DNA from three lines of SV40-transformed mouse cells. *Cell*, 25:547–559.
15. Colantuoni, V., Dailey, L., and Basilico, C. (1980): Amplification of integrated viral DNA sequences in polyoma virus-transformed cells. *Proc. Natl. Acad. Sci. USA*, 77:3850–3854.
16. Colby, W. W., and Shenk, T. (1982): Fragments of the simian virus 40 transforming gene facilitate transformation of rat embryo cells. *Proc. Natl. Acad. Sci.USA*, 79:5189–5193.
17. Conrad, S. E., and Botchan, M. R. (1982): Isolation and characterization of human DNA fragments

with nucleotide sequence homologies within the simian virus 40 regulatory region. *Mol. Cell. Biol.*, 2:949–965.

18. Deppert, W., Hanke, K., and Henning, R. (1980): Simian virus 40 T-antigen-related cell surface antigen: Serological demonstration on simian virus 40-transformed monolayer cells *in situ*. *J. Virol.*, 35:505–518.

19. Deppert, W., and Henning, R. (1980): SV40 T-antigen-related molecules on the surfaces of HeLa cells infected with adenovirus 2–SV40 hybrids and on SV40-transformed cells. *Cold Spring Harbor Symp. Quant. Biol.*, 44:225–234.

19a. Deppert, W., and Walter, G. (1982): Domains of Simian virus 40 large T-antigen exposed on the cell surface. *Virol.*, 122:56–70.

20. DiMaio, D., and Nathans, D. (1980): Cold-sensitive regulatory mutants of simian virus 40. *J. Mol. Biol.*, 140:129–142.

21. Dorn, A., Brauer, D., Fanning, E., and Knippers, R. (1982): Subclasses of simian virus 40 large tumor antigen: Partial purification and DNA binding properties of two subclasses of tumor antigen from productively infected cells. *Eur. J. Biochem.*, 128:53–62.

22. Fanning, E., Burger, C., and Gurney, E. G. (1981): Comparison of T antigen-associated host phosphoproteins from SV40-infected and -transformed cells of different species. *J. Gen. Virol.*, 55:367–378.

23. Fanning, E., Nowak, B., and Burger, C. (1981): Detection and characterization of multiple forms of simian virus 40 large T antigen. *J. Virol.*, 37:92–102.

24. Flyer, D. C., and Tevethia, S. S. (1982): Biology of simian virus 40 (SV40) transplantation antigen (TrAg). VIII. Retention of SV40 TrAg sites on purified SV40 large T antigen following denaturation with sodium dodecyl sulfate. *Virology*, 117:267–270.

25. Galanti, N., Jonak, G. J., Soprano, K. J., Floros, J., Kaczmarek, L., Weissman, S., Reddy, V. B., Tilghman, S. M., and Baserga, R. (1981): Characterization and biological activity of cloned simian virus 40 DNA fragments. *J. Biol. Chem.*, 256:6469–6474.

26. Galas, D. J., and Schmitz, A. (1978): DNase footprinting: A simple method for the detection of protein-DNA binding specificity. *Nucleic Acids Res.*, 5:3157–3170.

27. Ghosh, P. K., and Lebowitz, P. (1981): SV40 early mRNAs contain multiple 5′-termini upstream and downstream from a Hogness-Goldberg sequence. A shift in 5′-termini during the lytic cycle is mediated by large T-antigen. *J. Virol.*, 40:224–240.

28. Gilbert, W., Maxam, A., and Mirzabekov, A. (1976): Contacts between the lac repressor and DNA revealed by methylation. In: *Control of Ribosome Synthesis*, edited by N. O. Kjeldgaard and O. Maaloe, pp. 139–148. Academic Press, New York.

29. Gluzman, Y. (1981): SV40-transformed simian cells support the replication of early SV40 mutants. *Cell*, 23:175–182.

30. Goldman, N., Brown, M., and Khoury, G. (1981): Modification of SV40 T-antigen by poly ADP-ribosylation. *Cell*, 24:567–572.

31. Gooding, L. R. (1977): Specificities of killing by cytotoxic lymphocytes generated *in vivo* to syngeneic SV40 transformed cells. *J. Immunol.*, 118:920–927.

32. Gooding, L. (1979): Specificities of killing by T lymphocytes generated against syngeneic SV40 transformants: Studies employing recombinants within the H-2 complex. *J. Immunol.*, 122:1002–1008.

33. Gooding, L. R., Harlow, E., and McKay, R. (1983): Differential expression of T antigenic determinants on the surface of SV40-transformed cells. *J. Virol. (submitted)*.

34. Graessmann, A., Graessmann, M., Tjian, R., and Topp, W. C. (1980): Simian virus 40 small-t protein is required for loss of actin cable networks in rat cells. *J. Virol.*, 33:1182–1191.

35. Greenspan, D. S., and Carroll, R. B. (1981): Complex of simian virus 40 large tumor antigen and 48,000-dalton host tumor antigen. *Proc. Natl. Acad. Sci. USA*, 78:105–109.

36. Gurney, E. G., Harrison, R. O., and Fenno, J. (1980): Monoclonal antibodies against simian virus 40 T antigens: Evidence for distinct subclasses of large T antigen and for similarities among nonviral T antigens. *J. Virol.*, 34:752–763.

37. Hansen, U., Tenen, D. G., Livingston, D. M., and Sharp, P. A. (1981): T antigen repression of SV40 early transcription from two promoters. *Cell*, 27:603–612.

38. Harland, R. M., and Laskey, R. A. (1980): Regulated replication of DNA microinjected into eggs of *Xenopus laevis*. *Cell*, 21:761–771.

39. Harlow, E., Crawford, L. V., Pim, D. C., and Williamson, N. M. (1981): Monoclonal antibodies specific for simian virus 40 tumor antigens. *J. Virol.*, 39:861–869.

40. Harlow, E., Pim, D. C., and Crawford, L. V. (1981): Complex of simian virus 40 large T-antigen and host 53,000 molecular weight protein in monkey cells. *J. Virol.*, 37:564–573.

41. Hassell, J. A., Lukanidin, E., Fey, G., and Sambrook, J. (1978): The structure and expression of two defective adenovirus 2–simian virus 40 hybrids. *J. Mol. Biol.*, 120:209–247.

42. Henning, R., Lange-Mutschler, J., and Deppert, W. (1981): SV40-transformed cells express SV40 T antigen-related antigens on the cell surface. *Virology*, 108:325–337.

43. Hiscott, J., Murphy, D., and Defendi, V. (1980): Amplification and rearrangement of integrated SV40 DNA sequences accompany the selection of anchorage-independent transformed mouse cells. *Cell*, 22:535–543.

44. Hiscott, J. B., Murphy, D., and Defendi, V. (1981): Instability of integrated viral DNA in mouse cells transformed by simian virus 40. *Proc. Natl. Acad. Sci. USA*, 78:1736–1740.

45. Jay, G., Jay, F. T., Chang, C., Friedman, R. M., and Levine, A. S. (1978): Tumour-specific transplantation antigen: Use of the Ad2⁺ND1 hybrid virus to identify the protein responsible for simian virus 40 tumor rejection and its genetic origin. *Proc. Natl. Acad. Sci. USA*, 75:3055–3059.

46. Jessel, D., Landau, T., Hudson, J., Lalor, T., Tenen, D., and Livingston, D. M. (1976): Identification of regions of the SV40 genome which contain preferred SV40 T antigen binding sites. *Cell*, 8:535–545.

47. Kelly, T. J., Jr., and Lewis, A. M. (1973): Use of nondefective adenovirus-simian virus 40 hybrids for mapping the simian virus 40 genome. *J. Virol.*, 12:643–652.

47a. Klockmann, U., and Deppert, W. (1983): Acylation: A new post-translational modification specific for plasma membrane-associated Simian virus 40 large T-antigen. *FEBS LeH.*, 151:257–259.

48. Kress, M., May, E., Cassingena, R., and May, P. (1979): Simian virus 40-transformed cells express new species of proteins precipitable by anti-simian virus 40 tumour serum. *J. Virol.*, 31:472–483.

49. Kuchino, T., and Yamaguchi, N. (1975): Characterization of T antigen in cells infected with a temperature-sensitive mutant of simian virus 40. *J. Virol.*, 15:1302–1307.

50. Lane, D. P., and Crawford, L. V. (1980): The complex between simian virus 40 T antigen and a specific host protein. *Proc. R. Soc. Lond. [Biol.]*, 210:451–463.

51. Lane, D. P., and Hoeffler, W. K. (1980): SV40 large T shares an antigenic determinant with a cellular protein of molecular weight 68,000. *Nature*, 288:167–170.

52. Lanford, R. E., and Butel, J. S. (1979): Antigenic relationship of SV40 early proteins to purified large T polypeptide. *Virology*, 97:295–306.

53. Lange-Mutschler, J., and Henning, R. (1982): Cell surface binding affinity of simian virus 40 T-antigen. *Virology*, 117:173–185.

53a. Learned, R. M., Smale, S. T., Haltiner, M. M., and Tjian, R. (1983): Regulation of human ribosomal RNA transcription. *Proc. Natl. Acad. Sci. USA*, 80:(in press).

54. Lewis, A. M., Jr., and Martin, R. G. (1979): Oncogenicity of simian virus 40 deletion mutants that induce altered 17-kilodalton t-protein. *Proc. Natl. Acad. Sci. USA*, 76:4299–4302.

55. Lewis, A. M., and Rowe, W. P. (1973): Studies of non-defective adenovirus 2–simian virus 40 hybrid viruses. VIII. Association of simian virus 40 transplantation antigen with a specific region of the early viral genome. *J. Virol.*, 12:836–840.

56. Lovett, M., Clayton, C. E., Murphy, D., Rigby, P. W. J., Smith, A. E., and Chaudry, F. (1982): Structure and synthesis of a simian virus 40 super T-antigen. *J. Virol.*, 44:963–973.

57. Luborsky, S. W., and Chandrasekaran, K. (1980): Subcellular distribution of simian virus 40 T antigen species in various cell lines: The 56K protein. *Int. J. Cancer*, 25:517–527.

58. Manley, J. L., Fire, A., Cano, A., Sharp, P. A., and Gefter, M. L. (1979): DNA dependent transcription of adenovirus genes in a soluble whole-cell extract. *Proc. Natl. Acad. Sci. USA*, 77:3855–3859.

59. Marchionni, M. A., and Roufa, D. J. (1981): Replication of viral DNA sequences integrated within the chromatin of SV40-transformed Chinese hamster lung cells. *Cell*, 26:245–258.

60. Martin, R. G. (1981): The transformation of cell growth and transmogrification of DNA synthesis by simian virus 40. *Adv. Cancer Res.*, 34:1–68.

61. Martin, R. G., and Oppenheim, A. (1977): Initiation points for DNA replication in nontransformed and simian virus 40-transformed Chinese hamster lung cells. *Cell*, 11:859–869.

62. Martin, R. G., Setlow, V. P., Edwards, C. A. F., and Vembu, D. (1979): The roles of the simian virus 40 tumor antigens in transformation of Chinese hamster lung cells. *Cell*, 17:635–643.

63. May, E., Jeltsch, J.-M., and Gannon, F. (1981): Characterization of a gene encoding a 115K super T-antigen expressed by a SV40-transformed rat cell line. *Nucleic Acids Res.*, 9:4111–4128.

63a. May, E., Lasne, C., Prives, C., Borde, J., and May, P. (1983): Study of the functional activities concomitantly retained by the 115,000 Mr super T antigen, an evolutionary variant of Simian virus 40 large T antigen expressed in transformed rat cells. *J. Virol.*, 45:901–913.

64. May, P., Kress, M., Lange, M., and May, E. (1980): New genetic information expressed in SV40-transformed cells: Characterization of the 55K proteins and evidence for unusual SV40 mRNAs. *Cold Spring Harbor Symp. Quant. Biol.*, 44:189–200.

65. McCormick, F., Chaudry, F., Harvey, R., Smith, R., Rigby, P. W. J., Paucha, E., and Smith, A. E. (1980): T antigens of SV40-transformed cells. *Cold Spring Harbor Symp. Quant. Biol.*, 44:171–178.

66. McCormick, F., and Harlow, E. (1980): Association of a murine 53,000-dalton phosphoprotein with simian virus 40 large T antigen in transformed cells. *J. Virol.*, 34:213–224.

67. McCutchan, T. F., and Singer, M. F. (1981): DNA sequences similar to those around the simian virus 40 origin of replication are present in the monkey genome. *Proc. Natl. Acad. Sci. USA*, 78:95–99.

68. McKay, R. D. G. (1981): Binding of a simian virus 40 T antigen-related protein to DNA. *J. Mol. Biol.*, 145:471–488.

68a. Montemark, M., and Henning, R. (1983): Disaggregation and reconstitution of oligomeric complexes of Simian virus 40 large T-antigen. *J. Gen. Virol.*, 64:241–246.

68b. Montemark, M., and Henning, R. (1983): Self-assembly of Simian virus 40 large T antigen oligomers by divalent cations. *J. Virol.*, 45:531–538.

69. Mueller, C., Graessmann, A., and Graessman, M. (1978): Mapping of early SV40-specific functions by microinjection of different early viral DNA fragments. *Cell*, 15:579–585.

70. Mulligan, R. C., and Berg, P. (1981): Selection for animal cells that express the *Escherichia coli* gene coding for xanthine-guanine phosphoribosyl-transferase. *Proc. Natl. Acad. Sci. USA*, 78:2072–2076.

71. Myers, R. M., Rio, D. C., Robbins, A. K., and Tjian, R. (1981): SV40 gene expression is modulated by the cooperative binding of T antigen to DNA. *Cell*, 25:373–384.

72. Myers, R. M., and Tjian, R. (1980): Construction and analysis of simian virus 40 origins defective in tumor antigen binding and DNA replication. *Proc. Natl. Acad. Sci. USA*, 77:6491–6495.

73. Myers, R. M., Williams, R. C., and Tjian, R. (1981): Oligomeric structure of a simian virus 40 T antigen in free form and bound to DNA. *J. Mol. Biol.*, 148:347–353.

74. Oren, M., Winocour, E., and Prives, C. (1980): Differential affinities of simian virus 40 large tumor antigen for DNA. *Proc. Natl. Acad. Sci. USA*, 77:220–224.

75. Osborn, M., and Weber, K. (1975): SV40 T antigen, the A function and transformation. *Cold Spring Harbor Symp. Quant. Biol.*, 39:267–276.

76. Pfizenmaier, K., Trinchieri, G., Solter, D., and Knowles, B. B. (1978): Mapping of H-2 genes associated with T cell-mediated cytotoxic responses to SV40-tumour-associated specific antigens. *Nature*, 274:691–693.

76a. Pipas, J. M., Peden, K. W. C., and Nathans, D. (1983): Mutational analysis of Simian virus 40 large T antigen: Isolation and characterization of mutants with deletions in the T-antigen gene. *Mol. Cell. Biol.*, 3:203–213.

77. Polvino-Bodnar, M., and Cole, C. N. (1982): Construction and characterization of viable deletion mutants of simian virus 40 lacking sequences near the 3' end of the early region. *J. Virol.*, 43:489–502.

78. Postel, E. H., and Levine, A. J. (1976): The requirement of simian virus 40 gene A product for the stimulation of cellular thymidine kinase activity after viral infection. *Virology*, 73:206–215.

79. Potter, C., McLaughlin, B., and Oxford, J. (1969): SV40-induced T and tumor antigens. *J. Virol.* 4:574–579.

80. Prives, C., Barnet, B., Scheller, A., Khoury, G., and Jay, G. (1981): Discrete regions of simian virus 40 large T-antigen are required for nonspecific and viral origin-specific DNA binding. *J. Virol.*, 43:73–82.

81. Prives, C., Beck, Y., and Shure, H. (1980): DNA binding properties of simian virus 40 T-antigens synthesized *in vivo* and *in vitro*. *J. Virol.*, 33:689–696.

82. Rassoulzadegan, M., Cowie, A., Carr, A., Glaichenhaus, N., Kamen, R., and Cuzin, F. (1982): The roles of individual polyoma virus early proteins in oncogenic transformation. *Nature*, 300:713–718.

83. Teverthia, S. S., Teverthia, M. J., Lewis, A. J., Reddy, V. B., and Weissman, S. M. (1983):

Biology of Simian virus 40 (SV40) transplantation antigen (TrAg). IX. Analysis of TrAg in mouse cells synthesizing truncated SV40 large T antigen. *Virol. (in press).*

84. Reed, S. I., Ferguson, J., Davis, R. W., and Stark, G. R. (1975): T antigen binds to simian virus 40 DNA at the origin of replication. *Proc. Natl. Acad. Sci. USA*, 72:1605–1609.

85. Reich, N. C., and Levine, A. J. (1982): Specific interaction of the SV40-T-antigen-cellular p53 protein complex with SV40 DNA. *Virology*, 117:286–290.

86. Rio, D., Robbins, A., Myers, R., and Tjian, R. (1980): Regulation of simian virus 40 early transcription *in vitro* by a purified tumor antigen. *Proc. Natl. Acad. Sci. USA*, 77:5706–5710.

87. Rubin, H., Figge, J., Bladon, M. T., Chen, L. B., Ellman, M., Bikel, I., Farrell, M., and Livingston, D. M. (1982): Role of small t-antigen in the acute transforming activity of SV40. *Cell*, 30:469–480.

88. Sager, R., Anisowicz, A., and Howell, N. (1981): Genomic rearrangements in a mouse cell line containing integrated SV40 DNA. *Cell*, 23:41–50.

89. Santos, M., and Butel, J. S. (1982): Association of SV40 large tumor antigen and cellular proteins on the surface of SV40 transformed mouse cells. *Virology*, 120:1–17.

90. Scheller, A., Covey, L., Barnet, B., and Prives, C. (1982): A small subclass of SV40 T antigen binds to the viral origin of replication. *Cell*, 29:375–383.

91. Schutzbank, T., Robinson, R., Oren, M., and Levine, A. J. (1982): SV40 large tumor antigen can regulate some cellular transcripts in a positive fashion. *Cell*, 30:481–490.

92. Scott, M. R. D., and Rigby, P. W. J. (1983): Activation of mouse genes in SV40-transformed cells. *Cell, (submitted).*

93. Shalloway, D., Kleinberger, T., and Livingston, D. M. (1980): Mapping of SV40 replication origin region binding sites for the SV40 T antigen by protection against exonuclease III digestion. *Cell*, 20:411–422.

94. Shortle, D. R., Margolskee, R. F., and Nathans, D. (1979): Mutational analysis of the simian virus 40 replicon: Pseudorevertants of mutants with a defective replication origin. *Proc. Natl. Acad. Sci. USA*, 76:6128–6131.

95. Shortle, D., and Nathans, D. (1978): Local mutagenesis: A method for generating viral mutants with base substitutions in preselected regions of the viral genome. *Proc. Natl. Acad. Sci. USA*, 75:2170–2174.

96. Smith, A. E., Smith, R., and Paucha, E. (1979): Characterization of different tumor antigens present in cells transformed by simian virus 40. *Cell*, 18:335–346.

97. Soprano, K. J., Dev, V. G., Croce, C. M., and Baserga, R. (1979): Reactivation of silent rRNA genes by simian virus 40 in human-mouse hybrid cells. *Proc. Natl. Acad. Sci. USA*, 76:3885–3889.

97a. Soprano, K. J., Galanti, N., Jonak, G. J., McKercher, S., Pipas, J. M., Peden, K. W. C., and Baserga, R. (1983): Mutational analysis of Simian virus 40 T antigen: Stimulation of cellular DNA synthesis and activation of rRNA genes by mutants with deletions in the T-antigen gene. *Mol. Cell. Biol.*, 3:214–219.

98. Soprano, K. J., Jonak, G. J., Galanti, N., Floros, J., and Baserga, R. (1981): Identification of an SV40 DNA sequence related to the reactivation of silent rRNA genes in human>mouse hybrid cells. *Virology*, 109:127–136.

99. Soule, H. R., Lanford, R. E., and Butel, J. S. (1980): Antigenic and immunogenic characteristics of nuclear and membrane-associated simian virus 40 T antigen. *J. Virol.*, 33:887–901.

100. Soule, H. R., Lanford, R. E., and Butel, J. S. (1982): Detection of simian virus 40 surface-associated large tumor antigen by enzyme-catalyzed radioiodination. *Int. J. Cancer*, 29:337–344.

101. Spangler, G. J., Griffin, J. D., Rubin, H., and Livingston, D. M. (1980): Identification and initial characterization of a new low-molecular-weight virus-encoded T antigen in a line of simian virus 40-transformed cells. *J. Virol.*, 36:488–498.

102. Stringer, J. R. (1982): Mutant of simian virus 40 large T-antigen that is defective for viral DNA synthesis, but competent for transformation of cultured rat cells. *J. Virol.*, 42:854–864.

103. Tegtmeyer, P. (1972): Simian virus 40 deoxyribonucleic acid synthesis: The viral replicon. *J. Virol.*, 10:591–598.

104. Omitted in proof.

105. Tenen, D. G., Haines, L. L., and Livingston, D. M. (1982): Binding of an analog of the SV40 T antigen to wild type and mutant viral replication origins. *J. Mol. Biol.*, 157:473–492.

106. Tevethia, S. S., Blasecki, J. W., Waneck, G., and Goldstein, A. L. (1974): Requirement of

thymus-derived θ-positive lymphocytes for rejection of DNA virus (SV40) tumors in mice. *J. Immunol.*, 113:1417–1423.

107. Tevethia, S. S., Flyer, D. C., and Tjian, R. (1980): Biology of simian virus 40 (SV40) transplantation antigen (TrAg). VI. Mechanism of induction of SV40 transplantation immunity in mice by purified SV40 T antigen (D2 protein). *Virology*, 107:13–23.
108. Thummel, C. S., Burgess, T. L., and Tjian, R. (1981): Properties of simian virus 40 small t antigen overproduced in bacteria. *J. Virol.*, 37:683–697.
109. Thummel, C., Tjian, R., and Grodzicker, T. (1981): Expression of SV40 T antigen under control of adenovirus promoters. *Cell*, 23:825–836.
110. Tjian, R. (1978): The binding site on SV40 DNA for a T antigen-related protein. *Cell*, 13:165–179.
111. Tjian, R., Fey, G., and Graessmann, A. (1978): Biological activity of purified simian virus 40 T antigen proteins. *Proc. Natl. Acad. Sci. USA*, 75:1279–1283.
112. Tjian, R., Robbins, A., and Clark, R. (1980): Catalytic properties of the SV40 large T-antigen. *Cold Spring Harbor Symp. Quant. Biol.*, 44:103–111.
113. Tooze, J. (editor) (1981): *Molecular Biology of Tumor Viruses. Part 2. DNA Tumor Viruses*, revised ed. 2. Cold Spring Harbor Laboratory, Cold Spring Harbor, N.Y.
114. Topp, W. C., and Rifkin, D. B. (1980): The small-t protein of SV40 is required for loss of actin cable networks and plasminogen activator synthesis in transformed rat cells. *Virology*, 106:282–291.
115. Topp, W. C., Rifkin, D. B., and Sleigh, M. J. (1981): SV40 mutants with an altered small-t protein are tumorigenic in newborn hamsters. *Virology*, 111:341–350.
116. Trinchieri, G., Aden, D. P., and Knowles, B. B. (1976): Cell-mediated cytotoxicity to SV40-specific tumour-associated antigens. *Nature*, 261:312–314.
117. Van Roy, F., Fransen, L., and Fiers, W. (1981): Phosphorylation patterns of tumor antigens in cells lytically infected or transformed by simian virus 40. *J. Virol.*, 40:28–44.
118. Walter, G., Scheidtmann, K.-H., Carbone, A., Laudano, A. P., and Doolittle, R. F. (1980): Antibodies specific for the carboxy- and amino-terminal regions of simian virus 40 large tumor antigen. *Proc. Natl. Acad. Sci. USA*, 77:5197–5200.

Advances in Viral Oncology, Volume 3, edited by
George Klein. Raven Press, New York © 1983.

Structure and Function of Papillomavirus Genomes

Olivier Danos and Moshe Yaniv

*Tumor Viruses Unit, Department of Molecular Biology, Institut Pasteur,
75724 Paris Cedex 15, France*

Papovaviridae are small DNA tumor viruses that grow in the nuclei of higher-vertebrate cells and share common physicochemical features: an icosahedral protein capsid made of 72 capsomers (50), containing a double-stranded circular and superhelical DNA molecule (16) associated with cellular histones (29). The term papovavirus was proposed by Melnick (67), who composed it by associating the first two letters of the names of the three viruses known to show these characteristics: papillomavirus, polyomavirus, and vacuolating virus. A papillomavirus was first described by Shope (92) in 1933 as an infectious filterable agent recovered from large horny warts of wild cottontail rabbits; polyomavirus was shown by Gross in 1953 to produce tumor in C3H mice (40); the vacuolating simian virus 40 (SV40) was isolated by Sweet and Hilleman (99) in 1960. Two genera have been defined within the group. The papillomaviruses are distinguished from the polyomaviruses (polyoma, SV40, BKV) by the larger size of their capsids (55 nm versus 45 nm) and the higher complexity of their genomes (~8,000 base pairs versus ~5,200 base pairs).

Polyomaviruses are rarely, if ever, oncogenic for their natural host, whereas papillomaviruses induce benign tumors (warts) of the epithelium they colonize (skin or mucous membrane). These virally induced lesions of stratified epithelia are generally characterized by hypertrophy of dermal papillas, accompanied in some cases (bovine papillomavirus, deer and sheep fibromaviruses) by an underlying mesenchymal proliferation. The virus, which infects keratinocytes of the basal layer, is found to replicate in the upper keratinizing cells, and viral antigens are detected by immunofluorescence in the keratinized layer. See the work of Orth et al. (76) for a review. The warts are generally self-limiting and regress under the influence of the host immune system. Papillomavirus infection may occasionally lead to malignant transformation in natural and experimental systems. This has been observed for the Shope cottontail rabbit papillomavirus (CRPV) (88), bovine papillomaviruses (BPV) types 1, 2, and 4 (11,55), *Mastomys natalensis* papillomavirus (MnPV) (71), and human papillomavirus (HPV) type 5 (79–81).

Papillomaviruses show an exclusive tropism for epithelial cells (keratinocytes), and for a given host, each type of virus corresponds to a specific localization and/

or morphology of the lesion (12,58,76,80). No natural interspecies transmission of papillomaviruses has been observed, although a causative role for BPV1 and BPV2 in equine sarcoid has been strongly suggested (53,55).

A peculiarity of this family of viruses is its widespread heterogeneity. No serological reactivity has been observed between intact viruses from different species (26,62), but common antigenic determinants are evidenced between the denatured structural proteins (47,78). A large antigenic variation also exists for different types of papillomaviruses infecting the same organism (36,77,84). These interspecies and intraspecies variations reflect a large genetic heterogeneity. No hybridization has been detected, under standard conditions, between the DNAs of different papillomaviruses, but conserved regions of partial homologies (about 75%) have been located on the papillomavirus genomes using less stringent hybridization procedures (18,59). Rather than the serotype, the extent of DNA homology has been chosen as the criterion for papillomavirus classification (14): Two different types share less than 50% homology, and various subtypes or variants are defined by differences in the restriction enzyme cleavage patterns of their DNAs, with homology exceeding 50%. The actual characterization of 12 different types of human papillomaviruses, including more than 30 subtypes (51,80; G. Orth, *personal communication*), illustrates the outstanding diversity of papillomaviruses.

The molecular biology of polyomaviruses is today well known and studied. In contrast, such studies on papillomaviruses have been hampered by lack of an *in vitro* cell culture system in which the virus could be reproducibly propagated (10). However, the comprehension of papillomavirus biology would offer several points of interest. First, these viruses are capable of expressing their oncogenic potential in natural conditions, and thus they constitute an attractive system for *in vivo* analysis of virally induced carcinogenesis (76,80). Second, the close relationship between the viral cycle and the differentiation state of keratinocytes suggests that common regulatory mechanisms are involved, and studying virus–cell interactions could certainly help their elucidation. Finally, the maintenance in the host cell nucleus of the viral genome in a free episomal state (9,31,55,56,102) provides a model for studying fundamental properties of eukaryotic replicons and should permit the use of these viruses as vectors for the propagation and expression of foreign genes in the eukaryotic cell (23,91,108).

Despite the methodological barrier mentioned earlier, several model systems have proved useful during the past few years for the study of papillomavirus genome structure and expression. Briefly, these involve the following: (a) the domestic rabbit transplantable carcinomas derived from CRPV-induced carcinoma (49); (b) mouse, hamster, or bovine cell lines transformed with BPV (8,9,24,55,70); (c) the possibility of propagating papillomavirus genomes in bacterial cells by molecular cloning (19,41,44,51) and analyzing them by rapid DNA sequencing techniques (13,20,106).

We shall review here the latest advances in the study of papillomavirus molecular genetics, trying to focus on the clues they provide for an understanding of viral genome structure, evolution, expression, and multiplication in the host cell.

STRUCTURAL PROPERTIES OF PAPILLOMAVIRUSES

The Capsid

Early structural studies on papovavirus capsid were performed on Shope and human wart viruses (50). The roughly spherical structure observed by electron microscopy (Fig. 1a) has an icosahedral symmetry, with a triangulation number of seven, thus containing 72 capsomers. The diameter of the capsid is 55 nm (a value of 45 nm is found for polyomaviruses). This icosahedron is skewed to the left for the Shope virus and to the right for the human virus. The presence in a number of papillomavirus preparations of large open-ended cylinders (74) would argue for the existence of at least two types (or forms) of polypeptides as protomers. One would constitute the capsomers of the corners (pentons) and the other those of the faces (hexons). As a matter of fact, hexons by themselves can form flat sheets that can roll up to generate cylinders. However, this interpretation was recently challenged by Rayment et al. (87), who suggested that both the surface and the corners of polyomavirus capsid can be constituted by one protein subunit (VP1) associated in pentameric capsomers.

Two viral proteins and four histones of cellular origin (H2A, H2B, H3, H4) are reproducibly observed when disrupted virions are analyzed on SDS polyacrylamide gels. The estimated molecular masses of virus-specific proteins vary somewhat from one type of virus to another (Table 1) and are roughly 54 kilodaltons (Kd) for the major capsid protein (VP1), representing 75% of the total virus proteins, and 70 to 76 kd for the minor species (VP1') (27,29,36,66,78). Other minor bands, ranging from 85 to 45 Kd, are variably seen on gels, but whether they represent genuine viral proteins or artifacts due to degradation or contamination of the preparation is not clear. Meinke and Meinke (66) have purified the VP1 protein of BPV1 and have determined its amino acid composition. The ratio Asp + Asn + Glu + Gln/ Lys + Arg + His is found to be 1.68, a value that seems to be characteristic of the main structural component of papovavirus capsid (values of 2.17 and 1.76 are found for SV40 and polyoma, respectively).

Further studies will be required to elucidate the exact number, nature, and role of the viral polypeptides in the virion structure and morphogenesis. Immunological characterizations are currently in progress, and, as will be discussed later, the knowledge of viral genome organization at the level of DNA sequence brings in new elements.

The Viral Genome

The genetic information of papillomaviruses is carried by a double-stranded circular and superhelical DNA molecule enclosed in the capsid (Fig. 1c). This means a molecular weight of 5×10^6 (15,80), which represents about 12.5% of the total weight of the viral particle (Table 1). This size of the genome is confirmed by electron microscopy measurements (18) and establishment of the complete nucleotide sequences of HPV1 and BPV1 (20,106), whose respective lengths are

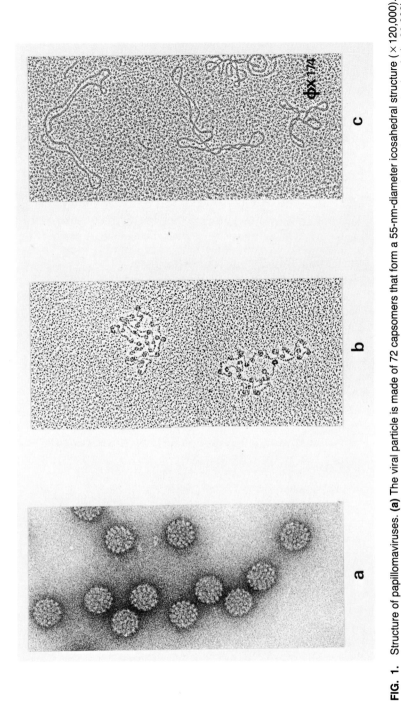

FIG. 1. Structure of papillomaviruses. **(a)** The viral particle is made of 72 capsomers that form a 55-nm-diameter icosahedral structure ($\times$120,000). **(b)** The viral DNA is associated with cellular histones in a minichromosome structure with a maximum number of 30 nucleosomes/molecule ($\times$80,000). **(c)** The virus genetic information is carried by a circular superhelical DNA molecule of about 5×10^6 daltons. ϕX174 DNA (replicative form) is shown as size standard ($\times$32,000). (Electron micrographs courtesy of O. Croissant.)

TABLE 1. *Structural features of papillomaviruses*

Virus	Genome size	G+C (%)	Capsid size (nm)	Major capsid protein		Minor capsid protein
				Estimated	Calculated	
HPV1	7,814 base pairs	40.3	55	54,000	57,570	76,000
BPV1	7,945 base pairs	45.3	55	53,500	55,490	70,500
CRPV	5.2×10^6 daltons	48–49.5	55	54,000	—	76,000

7,814 and 7,945 base pairs. The genome of BPV4, a papillomavirus associated with alimentary tract cancer in cattle, has been reported to be 10% smaller (11,46).

The G+C content of papillomavirus DNA is generally low (40.3% for HPV1, ~43% for canine oral papillomaviruses), the highest value being observed for CRPV (48%) (16,20). Sequence analysis of HPV1 DNA shows that the G+C content is not evenly distributed on the genome, as highly A+T-rich regions are evidenced (20). These easily melting sequences had been previously observed on HPV1 as being able to fix the bacteriophage T4 gene 32 protein (28).

The restriction maps of several papillomavirus DNAs have been established *(vide infra)*. Large inverted repeats occurring on HPV1 genomes have been observed by electron microscopy, and these structures were located on the physical map (35; O. Croissant, *personal communication*). Similar structures are also found in the BPV1 genome (105) and, with much more complex arrangement, on CRPV DNA (O. Croissant, *in preparation*).

Favre et al. (29) have shown that the viral DNA is associated with histones inside the capsid. This association in nucleosomes (a maximum number of 30 nucleosomes/molecules) forms a minichromosome structure (Fig. 1b) analogous to the one observed for SV40 and polyoma (17). The histones are of cellular origin and may have undergone covalent modifications (83).

MOLECULAR CLONING AND CHARACTERIZATION OF PAPILLOMAVIRUS GENOMES

Diversity of Papillomavirus Genomes

Until recently, all human warts were considered to be caused by the same virus. Comparative analyses by restriction endonuclease cleavage of viral DNA prepared from different isolates have demonstrated the existence of several types of viruses (34,51,76,77,79,80,105). This genetic heterogeneity of the papillomavirus family was further supported by the lack of hybridization between their nucleic acids, under stringent conditions (36,77,79,80). The numbers of different HPV types (with less than 50% DNA-DNA homologies as measured by reassociation kinetics and S1 digestion of the hybrid) and subtypes (bearing minor differences in the physical map) are increasing regularly. An outstanding diversity is found, especially for viruses associated with epidermodysplasia verruciformis (51,79,80). Variability has been observed for bovine viruses as well, and five types corresponding to different lesions and localizations have been analyzed for restriction enzyme cleavage patterns (11,12,54,84). Two distinct types of rabbit papillomaviruses are known: the Shope virus (CRPV) (92) and a virus associated with oral papillomatosis of domestic rabbits (82).

Molecular Cloning of Papillomavirus Genomes

Many of the characterizations of papillomavirus genomes became possible because of molecular cloning of the viral DNA in plasmidic vectors and subsequent propagation in *Escherichia coli* (19,22,41,44,51,102). Molecular cloning was obviously needed for several reasons: (a) It provides a never-ending source of material for molecular studies such as restriction mapping (19), detection of homologies (41), viral DNA probes (37,81,102), and DNA sequencing (13,20). This is a clear advantage when, for a number of types of viruses, only nanogram amounts of DNA are recoverable from the lesion (22,51). (b) It simplifies the procedure of viral DNA preparation, skipping the steps of biopsy and virus particle preparation that may result in loss or damage of material. (c) It ensures the purity of the viral DNA preparation, which otherwise could be composed of a mixture of several types of variants (36,52).

The construction of recombinant plasmids carrying subgenomic fragments of BPV1 has allowed Lowy et al. (63) to define the minimal portion of the genome required for *in vitro* tumorigenic transformation of mouse cells (NIH 3T3 and C127). The *Hind*III-*Bam*HI transforming fragment represents 69% of the entire genome (Fig. 2). Work in progress in our laboratory and several other laboratories makes use of papillomavirus genomes or subgenomic fragments propagated in bacterial

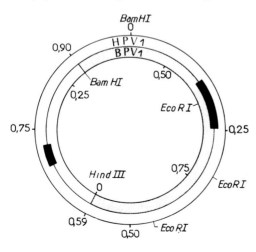

FIG. 2. Relative orientation of HPV1a and BPV1 physical maps. The stippled area represents the transforming fragment of the BPV1 genome. Regions of maximal homology *(black)* were mapped by electron microscopy observation of heteroduplexes. (Adapted from Croissant et al., ref. 18.)

vectors for *in vitro* mutagenesis, for functional tests of putative regulatory sequences, or for the preparation of molecular probes of defined viral segments.

Conserved Nucleotide Sequences Among Papillomavirus Genomes

Reassociation between heterologous DNA molecules can be detected under standard and optimal conditions (i.e., at 20 to 25°C below T_m) only for polynucleotides of closely related sequences. Two molecules with more than 15 to 20% nucleotide mismatches will not stably reassociate under these conditions (43). Thus, using classical procedures, no conserved sequences have been detected between papillomavirus genomes of different species (15) or types (36,77,79,80). This fact was in paradox with the existence of common antigenic determinants of CRPV and HPV1 (78), as well as with the probable common origin of papillomaviruses that argued for the existence of related polynucleotide sequences in their genomes. However, under less stringent conditions of hybridization (i.e., at 35 to 50°C below T_m), a certain degree of DNA homology was detected (59,78). With the help of the Southern (94) transfer technique it has been possible to locate conserved regions on the genomes of HPV1, HPV2, HPV4, BPV1, and CRPV (41,59). Electron microscopy observations of heteroduplexes have allowed more precise cartography of these 70 to 75% homologous segments (18) and the reciprocal orientation of the papillomavirus physical maps (Fig. 2). Two regions are conserved between HPV1 and BPV1, as well as in all papillomaviruses studied (O. Croissant, *personal communication*). The first lies in the 69% transforming fragment of BPV1 and represents about 10% of the whole genome. The second segment of homology (~4% of genome length) is located in a diametrically opposed position in the physical map and should represent sequences coding for structural polypeptides. These homologies are entirely confirmed by comparison of the DNA sequences of HPV1 and BPV1 (Figs. 5 and 7).

STATE AND EXPRESSION OF PAPILLOMAVIRUS GENOMES IN THE HOST CELL

As already mentioned, there is no *in vitro* system in which a lytic cycle of papillomaviruses can be observed. Thus, until now, expression and multiplication of their genomes have been studied mostly in rather atypical systems in which the host cell is stably transformed by the virus, without apparent production of viral antigens or particles. Only the CRPV-induced transplantable carcinoma VX7 is known to produce a small amount of viral antigens (78). Two fundamental properties of papillomaviruses have emerged from these studies: (a) They behave as true replicons in the transformed host cell, in which they are maintained as free episomes. (b) Only one strand of the viral DNA is transcribed. These two properties differ from polyomaviruses whose DNA is integrated in the chromosomes of the transformed cells and where both strands of the viral DNA are transcribed in the lytic cycle.

State of Viral DNA

Replicating viral DNA can be observed by *in situ* hybridization with ^{32}P-labeled cRNA probes on sections of papilloma induced by HPV or CRPV (75,76,80). Multiple DNA copies are also detected by reassociation kinetics in non-virus-producing neoplasms as domestic rabbit carcinomas and papillomas induced by CRPV (96), or as equine sarcoid tumors, in which Lancaster et al. (53) have demonstrated the presence of BPV sequences.

The state of the BPV DNA in sarcoid tumors has been investigated by Lancaster and Olson (55,56) and Amtmann et al. (1), who detected only free episomic forms migrating on agarose gels as authentic BPV virion DNA. There is no evidence for integration of viral DNA into the host chromosome, and the oncogenic process seems to be mediated solely by free episomal molecules present in the transformed equine cells at roughly 50 copies. One of the tumors analyzed contained an additional class of BPV1 DNA molecule bearing a deletion in the small BamHI-HindIII fragment, not required for transformation (11). Similarly, Favre et al. (31) have shown that the CRPV DNA is maintained in an extrachromosomal state in VX2 and VX7 transplantable carcinomas, with respective copy numbers of about 40 and 440. The DNA molecules are in a concatenated state, forming high-molecular-weight complexes that are transformed into unit-length linear molecules by cleavage with a single-cut restriction enzyme. Large multimeric circles have been shown to predominate in domestic rabbit carcinomas (104). In the VX7 carcinomas, deleted molecules lacking 10% of the genome are present together with the intact ones (31). HPV5 DNA present in squamous cell carcinomas from patients with epidermodysplasia verruciformis (79,80) is unintegrated as well, and deleted molecules have also been detected (81).

Besides the naturally occurring neoplasms, it has been possible to establish papillomavirus-transformed cell lines (a) from natural or experimentally induced BPV tumors of cattle, horses (55,56), and hamsters (9,70), (b) after BPV infection of mouse fibroblasts (55,56) or bovine tissue culture (69), (c) after transfection of mouse (60) or rat (107,108) fibroblasts with BPV DNA using the calcium phosphate coprecipitation technique (39), and (d) from transplantable carcinomas containing CRPV genomes (65; E. George, *personal communication*).

In all the cases studied, viral DNA has been found unlinked to the cellular DNA, more often in the form of high-molecular-weight catenated structures (60), with a variable copy number ranging from 10 for some transfected mouse cell lines (60) to 500 for the established hamster tumor cell lines (19,70). Such catenated structures may represent replication intermediates (97). Reconstitution experiments have shown that the limit of detection of an integrated genome would be 0.1 to 0.2 genome equivalent/cell (60). Recently, La Porta and Taichman (57) observed vegetative replication of HPV1 as a stable episome in cultured epidermal keratinocytes for periods up to 4 months (eight passages); 50 to 200 copies of free viral DNA were observed, and the cells were apparently nontransformed.

Nevertheless, some evidence for integration of viral DNA in addition to free episomal forms has been reported for BPV1 in hamster tumor cell lines (19) and for CRPV in domestic rabbit papillomas and carcinomas (102,104) and in transplantable carcinomas (65). Furthermore, when a recombinant plasmid carrying the BPV genome linked to the herpes simplex thymidine kinase (tk) gene is introduced in mouse or rat tk⁻ cells, all the BPV sequences seem to be integrated (64). But these cases seem to be exceptional, and further analysis of the integration pattern is required. As a general rule, integration of viral DNA is not essential for the cellular transformation processes mediated by papillomaviruses.

As a putative determinant of gene expression [for a review, see Ehrlich and Wang (25)], DNA methylation on cytosine residues of dinucleotide CpG has been investigated by restriction enzyme analysis (7). BPV DNA in transformed bovine cell lines or in hamster tumors does not show any methylation of CpG sites (85; M. H. Moar et al., *in preparation*), whereas CRPV genome is methylated in domestic rabbit carcinomas as well as in transplantable carcinomas, and more partially in papillomas (F. O. Wettstein, *personal communication*). Two methylation sites of CRPV genome remain unmethylated in any case. On HVP1 virion DNA, one of the four *Hpa*II sites (CCGG) is methylated in 40% of the viral DNA population (19). One cannot draw from this result any clear correlation between the extent of methylation and the low level of viral genome expression observed in the transformed cells *(vide infra)*.

Transcription of Papillomavirus Genomes

Transcripts complementary to the CRPV genome have been detected by reassociation kinetics in virus-producing papilloma of cottontail rabbits and in noninvading malignant tumors of domestic rabbits (103). Only small portions (about 10%) of the viral DNA sequences are transcribed in these lesions. In transplantable carcinomas, specific transcripts can be detected by Northern blott procedures (100) and hybridization with a viral probe (E. Georges, *personal communication*; F. O. Wettstein, *personal communication*). The major polyadenylated RNAs are of 1,300 and 2,000 bases, and their precise mapping is in progress.

Transcription of BPV1 genome has been studied by Heilman et al. (42) and Amtmann and Sauer (3) in transformed mouse cells. Five transcripts complementary to a single DNA strand and sharing common polyadenylated termini have been detected in whole-cell RNA preparations. The three major ones are 1,050, 1,150, and 1,700 bases long, and the two others are 3,800 and 4,050 bases long. Figure 3 shows the positions of these transcripts on the BPV1 genome. All are contained within the 69% transforming fragment. Nuclease S1 analysis (5) of the three major transcripts did not show any internal splicing event. However, the presence of a common 3′ terminus suggests that these transcripts are produced by differential removal of leader sequences from a large mRNA precursor. Considering the papillomavirus structure revealed by DNA sequences (20), and the location of putative control regions *(vide infra)*, this precursor could be the minor 4,050-base species

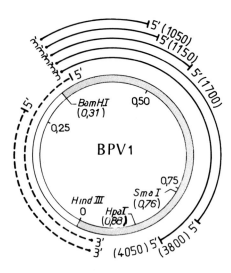

FIG. 3. Transcription map of BPV1 genome. The stippled area represents the transforming fragment of the BPV1 genome. Polyadenylated mRNAs detected in transformed cell lines (3,42) are drawn as continuous lines. Transcripts from the nontransforming region (3; P. Howley, *personal communication*) are shown as dotted lines.

that represents less than 5% of total viral RNA. This hypothesis is further supported by the common hybridization of all transcripts to an *Hpa*I-*Sma*I probe (Fig. 3) (3).

In BPV1-induced hamster tumors, two major species of RNA, 1,300 and 1,100 bases long, were found (3,33; U. K. Freese, *personal communication*), together with three minor species of 1,800, 1,600, and 1,000 bases (3). All these transcripts are complementary to the 69% transforming fragment. BPV1 genome propagated in bovine conjunctival or palate cell lines is also transcribed in at least four RNA species, whose sizes range from 3,800 to 1,100 bases (M. H. Moar, *personal communication*). In the peripheral part of bovine fibropapillomas, where viral antigens are expressed, two additional RNA species of about 2,000 and 3,000 bases were detected (3; P. Howley, *personal communication*). These transcripts should code for the viral structural proteins (Fig. 3).

As observed for CRPV-transformed cells, the rate of transcription of BPV1 DNA in mouse cells is very low, about 0.006 to 0.01% of the polyadenylated RNA pool of the cells (42). Such a weak expression of BPV sequences, contrasting with the high copy number, is also observed in simian COS cells (93), propagating up to 2.5×10^5 copies of the viral genome linked to the SV40 origin of replication (108). Activation of BVP1 transcription in mouse embryo fibroblasts is observed after treatment with the tumor-promoting agent 12-*O*-tetradecanoyl phorbol-13-acetate (TPA) (2). It should be noted that the combination of viral infection with an environmental carcinogen (bracken fern, ultraviolet light, polycyclic hydrocarbons) has long been invoked in the etiology of papillomavirus-induced tumors (45,76,80).

Nothing is yet known about the mode of regulation of papillomavirus gene expression, but examination of DNA sequences has indicated putative control regions *(vide infra)* (Fig. 5). Lusky et al. (64) have shown that a 2.9-kb *Bam*HI-*Bgl*II fragment of BPV1 possesses an enhancer activity on gene expression similar to the one observed for the 72-base-pair repeat of SV40 (4).

SEQUENCE STUDIES AND ORGANIZATION OF PAPILLOMAVIRUS GENOMES

Another helpful tool for understanding papillomavirus structure and biology is determination of the nucleotide sequences of their genomes. These sequences should provide information on the different polypeptides coded by the virus and information on putative control regions. Furthermore, elucidation of the genome organization can prove useful in providing the information for chemical synthesis of virus-specific epitopes for immunological characterization of unknown viral proteins (98,101). The structure of the regulatory regions and signals on the genome should bring new insights into the interaction of the virus with the host cell.

Structure of the HPV1a Genome

The complete nucleotide sequence of the HPV1a genome has been determined in our laboratory (20). This human virus was originally chosen because it was used as the prototype for physicochemical characterization of papillomavirus *(vide supra)*. The sequence was established starting with pBR322-cloned DNA (19), subcloning of genomic fragments in M13 vectors (68,90), and direct sequencing of the M13-HPV1a recombinants with Sanger's dideoxy technique (89). The genome is 7,814 nucleotides long, and the first nucleotide of the numbering system is the internal thymidine of the unique *Bam*HI site, previously chosen as origin of the physical map (30).

Figure 4 presents the organization of the HPV1a genome deduced from the nucleotide sequence. In contrast to the situation with polyomaviruses (32,93), the genetic information of the virus seems to be coded only by one DNA strand. This is consistent with the mapping of BPV1 transcripts presented in Fig. 3. No homology has been found between HPV1a and polyoma on SV40, neither at the nucleotide sequence level nor between the proteins. The possibility of orienting HPV1a and BPV1 genomes (18), the existence of a 69% transforming fragment of BPV1 DNA (63), and the distribution of open reading frames and control signals (polyadenylation sites, putative promoters for RNA polymerase II) allow the definition of two functional regions on the HPV1a genome.

The late region contains genes L1 and L2 that are likely to code for structural polypeptides. The calculated molecular weight for the L1-encoded protein is 57,569 d, which reasonably matches the estimated 54 kd for the virion major protein. In addition, the deduced amino acid composition for L1 resembles that of BPV1 VP1 protein (66). The only common feature of L1 and L2 proteins with polyomavirus capsid proteins VP2 and VP3 is their highly basic C terminus, which has been proposed as a site of protein–DNA interaction in the virion (32).

In the early region, which corresponds to the BPV1 transforming fragment, we found two major open reading frames starting with a methionine codon (E1 and E2), together with several small ones, whose role as small exons remains uncertain in the absence of any results about HPV1a transcription. Nevertheless, the conservation in the BPV1 genome of the small open reading frame E6 (106), with

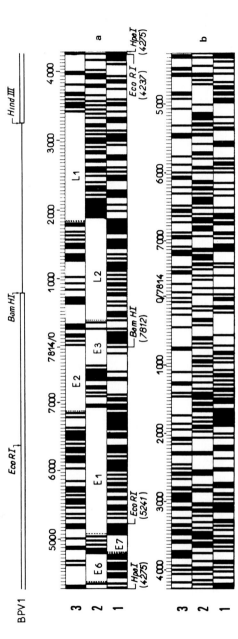

FIG. 4. Distribution of the termination codons on the HPV1a genome. Diagrams **a** and **b** show the distributions of the termination codons on sense and anti-sense strands, respectively, starting from the *HpaI* site at position 4,275. From left to right, the sequence is read 5′ to 3′. Groups of 10 codons are observed in each of the three reading frames, and a vertical bar is drawn when at least one termination codon occurs among them. Large open reading frames starting with ATG (*dotted vertical bars*) are seen on the sense strand only (**a**). A schematic representation of the BPV1 genome, oriented relative to HPV1a, is given in the top of the figure. The *BamHI-HindIII* 69% transforming fragment is depicted as a solid bar.

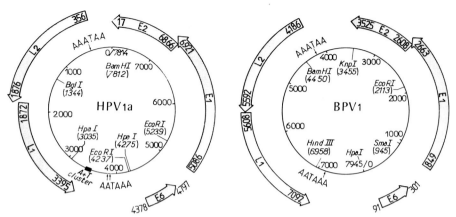

FIG. 5. Genome organization of HPV1a and BPV1. Viral genes are depicted as arrows in which the positions of start and stop codons are indicated.

similar amino acid distribution, suggests that this region is indeed coding (Fig. 5). E1 and E2 can code, respectively, for 612- and 322-amino-acid-long polypeptides, but no such specific viral proteins have been characterized so far in papillomavirus-infected or -transformed cells (9). The E2 coding region contains two stretches of homology with the consensus sequence of the human Alu family of ubiquitous repeats (21), between positions 7,560 and 7,700. The codon usage in E2 is somewhat different from that of other genes, and the possible cellular origin of this gene is under investigation.

Comparison of HPV1 and BPV1 Sequences

The nucleotide sequence of BPV1 has also been determined recently (106), and the genetic organization of this virus is very similar to that described for HPV1a (Fig. 5). The same is true for the genome of HPV6b, a virus found in human genital lesions (22), whose sequence has recently been determined (E. Schwarz, *personal communication*). Comparison of papillomavirus DNA sequences (HPV1a, BPV1, HPV6b, and CRPV; this work is in progress in our laboratory) will allow us to answer several questions: (a) which are the conserved open reading frames? The answer will point out genuine papillomavirus genes or exons. (b) Which are the conserved amino acid sequences in the encoded proteins? This information will permit us to discriminate between conserved antigenic determinants hidden in the protein tertiary structure that are revealed after denaturation (47,78) and variable antigenic motives of the surface that cause papillomavirus antigenic diversity. (c) How do the control sequences for gene expression differ? This could shed light on papillomavirus oncogenicity and host restriction. (d) What is the molecular basis of papillomavirus diversity? Comparison of genomic sequences will help to elucidate mechanisms of variability (between different types of viruses) and evolution (between viruses infecting different species).

An overall computer-based graphic comparison between HPV1a and BPV1 genomes is shown in Fig. 6. The two genomes can be perfectly aligned, and the maximal homologies are found in the coding sequences E1, E2, L1, and L2.

This matrix comparison also indicates that the extra 130 base pairs of BPV1 are not distributed throughout the sequence, but correspond to an insertion at about position 400 on the HPV1a sequence.

The E1 and L1 protein sequences from both genomes are compared in Fig. 7. The sequence conservation shown here is striking in view of the small amount of biochemically detectable homology between the two genomes (18,59). Actually,

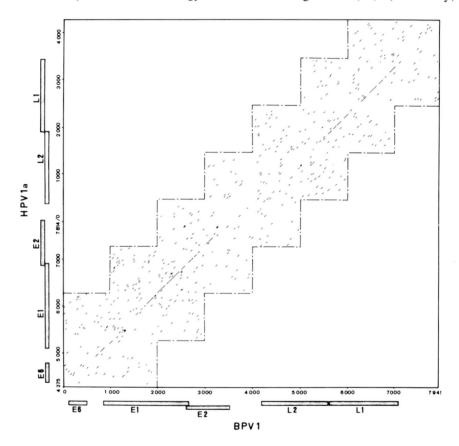

FIG. 6. Matrix comparison of HPV1a and BPV1 DNA sequences. Abscissa and ordinate represent BPV1 and HPV1a DNA sequences, respectively. The origin of the axis corresponds to the *Hpa*I site of BPV1 (position 1) and HPV1a (position 4,275). The two sequences were compared using the program PBASCOMP, which calculates a matrix of homologies for successive groups of 10 nucleotides. The level of homology used is 70%. The output shown here is the result of a second filtration performed by the program PBASCOMP, where only the most significant homologies are shown (i.e., with an overall level of at least 50% on 50 nucleotides). Only regions around the diagonal were compared, and the figure is redrawn from original computer output.

most of the changes in the DNA sequences affect the third base of codons, thus preserving the same amino acid sequence, because of the degeneracy of the genetic code. This alignment also evidences preferentially conserved domains in E1 and L1 proteins. Comparison of the C-terminal parts of E1 protein from HPV1a and HPV6b shows that the same peptides are conserved between HPV1a, BPV1, and HPV6b (E. Schwarz, *personal communication*).

The structure of the putative regulatory region upstream from the early genes for both viruses is conserved as well. Possible signals for the polymerase II transcription are found (20) together with palindromic structures and short direct repeats. The polyadenylation signals are also similarly positioned relative to the coding regions, in the two DNA sequences (Fig. 5). Thus far, there is no evidence for the localization of an origin of replication on papillomavirus genomes, although experiments are in progress to select a genomic fragment that will allow autonomous replication of a selectable marker in cells transformed by BPV1 (6,61).

USE OF PAPILLOMAVIRUSES AS EUKARYOTIC VECTORS

The ability of papillomavirus genomes to proliferate in the nucleus of the eukaryotic cell as free episomes *(vide supra)* has made them attractive candidates for eukaryotic vectors. Papillomavirus-based vectors could theoretically propagate a fragment of foreign DNA in the recipient cell without integration in the host or carrier DNA. Thus, the environment of genes cloned in papillomaviruses could be closely controlled. This would allow a higher reproducibility of transfection and expression experiments. Until now, BPV1 has been mainly chosen to test the efficiency of papillomaviruses as vectors, because the use of BPV1 69% transforming fragment (BPVT69) as vector leads to direct selection of transfected cells by their transformed phenotype. If prokaryotic sequences allowing replication in *E. coli* (such as plasmid pBR322) could be stably introduced in BPV vectors without interfering with the replication in the eukaryotic cell, this would provide an ideal shuttle vector. With such a vector, all constructions and *in vitro* mutagenesis steps could be done in bacteria, with expression or phenotypical tests in the recipient eukaryotic cell.

Several genes linked to the BPVT69 have already been successfully propagated as extrachromosomal elements in mouse cells. Production of authentic rat preproinsulin (91) (Fig. 8), human interferon (23), and human growth hormone (23) has been observed. Furthermore, hormonal regulation of the Harvey sarcoma virus *ras* gene, placed under the control of mouse mammary tumor virus (MMTV) long terminal repeat and linked to the BPVT69, can be monitored (G. Hager, *personal communication*). Gene dosage effects on the toxicity of cadmium can be also studied with the BPVT69 human metallothioneine I gene multicopy episome in mouse transformed cells (M. Karin, *personal communication*).

A limitation of the BPVT69 vector system is the dependence on the transformed

```
BPV1      MALWQQGQ KLYLPPTPVSKVLCSETYVQRKSIFYHAETERLLTIGHPYYPVSI   53
HPV1   MYNVFQMAVWLPAQNKFYLPPQPITRILSTDEYVTRTNLFYHATSERLLLVGHPLFEISS   60

       GAKTV  PKVSANQYRVFKIQLPDPNQFALPDRTVHNPSKERLVWAVIGVQVSRGQPLGG  111
       NQTVTIPKVSPNAFRVFRVRFADPNRFAFGDKAIFNPETERLVWGLRGIEIGRGQPLGI  119

       TVTGHPTFNALLDAENVNRKVTTQTTDDRKQ TGLDAKQQQILLLGCTPAEGEYWTTARP  170
       GITGHPLLMKLDDAENPTNYINTHANGDSRQNTAFDAKQTQMFLVGCTPASGEHWTSSRC  179

       CVTDRLENGACPPLELKNKHIEDGDMMEIGFGAANFKEINASKSDLPLDIQNEICLYPDY  230
       PGEQVKL GDCPRVQMIESVIEDGDMMDIGFGAMDFAALQQDKSDVPLDVVQATCKYPDY  238

  L1   LKMAEDAAGNSMFFFARKEQVYVRHIWTRGGS EKEAPTTDFYLKNNKGDATLKIPSVH  288
       IRMNHEAYGNSMFFFARREQMYTRHFFTRGGSVGDKEAVPQSLYLTADAEPRTTLATTNY  298

       FGSPSGSLVSTDNQIFNRPYWLFRAQGMNNGIAWNNLLFLTVGDNTRGTNLTISVASDGT  348
       VGTPSGSMVSSDVQLFNRSYWLQRCQGQNNGICWRNQLFITVGDNTRGTSLSISMKNNAS  358

       PLTEYDSSKFNVYHRHMEEYKLAFILELCSVEITAQTVSHLQGLMPSVLENWEIGV QPP  407
       TTYSNANFNDFLRHTEEFDLSFIVQLCKVKLTPENLAYIHTMDPNILEDWQLSVSQPP  416

       TSSILEDTYRYIE SPATKCASNVIPAKE DPYAGFKFWNIDLKEKLSLDLDQFPLGRRF  465
       TNP LEDQYRFLGSSLAAKCPEQAPPEPQTDPYSQYKFWEVDLTERMSEQLDQFPLGRKF  475

       LAQQG  AGCSTVRKRRISQKTSSKPAKKKKK                              495
       LYQSGMTQRTATSSTTKRKTVRVSTS  AKRRRKA                          508

BPV1   MANDKGSNWDSGLGCSYLLTEA ECESDKENEEPGAGVELSVESDRYDSQDEDFVDNASV   59
HPV1   MADNKGTEND        WFLVEATDCEETLEETSLGDLDNVSCVSDLSDLLDE  APQ   49

       FQGNHLEVFQALEKKAGEEQILNLKRKVLGSSQNSSGSEA          SETPVKRR  107
       SQGNSLELFHKQESLESEQELNALKRKLLYSPQARSADETDIASISPRLETISITKQDKK  109

       KSGAKRR LFAENEANRVLTPLQVQGEGEGRQELNEEQAISHLHLQLVKSKNA     T  160
       R   YRRQLFSQDDSGLELSLLQDETENIDESTQVDQQQKEHTGEVGAAGVNILKASNIR  166

       VFKLGLFKSLFLCSFHDITRLFKNDKTTNQQWVLAVFGLAEVFFEASFELLKKQCSFLQM  220
       AALLSRFKDTAGVSFTDLTRSYKSNKTCCGDWVLAVWGVRENLIDSVKELLQTHCVYIQL  226

       QKRSHEGGTCAVYLICFNTAKSRETVRNLMANTLNVREECLMLQPAKIRGLSAALFWFKS  280
       EHAVTEKNRFLFLLVRFKAQKSRETVIKLITTILPVDASYILSEPPKRRSVAAALFWYKR  286

  E1   SLSPATLKHGALPEWIRAQTTL NESLQTEK FDFGTMVQWAYDHKYAEESKIAYEYALA  338
       SMSSTVFTWGTTLEWI AQQTLINHQLDSESPFELCKMVQWAYDNGHTEECKIAYYYAVL  345

       AGSDSNARAFLATNSQAKHVKDCATMVRHYLRAETQALSMPAYIKARCKLATGEGS  WK  396
       ADEDENARAFLSSNSQAKYVKDCAQMVRHYLRAEMAQMSMSEWIFR  KLDNVEGSGNWK  403

       SILTFFNYQNIELITFINALKLWLKGIPKKNCLAFIGPPNTGKSMLCNSLIHFLGGSVLS  456
       EIVRFLRFQEVEFISFMIAFKDLLCGKPKKNCLLIFGPPNTGKSMFCTSLLKLLGGKVIS  463

       FANHKSHFWLASLADTRAALVDDATHACWRYFDTYLRNALDGYPVSIDRKHKAAVQIKAP  516
       YCNSKSQFWLQPALDAKIGLLDDATKPCWDYMDIYMRNALDGNTICIDLKHRAPQQIKCP  523

       PLLVTSNIDVQAEDRYLYLHSRVQTFRFEQPCTDESGEQP FNITDADWKSFFVRLWGRL  575
       PLLITSNIDVKSDTCWMYIHSRISAFKFAHEFPFKDNGDPGFSLTDENWKSFFERFWQQL  583

       DLIDEEEDSEEDGDSMRTFTCSARNTNAVD                               605
       ELSDQ EDEGNDGKPQOSLRLTARAANEPI                               612
```

phenotype of the cell. Experiments are restricted to the use of BPV-transformable recipient cells. For these reasons, attempts have been made to use the self-replicating capacity of BPV sequences in conjunction with a dominant marker, whose expression can be selected in a wide range of cells (6,61,108). Such BPV vectors contain the *E. coli* xanthine guanine phosphoribosyl transferase *(gpt)* gene, placed under the control of SV40 early promoter. Expression of the *gpt* gene in eukaryotic cells allows the use of xanthine as substrate for the purine salvage pathway. Cells provided with xanthine are thus able to grow in the presence of mycophenolic acid, which normally inhibits purine synthesis (MAX selective medium) (72,73). The use of bacterial phosphotransferases encoded in transposon Tn5 (48), which confers to the eukaryotic cell resistance to the cytotoxic compound G418 (95), is also being examined (P. Howley, *personal communication*; F. Cuzin, *personal communication*; M. Lusky, *personal communication).*

Another problem associated with the use of BPV as vector is the poor maintenance of prokaryotic sequences as pBR322 linked to the free replicating molecules. Rearrangements and deletions of both viral and bacterial sequences frequently occur when DNA is introduced in the cell without removing the bacterial part (6,23,77; I. Giri, *unpublished observations).* Moreover, the association with pBR322 dramatically reduces the efficiency of transfection by the calcium phosphate coprecipitation technique (6,107). Thus, such plasmids cannot be conveniently used to shuttle genes between bacteria and eukaryotic cells. Despite this, Binetruy et al. have reported a successful shuttle when the high-transfer-efficiency technique of protoplast fusion is used (86). Di Maio et al. (23) have observed that the presence in a BPV-derived recombinant plasmid of a 7.6-kb fragment of DNA from the human β-globin gene cluster enhances both transfection efficiency and maintenance in the host cell of an intact molecule. This episome can be efficiently established back in bacteria. The role of the β-globin fragment is not understood, but it points out that other "stabilizing" elements are required for the construction of operational BPV vectors.

CONCLUSION

We have presented here recent advances in the understanding of papillomavirus genome structures and the control of their expression. The genetic studies that have been such powerful tools for the comprehension of SV40 and polyoma biology have not been possible here because of the lack of a cell culture system. We have reviewed the specific interests of papillomavirus studies, because these viruses

FIG. 7. Alignment of L1 and E1 protein sequences of BPV1 and HPV1a. The primary structures of L1 and E1 proteins of BPV1 and HPV1a are shown. Homologous amino acids are bracketed, and gaps are introduced to maximize homologies. In the L1 proteins, about 45% of the amino acids are conserved, and 30% of the remaining changes are conservative. In the E1 proteins, about 41% of the amino acids are conserved, and 16% of the remaining changes are conservative. The designations of the amino acids are as follows: A, Ala; R, Arg; N, Asm; D, Asp; C, Cys; Q, Gln; E, Glu; G, Gly; H, His; I, Ile; L, Leu; K, Lys; M, Met; F, Phe; P, Pro; S, Ser; T, Thr; W, Trp; Y, Tyr; V, Val.

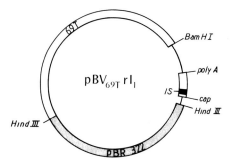

FIG. 8. Use of BPV1 transforming fragment as a eukaryotic cloning vector. The structure of a recombinant plasmid carrying the rat preproinsuline gene is shown (91). The *Hind*III-*Bam*HI transforming fragment of BPV1 (69T) allows the propagation and expression of the rat gene in mouse C127 cells, after excision of pBR322 bacterial sequences. The preproinsuline gene is transcribed, polyadenylated, and spliced using the rat control sequences (I.S: rat preproinsuline intervening sequence).

interact with terminally differentiating cells, behave as true autonomous eukaryotic replicons, can express their oncogenic potential in natural conditions, and could be used as eukaryotic viral vectors. The incoming data of the past few years have left people in the field with great expectations. The next step is certainly the characterization of early gene products revealed by the DNA sequences, to be followed by a search for molecular mechanisms of virus–cell interactions.

ACKNOWLEDGMENTS

We are grateful to O. Croissant for the gift of electron microscopy photography. We are indebted to all our colleagues who communicated to us unpublished information for the completion of this review, to B. Caudron (Unité de Calcul, Institut Pasteur) for advice in computer analysis of sequence data, and to C. Maczuka for her help in the preparation of the text. This work was supported by grants from C.N.R.S. (ATP Biologie moléculaire du gène and LA 0270), I.N.S.E.R.M. (PRC 118011), and the Fondation pour la Recherche Médicale Française.

REFERENCES

1. Amtmann, E., Müller, H., and Sauer, G. (1980): Equine connective tissue tumors contain unintegrated bovine papillomavirus DNA. *J. Virol.*, 35:962–964.
2. Amtmann, E., and Sauer, G. (1982): Activation of non-expressed bovine papillomavirus genomes by tumour promoters. *Nature*, 296:675–677.
3. Amtmann, E., and Sauer, G. (1982): Bovine papillomavirus transcription: Polyadenylated RNA species and assessment of the direction of transcription. *J. Virol.*, 43:59–66.
4. Banerji, J., Rusconi, S., and Schaffner, W. (1981): Expression of a β-globin gene is enhanced by remote SV40 DNA sequences. *Cell*, 27:299–308.
5. Berk, A. J., and Sharp, P. A. (1977): Sizing and mapping of early adenovirus mRNA's by gel electrophoresis of S1 endonuclease digested hybrids. *Cell*, 12:721–732.
6. Binetruy, B., Rautmann, G., Meneguzzi, G., Breathnach, R., and Cuzin, F. (1982): Bovine papillomavirus 1-pBR322 recombinants as eukaryotic vectors. In: *Eukaryotic Viral Vectors*, edited by Y. Gluzman, pp. 87–92. Cold Spring Harbor Laboratory, Cold Spring Harbor, N.Y.
7. Bird, A. P., and Southern, E. M. (1978): Use of restriction enzymes to study eukaryotic DNA methylation. I. The methylation pattern in ribosomal DNA from *Xenopus laevis*. *J. Mol. Biol.*, 118:27–47.
8. Boiron, M., Thomas, M., and Chenaille, P. (1965): A biological property of deoxyribonucleic acid extracted from bovine papilloma virus. *Virology*, 26:150–153.
9. Breitburd, F., Favre, M., Zoorob, R., Fortin, D., and Orth, G. (1981): Detection and character-

ization of viral genomes and search for tumoral antigens in two hamster cell lines derived from tumor induced by bovine papillomavirus type 1. *Int. J. Cancer*, 27:693–702.

10. Butel, J. S. (1972): Studies with human papillomavirus modeled after known papovavirus systems. *J. Natl. Cancer Inst.*, 48:285–299.

11. Campo, M. S., Moar, M. H., Jarrett, W. F. H., and Laird, H. M. (1980): A new papillomavirus associated with alimentary cancer in cattle. *Nature*, 286:180–182.

12. Campo, S. M., Moar, M. H., Laird, H. M., and Jarrett, W. F. H. (1981): Molecular heterogeneity and lesion specificity of cutaneous bovine papillomaviruses. *Virology*, 113:323–335.

13. Clad, A., Gissmann, L., Meier, B., Freese, U. K., and Schwarz, E. (1981): Molecular cloning and partial nucleotide sequence of human papillomavirus type 1a DNA. *Virology*, 118:254–259.

14. Coggin, J. R., Jr., and zur Hausen, H. (1979): Workshop on papillomaviruses and cancer. *Cancer Res.*, 39:545–546.

15. Crawford, L. V. (1965): A study of human papillomavirus DNA. *J. Mol. Biol.*, 13:362–372.

16. Crawford, L. V. (1969): Nucleic acids of tumor viruses. *Adv. Virus Res.*, 14:89–152.

17. Crémisi, C., Pignatti, P. F., Croissant, O., and Yaniv, M. (1976): Chromatin-like structures in polyomavirus and simian virus 40 lytic cycle. *J. Virol.*, 17:204–211.

18. Croissant, O., Testanière, V., and Orth, G. (1982): Mise en évidence et localisation de régions conservées dans les génomes du papillomavirus humain 1a et du papillomavirus bovin 1 par analyse d'"hétéroduplex" au microscope électronique. *C. R. Acad. Sci. (Paris)*, 294:581–586.

19. Danos, O., Katinka, M., and Yaniv, M. (1980): Molecular cloning refined physical map and heterogeneity of methylation sites of papillomavirus type 1a DNA. *Eur. J. Biochem.*, 109:457–461.

20. Danos, O., Katinka, M., and Yaniv, M. (1982): Human papillomavirus 1a DNA sequence: A novel type of genome organization among papovaviridae. *EMBO Journal*, 1:231–236.

21. Deininger, P. L., Jolly, D. J., Rubin, C. M., Friedmann, T., and Schmid, C. W. (1981): Base sequence studies of 300 nucleotide renatured repeated human DNA clones. *J. Mol. Biol.*, 151:17–33.

22. De Villiers, M., Gissmann, L., and zur Hausen, H. (1981): Molecular cloning of viral DNA from human genital warts. *J. Virol.*, 40:932–935.

23. Di Maio, D., Treisman, R., and Maniatis, T. (1982): A bovine papillomavirus vector which propagates as a plasmid in both mouse and bacterial cells. *Proc. Natl. Acad. Sci. USA*, 79:4030–4034.

24. Dvoretzky, I., Shober, R., Chattopadhayay, S. K., and Lowy, D. R. (1980): A quantitative *in vitro* focus assay for bovine papillomavirus. *Virology*, 103:369–375.

25. Ehrlich, M., and Wang, R. Y. H. (1981): 5-Methylcytosine in eukaryotic DNA. *Science*, 212:1350–1357.

26. Favre, M., Breitburd, F., Croissant, O., and Orth, G. (1974): Hemagglutinating activity of bovine papillomavirus. *Virology*, 60:572–578.

27. Favre, M., Breitburd, F., and Orth, G. (1975): Structural polypeptides of rabbit, bovine and human papillomaviruses. *J. Virol.*, 15:1239–1247.

28. Favre, M., Orth, G., Croissant, O., and Yaniv, M. (1975): Human papillomavirus DNA: Physical map. *Proc. Natl. Acad. Sci. USA*, 72:4810–4814.

29. Favre, M., Breitburd, F., Croissant, O., and Orth, G. (1977): Chromatin-like structures obtained after alkaline disruption of bovine and human papillomaviruses. *J. Virol.*, 21:1205–1209.

30. Favre, M., Orth, G., Croissant, O., and Yaniv, M. (1977): Human papillomavirus DNA: Physical mapping of the cleavage sites of *Bacillus amyloliquefaciens* (*Bam*I) and *Haemophilus parainfluenzae* (*Hpa*II) endonucleases and evidence for partial heterogeneity. *J. Virol.*, 21:1210–1214.

31. Favre, M., Jibard, N., and Orth, G. (1982): Restriction mapping and physical characterization of the cottontail rabbit papillomavirus genome in transplantable VX2 and VX7 domestic rabbit carcinomas. *Virology*, 119:298–309.

32. Fiers, W., Contreras, R., Haegeman, G., Rogiers, R., van de Voorde, A., van Heuverswys, H., van Herreveghe, J., Volckaert, G., and Ysebaert, M. (1978): Complete nucleotide sequence of SV40 DNA. *Nature*, 273:113–120.

33. Freese, U. K., Schulte, P., and Pfister, H. (1982): Bovine papillomavirus-induced tumor contains a virus specific transcript. *Virology*, 117:257–261.

34. Gissmann, L., and zur Hausen, H. (1976): Human papillomavirus DNA: Physical mapping and genetical heterogeneity. *Proc. Natl. Acad. Sci. USA*, 73:1310–1313.

35. Gissmann, L., and zur Hausen, H. (1977): Inverted repetitive sequences in human papillomavirus 1 (HPV-1) DNA. *Virology*, 83:271–276.
36. Gissmann, L., Pfister, H., and zur Hausen, H. (1977): Human papillomaviruses (HPV): Characterization of 4 different isolates. *Virology*, 76:569–580.
37. Gissmann, L., de Villiers, E. M., and zur Hausen, H. (1982): Analysis of human genital warts (condylomata acuminata) and other genital tumors for human papillomavirus type 6 DNA. *Int. J. Cancer*, 29:143–146.
38. Gluzman, Y. (1981): SV40 transformed simian cells support the replication of early SV40 mutants. *Cell*, 23:175–182.
39. Graham, F. L., and van der Eb, A. J. (1973): Transformation of rat cells by DNA of human adenovirus S. *Virology*, 54:536–539.
40. Gross, L. (1953): A filterable agent, recovered from Ak leukemic extracts, causing salivary gland carcinomas in C3H mice. *Proc. Soc. Exp. Biol. Med.*, 83:414–421.
41. Heilman, C. A., Law, M. F., Israel, M. A., and Howley, P. M. (1980): Cloning of human papillomavirus genomic DNAs and analysis of homologous polynucleotide sequences. *J. Virol.*, 36:395–407.
42. Heilman, C. A., Engel, L., Lowy, D. R., and Howley, P. M. (1982): Virus specific transcription in bovine papillomavirus-transformed mouse cells. *Virology*, 119:22–34.
43. Howley, P. M., Israel, M. A., Law, M. F., and Martin, M. A. (1979): A rapid method for detecting and mapping homology between heterologous DNAs. Evaluation of polyomavirus genomes. *J. Biol. Chem.*, 254:4876–4883.
44. Howley, P. M., Law, M. F., Heilman, C., Engel, L., Alonso, M. C., Israel, M. A., Lowy, D. R., and Lancaster, W. D. (1980): Molecular characterization of papillomavirus genomes. In: *Viruses in Naturally Occurring Cancers, Cold Spring Harbor Conferences on Cell Proliferation, Vol. 7*, edited by M. Essex, G. Todaro, and H. zur Hausen, pp. 233–248. Cold Spring Harbor Laboratory, Cold Spring Harbor, N.Y.
45. Jarrett, W. F. H., McNeil, P. E., Grimshaw, W. T. R., Selman, I. E., and McIntyre, W. I. M. (1978): High incidence area of cattle cancer with a possible interaction between an environmental carcinogen and a papillomavirus. *Nature*, 274:215–217.
46. Jarrett, W. F. H., McNeil, P. E., Laird, H. M., O'Neil, B. W., Murphy, J., Campo, M. S., and Moar, M. H. (1980): Papillomaviruses in benign and malignant tumors of cattle. In: *Viruses in Naturally Occurring Cancers, Cold Spring Harbor Conferences on Cell Proliferation, Vol. 7*, edited by M. Essex, G. Todaro, and H. zur Hausen, pp. 215–222. Cold Spring Harbor Laboratory, Cold Spring Harbor, N.Y.
47. Jenson, A. B., Rosenthal, J. R., Olson, C., Pass, F., Lancaster, W. D., and Shah, K. (1980): Immunological relatedness of papillomaviruses from different species. *J. Natl. Cancer Inst.*, 64:495–500.
48. Jorgenser, A., Rothstein, S. J., and Reznikoff, W. S. (1979): A restriction enzyme cleavage map of Tn5 and location of a region encoding neomycin resistance. *Mol. Gen. Genet.*, 177:65–72.
49. Kidd, J. G., and Rous, P. (1940): A transplantable rabbit carcinoma originating in a virus-induced papilloma and containing the virus in masked or altered form. *J. Exp. Med.*, 71:813–837.
50. Klug, A., and Finch, J. T. (1965): Structure of viruses of the papilloma-polyoma type. I. Human wart virus. *J. Mol. Biol.*, 11:403–423.
51. Kremsdorf, D., Jablonska, S., Favre, M., and Orth, G. (1982): Biochemical characterization of two types of human papillomaviruses associated with epidermodysplasia verruciformis. *J. Virol.*, 43:436–447.
52. Krzyzek, R. A., Watts, S. L., Anderson, D. L., Faras, A. J., and Pass, F. (1980): Anogenital warts contain several distinct species of human papillomavirus. *J. Virol.*, 36:236–244.
53. Lancaster, W. D., Olson, C., and Meinke, W. (1977): Bovine papillomavirus: Presence of virus-specific DNA sequences in naturally occurring equine tumors. *Proc. Natl. Acad. Sci. USA*, 74:524–528.
54. Lancaster, W. D. (1979): Physical maps of bovine papillomaviruses type 1 and type 2 genomes. *J. Virol.*, 32:684–687.
55. Lancaster, W. D., and Olson, C. (1980): State of bovine papillomavirus DNA in connective-tissue tumors. In: *Viruses in Naturally Occurring Cancers, Cold Spring Harbor Conferences on Cell Proliferation, Vol. 7*, edited by M. Essex, G. Todaro, and H. zur Hausen, pp. 223–232. Cold Spring Harbor Laboratory, Cold Spring Harbor, N.Y.
56. Lancaster, W. D. (1981): Apparent lack of integration of bovine papillomavirus DNA in virus

induced equine and bovine tumor cells and virus-transformed mouse cells. *Virology*, 108:251–255.

57. La Porta, R. F., and Taichman, L. B. (1982): Human papilloma viral DNA replicates as a stable episome in cultured epidermal keratinocytes. *Proc. Natl. Acad. Sci. USA*, 79:3393–3397.

58. Laurent, L., Kienzler, J. L., Croissant, O., and Orth, G. (1982): Two anatomoclinical types of warts with plantar localization: Specific cytopathogenic effects of papillomavirus type 1 (HPV1) and type 2 (HPV2). *Arch. Dermatol. Res.*, 274:101–111.

59. Law, M. F., Lancaster, W. D., and Howley, P. M. (1979): Conserved polynucleotide sequences among the genomes of papillomaviruses. *J. Virol.*, 32:199–207.

60. Law, M. F., Lowy, D. R., Dvoretzky, T., and Howley, P. M. (1981): Mouse cells transformed by bovine papillomavirus contain only ectrachromosomal viral DNA sequences. *Proc. Natl. Acad. Sci. USA*, 78:2727–2731.

61. Law, M. F., Howard, B., Sarver, N., and Howley, P. M. (1982): Expression of selective traits in mouse cells transformed with a BPV DNA-derived hybrid molecule containing *Escherichia coli gpt*. In: *Eukaryotic Viral Vectors*, edited by Y. Gluzman, pp. 79–85. Cold Spring Harbor Laboratory, Cold Spring Harbor, N.Y.

62. Le Bouvier, G. L., Sussman,M., and Crawford, L. V. (1966): Antigenic diversity of mammalian papillomaviruses. *J. Gen. Microbiol.*, 45:497–501.

63. Lowy, D. R., Dvoretzky, I., Shober, R., Law, M. F., Engel, L., and Howley, P. M. (1980): In vitro tumorigenic transformation by a defined subgenomic fragment of bovine papillomavirus DNA. *Nature*, 287:72–74.

64. Lusky, M., Berg, L., and Botchan, M. (1982): Enhancement of tk transformation by sequence of bovine papillomavirus. In: *Eukaryotic Viral Vectors*, edited by Y. Gluzman, pp. 87–92. Cold Spring Harbor Laboratory, Cold Spring Harbor, N.Y.

65. McVay, P., Fretz, M., Wettstein, F. O., Stevens, J., and Ito, Y. (1982): Integrated Shope virus DNA is present and transcribed in the transplantable rabbit tumor VX7. *J. Gen. Virol.*, 60:271–278.

66. Meinke, W., and Meinke, G. C. (1981): Isolation and characterization of the major capsid protein of bovine papillomavirus type 1. *J. Gen. Virol.*, 52:15–24.

67. Melnick, J. L. (1962): Papova virus group. *Science*, 135:1128–1131.

68. Messing, J., Crea, R., and Seeburg, P. H. (1981): A system for shotgun DNA sequencing. *Nucleic Acids Res.*, 9:309–321.

69. Moar, M. H., Campo, S. M., Laird, H. M., and Jarrett, W. F. H. (1981): Persistence of non-integrated viral DNA in bovine cells transformed *in vitro* by bovine papillomavirus type 2. *Nature*, 293:749–751.

70. Moar, M. H., Campo, S. M., Laird, H. M., and Jarrett, W. F. H. (1981): Unintegrated viral DNA sequences in a hamster tumor induced by bovine papillomavirus. *J. Virol.*, 39:945–949.

71. Müller, H., and Gissmann, L. (1978): *Mastomys natalensis* papilloma virus (MnPV), the causative agent of epithelial proliferations: Characterization of the virus particle. *J. Gen. Virol.*, 41:315–323.

72. Mulligan, R. C., and Berg, P. (1980): Expression of a bacterial gene in mammalian cells. *Science*, 209:1422–1427.

73. Mulligan, R. C., and Berg, P. (1981): Selection for animal cells that express the *Escherichia coli* gene coding for xanthine-guanine phosphoribosyl transferase. *Proc. Natl. Acad. Sci. USA*, 78:2072–2076.

74. Noyes, W. F. (1964): Structure of the human wart virus. *Virology*, 23:65–72.

75. Orth, G., Jeanteur, P., and Croissant, O. (1971): Evidence for and localization of vegetative viral DNA replication by autoradiographic detection of RNA-DNA hybrids in sections of tumors induced by Shope papillomavirus. *Proc. Natl. Acad. Sci. USA*, 68:1876–1880.

76. Orth, G., Breitburd, F., Favre, M., and Croissant, O. (1977): Papillomaviruses: A possible role in human cancer. In: *Cold Spring Harbor Conferences on Cell Proliferation, Vol. 4*, edited by H. H. Hiatt, J. D. Watson, and J. A. Winsten, pp. 1043–1068. Cold Spring Harbor Laboratory, Cold Spring Harbor, N.Y.

77. Orth, G., and Favre, M. (1977): Characterization of a new type of human papillomavirus that causes skin wart. *J. Virol.*, 24:108–120.

78. Orth, G., Breitburd, F., and Favre, M. (1978): Evidence for antigenic determinants shared by the structural polypeptides of (Shope) rabbit papillomavirus and human papillomavirus type 1. *Virology*, 91:243–255.

79. Orth, G., Jablonska, S., Favre, M., Croissant, O., Jenzabek-Chozelska, M., and Rzesa, G. (1978): Characterization of two types of human papillomaviruses in lesions of epidermodysplasia verruciformis. *Proc. Natl. Acad. Sci. USA*, 75:1537–1541.
80. Orth, G., Favre, M., Breitburd, F., Croissant, O., Jablonska, S., Obalek, S., Jarzabek-Chorzelska, M., and Rzesa, G. (1980): Epidermodysplasia verruciformis: A model for the role of papillomavirus in human cancer. In: *Viruses in Naturally Occurring Cancers, Cold Spring Harbor Conferences on Cell Proliferation, Vol. 7*, edited by M. Essex, G. Todaro, and H. zur Hausen, pp. 259–282. Cold Spring Harbor Laboratory, Cold Spring Harbor, N.Y.
81. Ostrow, R. S., Bender, M., Niimura M., Seki, T., Kawashima, M., Pass, F., and Faras, A. J. (1982): Human papillomavirus DNA in cutaneous primary and metastasized squamous cell carcinomas from patients with epidermodysplasia verruciformis. *Proc. Natl. Acad. Sci. USA*, 79:1634–1638.
82. Parson, R. J., and Kidd, J. G. (1943): Oral papillomatosis of rabbits: A virus disease. *J. Exp. Med.*, 77:233–250.
83. Pfister, H., and zur Hausen, H. (1978): Characterization of proteins of human papillomaviruses (HPV) and antibody response to HPV1. *Med. Microbiol. Immunol.*, 166:13–19.
84. Pfister, H., Linz, U., Gissmann, L., Huchthausen, B., Hoffmann, D., and zur Hausen, H. (1979): Partial characterization of a new type of bovine papilloma viruses. *Virology*, 96:1–8.
85. Pfister, H., Fink, B., and Thomas, C. (1981): Extrachromosomal bovine papillomavirus type 1 DNA in hamster fibromas and fibrosarcomas. *Virology*, 115:414–418.
86. Rassoulzadegan, M., Binetruy, B., and Cuzin, F. (1982): High frequency of gene transfer after fusion between bacteria and eukaryotic cells. *Nature*, 295:257–259.
87. Rayment, I., Baker, T. S., Caspar, D. L. D., and Murakami, W. T. (1982): Polyoma virus capsid structure at 22,5 Å resolution. *Nature*, 295:110–115.
88. Rous, P., and Beard, J. W. (1935): The progression to carcinoma of virus-induced rabbit papillomas (Shope). *J. Exp. Med.*, 62:523.
89. Sanger, F., Nicklen, S., and Coulson, A. R. (1977): DNA sequencing with chain-terminating inhibitors. *Proc. Natl. Acad Sci. USA*, 74:5463–5467.
90. Sanger, F., Coulson, A. R., Barrell, B. G., Smith, A. J. H., and Roe, B. A. (1980): Cloning in single-stranded bacteriophage as an aid to rapid DNA sequencing. *J. Mol. Biol.*, 143:161–178.
91. Sarver, N., Gruss, P., Law, M. F., Khoury, G., and Howley, P. M. (1981): Bovine papilloma virus deoxyribonucleic acid: A novel eukaryotic cloning vector. *Mol. Cell. Biol.*, 1:486–496.
92. Shope, R. E. (1933): Infectious papillomatosis of rabbit. *J. Exp. Med.*, 58:607–624.
93. Soeda, E., Arrand, J. R., Smolar, N., Walsh, J. E., and Griffin, B. E. (1980): Coding potential and regulatory signals of the polyoma virus genome. *Nature*, 2832:445–453.
94. Southern, E. M. (1975): Detection of specific sequences among DNA fragments separated by gel electrophoresis. *J. Mol. Biol.*, 98:503–517.
95. Southern, P., and Berg, P. (1982): Mammalian cell transformation with SV40 hybrid plasmid vectors. In: *Eukaryotic Viral Vectors*, edited by Y. Gluzmann, pp. 41–45. Cold Spring Harbor Laboratory, Cold Spring Harbor, N.Y.
96. Stevens, J. G., and Wettstein, F. O. (1979): Multiple copies of Shope virus DNA are present in cells of benign and malignant non-virus producing neoplasms. *J. Virol.*, 30:891–898.
97. Sundin, O., and Varshavsky, A. (1980): Terminal stages of SV40 DNA replication proceed via multiply intermined catenated dimers. *Cell*, 21:103–114.
98. Sutcliffe, J. G., Shinnick, T. M., Green, N., Liu, L. T., Niman, H. L., and Lerner, R. A. (1980): Chemical synthesis of a polypeptide predicted from nucleotide sequence allows detection of a new retroviral gene product. *Nature*, 287:801–805.
99. Sweet, B. H., and Hilleman, M. R. (1960): The vacuolating virus SV40. *Proc. Soc. Exp. Biol. Med.*, 105:420–427.
100. Thomas, P. S. (1980): Hybridization of denatured RNA and small DNA fragments transferred to nitrocellulose. *Proc. Natl. Acad. Sci. USA*, 77:5201–5205.
101. Walter, G., Scheidtmann, K. H., Carbone, A., Laudano, A. P., and Doolittle, R. F. (1980): Antibodies specific for the carboxy- and amino-terminal regions of simian virus 40 large tumor antigen. *Proc. Natl. Acad. Sci. USA*, 77:5197–5200.
102. Wettstein, F. O., and Stevens, J. G. (1980): Distribution and state of viral nucleic acid in tumors induced by Shope papilloma virus. In: *Viruses in Naturally Occurring Cancers, Cold Spring Harbor Conferences on Cell Proliferation, Vol. 7*, edited by M. Essex, G. Todaro, and H. zur Hausen, pp. 301–307. Cold Spring Harbor Laboratory, Cold Spring Harbor, N.Y.

103. Wettstein, F. O., and Stevens, J. G. (1981): Transcription of the viral genome in papillomas and carcinomas induced by the Shope virus. *Virology*, 109:448–451.
104. Wettstein, F. O., and Stevens, J. G. (1982): Variable-sized free episomes of Shope papilloma virus DNA are present in all non-virus producing neoplasms and integrated episomes are detected in some. *Proc. Natl. Acad. Sci. USA*, 79:790–794.
105. zur Hausen, H. (1981): Papilloma viruses: In: *DNA Tumor Viruses—Molecular Biology of Tumor Viruses, Part 2*, ed. 2, edited by J. Tooze, pp. 371–382. Cold Spring Harbor Laboratory, Cold Spring Harbor, N.Y.
106. Chen, E. Y., Howley, P. M., Levinson, A. D., and Seeburg, P. H. (1982): The primary structure and genetic organization of the bovine papillomavirus type I genome. *Nature*, 299:529–534.
107. Binetruy, B., Meneguzzi, G., Breathnach, R., and Cuzin, F. (1983): Recombinant DNA molecules comprising bovine papillomavirus type I DNA linked to plasmid DNA are maintained in a plasmidal state both in rodent fibroblasts and in bacterial cells. *(in press)*.
108. Giri, I., Jouanneau, J., and Yaniv, M. (1983): Comparative studies of the expression of linked E. *coli. gpt* gene and BPV-1 DNAs in transfected cells. *Virology, (in press)*.

Advances in Viral Oncology, Volume 3, edited by
George Klein. Raven Press, New York © 1983.

Molecular Biology of Adenovirus Transformation

Ulf Pettersson and Göran Akusjärvi

Department of Medical Genetics, The Biomedical Center, S-751 23 Uppsala, Sweden

During the past decade the adenoviruses have attracted considerable attention, not because of their clinical significance but rather because they have become important tools in fundamental biological research. Both the papovaviruses and the adenoviruses have been extensively used as model systems to study the organization and expression of eukaryotic genes. A vast amount of knowledge has been accumulated concerning the structures of several DNA virus genomes, and we know today the entire nucleotide sequences of several papovavirus genomes (309). Many properties that are unique to the eukaryotic organisms were first discovered through studies of animal DNA viruses and were later shown to be shared by the more complex eukaryotes. The splicing phenomenon, for instance, was first discovered in the adenovirus system (22,42,64,147,150,180) and then later demonstrated to be a common property of all higher eukaryotes; for a review, see Breatnach and Chambon (30).

The small DNA viruses, like the papovaviruses and the adenoviruses, have also played an important role in cancer research because they provide one of the simplest model systems, allowing the identification of genes and gene products implicated in transformation. It was discovered two decades ago (130,310) that adenoviruses cause tumors when injected into newborn hamsters and rats. Since then, a vast amount of work has been devoted to studies of the structure and expression of adenovirus transforming genes. The fundamental properties of the adenovirus system have been reviewed (79), and this chapter will focus mainly on results that have been reported since that publication. Adenovirus research, like research in many other fields in biological research, has made a quantum leap during the past years because of the availability of new tools in DNA technology. DNA sequencing, molecular cloning, and the development of *in vitro* systems for transcription and DNA replication are the tools that have been of most importance. More than half of the sequence of the 36,000-base-pairs-long human adenovirus genome is known today, and the entire sequence will undoubtedly be known by the time this chapter reaches print. Thanks to molecular cloning, adenovirus DNA fragments can be produced in large quantities for structural and genetic studies, and in addition cDNA copies of many spliced mRNAs have been constructed in order to determine their structure at the molecular level. Cloned restriction enzyme fragments are also being used to change specifically the nucleotide sequences of defined regions in the adenovirus genome, thereby generating mutations at strategic locations in the DNA.

In the past, the adenoviruses have been of importance in that they contributed to our current understanding of eukaryotic gene structure and expression. Today, genes can be isolated from complex eukaryotic organisms, and it could be argued that the animal DNA viruses are no longer required as models for detailed structural studies of genes and their function. It is, however, in our opinion, clear that simple model systems will be required in order to understand the complex and sophisticated details of gene regulation and cell transformation. It is thus likely that the adenoviruses will continue to serve as important research tools in the future.

THE ADENOVIRUS FAMILY

The adenovirus genus comprises more than 80 different serotypes, 39 of which are human isolates (216,329,337; G. Wadell, *personal communication*). Adenoviruses have been isolated from a variety of animal species, ranging from frogs to humans. Most serotypes, except the avian, share a common group-specific antigen that is an important marker in classification, and in addition all adenoviruses have the same basic morphology (Fig. 1). The genomes of the mammalian adenoviruses consist of 35 to 36 kilobases (kb) (108,313), whereas those of the avian adenoviruses are significantly larger, comprising some 45 kb (19,168). Although few adenovirus genomes of animal origin have been studied in detail, it appears likely that they all have the same basic structure and that they stem from a common ancestor. The human adenoviruses, which have been studied most thoroughly, are currently being subdivided into seven subgenera or subgroups (groups A–G) (216,329,337; G. Wadell, *personal communication*). Originally, Huebner (129) subdivided the human serotypes into three groups on the basis of their oncogenic properties. Group A comprises the highly oncogenic serotypes, being those that rapidly and with high frequency induce tumors in newborn hamsters. Members of group B, or the weakly oncogenic serotypes, induce tumors after a longer latency period and with a lower frequency. Once established, however, it appears that adenovirus tumors have similar properties regardless of which serotype has induced the tumor. The remaining adenovirus serotypes do not give rise to tumors in animals and hence are classified as nononcogenic. They were originally classified as a single subgroup but were later found to be heterogeneous and therefore were subdivided into subgroups C and D (202). Subgroup E includes a single member, serotype 4 (112,329), whereas subgroups F and G comprise a newly discovered group of enteric adenoviruses that are difficult to propagate in tissue culture (329; G. Wadell, *personal communication*). The latter serotypes have for natural reasons been studied much less intensively. Therefore, most of our current knowledge of the adenoviruses stems from studies of the human serotypes 2 and 5, which belong to the nononcogenic subgroup C and which can be considered as the prototypes for the human adenovirus family. Members within each subgroup have immunologically cross-reacting tumor antigens and in most cases are closely related, as judged by DNA sequence homology

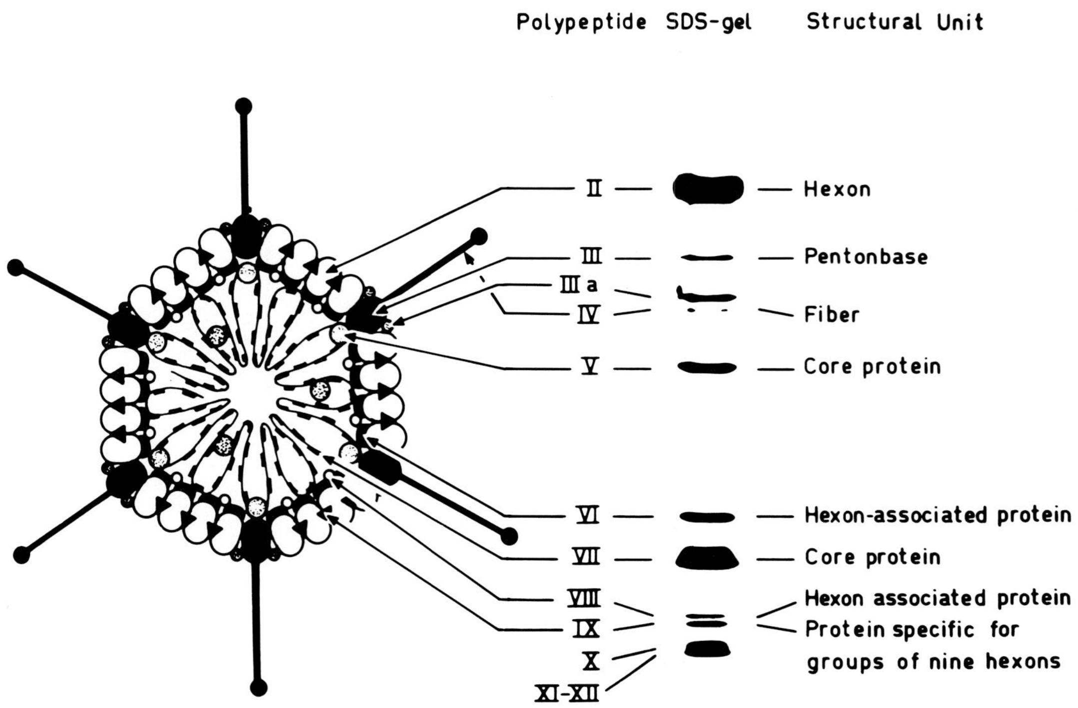

FIG. 1. A model of the adenovirus particle showing the proposed locations of different polypeptides. The locations of the hexon, the penton base, the fiber, and the core proteins are known, whereas the assignments of the remaining polypeptides are tentative. The polypeptide pattern as revealed by SDS polyacrylamide gel electrophoresis is also shown. (Adapted from Persson and Philipson, ref. 232.)

(93,107,159–161,189), as opposed to members of different subgroups that usually share little sequence homology (5–25%). When the genomes of different human subgroup members have been compared, it has been observed that each subgroup has its characteristic GC content (107,241,242).

From a medical point of view, the adenoviruses play a subordinate role. Most serotypes cause either inapparent or mild respiratory tract infections, whereas the human serotype 8 gives rise to keratoconjunctivitis, and some others cause enteric infections. A large fraction of the human population carries antibodies against several adenovirus serotypes, in many cases as the result of inapparent infections.

THE VIRION

The structure of the adenovirus particle is illustrated in Fig. 1; for more detailed reviews, see Ginsberg (90) and Philipson (238). The capsid consists of 252 capsomers; 240 hexons form the facets of the icosahedron, and 12 pentons are located at the corners of the capsid. The pentons consist of the penton base or the vertex capsomer and a noncovalently attached protein, known as the fiber. The fiber functions as the attachment organ for the adenovirus particle by binding to the receptors on the surface of the host cell (186,239). Adenoviruses belonging to different subgroups have fibers of different lengths (215). It has also been shown that avian serotypes have two fibers extending from each vertex (168). The total molecular weight of the adenovirus particle is approximately 175×10^6, and the virion is a complex structure composed of at least 10 different polypeptides (76,190) (Fig. 1). Polypeptides VI, VII, and VIII are synthesized as precursors that are trimmed by a protease during virus maturation (12,26). It is of interest that the adenovirus DNA, unlike the DNA of the papovaviruses, carries its own histonelike proteins (polypeptides V and VII) inside the virus particle (49,167,244,245). Early after infection the adenovirus chromatin changes into a nucleosomal structure, probably by replacement of the viral core proteins with cellular histones (276,304). At late times of infection, when viral DNA replication provides an excess of DNA for virus assembly, the DNA becomes associated again with the viral core proteins. The viral DNA appears to enter a preformed capsid (66,297), and packaging of the DNA starts from the left-hand end.[1] A short sequence has been identified near the left end that is required for encapsidation (121).

THE ADENOVIRUS GENOME AND ITS
FUNCTIONAL ORGANIZATION

The topography of the adenovirus chromosome has been studied in great detail using several modern techniques. Early results, using liquid hybridization between cytoplasmic RNA and the separated strands of restriction fragments of adenovirus DNA, demonstrated that early RNA is transcribed from four widely separated

---

[1]The left-hand end of the adenovirus genome is defined as the end that is GC-rich and carries the genes required for transformation.

regions of the genome (217,240,277,288), designated E1 to E4. Regions E1 and E3 are transcribed from the viral r strand,[2] whereas regions E2 and E4 are transcribed from the viral l strand (Fig. 2). More detailed mapping of promoters by nascent chain analysis (75), ultraviolet inactivation of transcription (23), DRB inhibition of transcription (275), direct sequence analysis of the capped 5′ ends of mRNAs (7,18), and more recently *in vitro* transcription (78,196) has shown that all early and late transcription units are preceded by an initiation site for RNA polymerase II. Further studies have shown that region E1 can be subdivided into two separate transcription units, E1A and E1B (275,341).

So far, eight transcription units have been identified on the adenovirus genome. In addition to the five early transcription units that were described earlier, there exist the major late transcription unit and two transcription units for mRNAs expressed at intermediate times of infection. The promoter for the major late transcription unit is located at map coordinate 16.5 (4,94,352), and it directs the synthesis of the mRNAs for all virion polypeptides, with the exception of polypeptide IX (180,237). Although polypeptide IX is a structural polypeptide of the virion (76,190), its synthesis is regulated from an independent promoter located within the early region E1B (9,341) (Fig. 2). Polypeptide IVa_2 serves as a maturation protein during adenovirus morphogenesis (226), and its mRNA is transcribed from the viral l strand using a promoter located immediately to the left of the major late promoter (43,45) (Fig. 2). Both polypeptides IX and IVa_2 are usually referred to as intermediate polypeptides, because they accumulate before and independent of viral DNA replication (45,226).

The schematic structure of the mRNAs that are encoded by the eight adenovirus transcription units is illustrated in Fig. 2. This figure is a compilation of data obtained by electron microscopy, S1 nuclease analysis, DNA sequence analysis, and molecular cloning. A multitude of differently spliced mRNAs are generated from all the early and late transcription units by processing the primary transcripts in different fashions. It has been possible in some cases (but not all cases) to correlate the different mRNAs with specific proteins.

Region E2 differs from the other adenovirus transcription units by using alternative promoter sites for initiation of transcription (44) (Fig. 2). One promoter, located at coordinate 75, is preferentially used at early times of infection. During the switch from early to late phase, a promoter shift occurs, so that the E2 mRNAs are preferentially transcribed from an alternative promoter, located at coordinate 72. The promoter shift requires viral protein synthesis, suggesting that the E2 transcription unit is regulated by one or more viral gene products.

It was recently shown that the E2 promoter at intermediate and late times after infection also transcribes the region between map coordinates 29.5 and 11.2 into mRNA (294). Because these mRNAs are transcribed from the same promoter as the mRNAs in region E2, this novel region has been designated E2B, in contrast

---

[2]The r strand is the strand of the adenovirus DNA that is transcribed in the rightward direction, as opposed to the l strand, which is transcribed in the leftward direction.

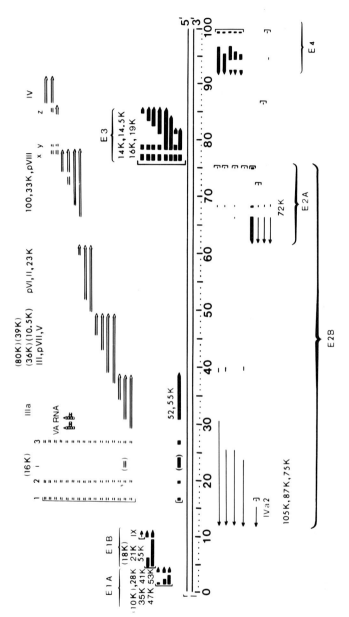

FIG. 2. Schematic drawing showing the principal organization of the adenovirus type 2 genome. Arrowheads show the locations of 3' ends of the mRNAs, and the promoter sites are indicated with brackets. Selected polypeptides that have been assigned to different regions are indicated. Thick lines represent mRNAs that are expressed early after infection, in the absence of viral DNA replication. Open arrows indicate sequences present in late mRNA. Thin lines indicate mRNAs that are expressed at intermediate and late times after infection. Five separate cotermination families of late mRNA are present. The three segments that are spliced together to form the tripartite leader (1, 2, 3) are also shown, as well as the location of the i leader. Two small RNAs, VA RNAI and VA RNAII, map around position 30. (Adapted from Chow et al., ref. 45.)

to the E2A region, which is located between map coordinates 61 and 75 (Fig. 2). So far, four differently spliced mRNAs have been identified from region E2B by electron microscopy (294).

The transcription late after infection is in many respects different from that observed early after infection; at late times the major late adenovirus promoter generates a primary transcript consisting of approximately 28,000 nucleotides (75) that is then spliced in different fashions to generate the mRNAs for all proteins present in the viral capsid, with the exception of polypeptide IX (21,43,180,237). Two mRNAs for nonstructural polypeptides with molecular weights of 100K and 33K are also transcribed from the major late promoter (43,180). The late mRNAs are generated by a characteristic splicing pattern (Fig. 2); three short segments with a combined length of 203 nucleotides, derived from map coordinates 16.5, 19.6, and 26.6, are joined to form a common tripartite leader sequence that then is attached to the different mRNA bodies (3,4,22,42,349). As a consequence, all mRNAs from the major late transcription unit will have identical 5′ ends. The tripartite leader does, however, not encode any AUG triplets (3,349), and consequently the late proteins will have unique N-terminal sequences.

There are a few exceptions to this general pattern of mRNA formation; certain mRNAs contain an additional leader segment, designated the i leader, which is encoded by a DNA segment located around map position 22 (6,45,325). The i leader contributes an AUG triplet followed by an open translational reading frame encoding a hypothetical 16K polypeptide, and it has been demonstrated that translation of mRNAs containing the i leader gives rise to a small protein whose function is unknown (6,97,181,325). Furthermore, the fiber mRNA is sometimes connected with additional leader segments, designated x, y, and z (41) (Fig. 2). Experimental proof exists that the addition of the y leader does not alter the coding capacity of the fiber mRNA (65), and this is expected, because the y leader does not contain AUG triplets (311,349). The DNA sequence of the z leader has also been determined, and the result shows that the z leader contributes an AUG triplet followed by a short translational reading frame (311). Whether or not the z leader alters the coding capacity of the fiber mRNA has not yet been tested experimentally.

Besides having a common 5′ leader sequence, many of the late mRNAs share poly(A) addition sites (203,209,351). Within the major late transcription unit, five major poly(A) addition sites have been identified, and this allows the late mRNAs to be divided into five 3′ coterminal families designated L1 to L5 (Fig. 2). The 3′ ends of the mRNAs are not generated by termination of transcription at the five poly(A) addition sites. Instead, transcription continues beyond the poly(A) site, and the 3′ end is generated by an endonucleolytic cleavage followed by posttranscriptional addition of the poly(A) tail (85). Selection of one of the poly(A) addition sites usually precedes the leader–body splice (210), although poly(A) addition does not seem to be a prerequisite for the splicing event (350). The fact that many late adenovirus mRNAs share common 3′ ends means that they are structurally polycistronic, although in a functional sense they are monocistronic. For example, the pVI mRNA (Fig. 2) contains the structural information for the pVI, the hexon, and the 23K polypeptides (7,8,43). However, as is the case for eukaryotic mRNAs in general, the first AUG following the capped 5′ end is used for initiation of translation (155). In this way the pVI polypeptide will be the only translated product from the pVI mRNA, although it encodes two additional polypeptides.

The term "major late promoter" is in one respect inappropriate for the promoter located at map position 16.5, because it has been shown that this promoter is also active at early times of infection (6,45,86,146,181), selectively producing mRNAs encoding a 52K/55K protein and a 13.5K polypeptide (181). Furthermore, studies using protein synthesis inhibitors have indicated that the major late promoter may be the first promoter activated during a lytic infection (181). The regulation of the major late promoter at different times after infection will be discussed later.

VIRUS-ASSOCIATED RNAs

The adenovirus genome encodes two low-molecular-weight RNAs, the so-called virus-associated (VA) RNAs (192,194,195,235,251,302,335). The VA RNAs are synthesized following different kinetics during lytic infection (302); at early times, both RNA species accumulate. After the onset of viral DNA replication, however, the synthesis of VA RNAII levels off, whereas the synthesis of VA RNAI increases, and it becomes the most prominent RNA species synthesized at late times after infection (302). The two VA RNAs do not suffer posttranscriptional processing at their 5′ termini (302,335), suggesting that they are initiated at separate promoters. They are transcribed from the viral r strand (192,235), and their genes have been mapped as two tandem transcription units located between map coordinates 29 and 30 on the ad2 genome (Fig. 2) (5,192,194,235,302). Sequence studies of the VA RNAs and their genes (5,34,35,218) have shown that VA RNAI is heterogeneous, ranging between 157 and 160 nucleotides in length. The heterogeneity is due to two alternative start sites for transcription (separated by 3 nucleotides) and the termination of transcription, which occurs heterogeneously within a cluster of T residues. A spacer of about 98 nucleotides separates the termination signal for the VA RNAI transcription from the initiation site for VA RNAII (5). The length of VA RNAII ranges between 158 and 163 nucleotides as a result of a heterogeneous 3′ end (5).

The VA RNAs are unique among adenovirus genes, being synthesized by RNA polymerase III (246, 302, 334, 335). The control region for VA RNAI transcription has been studied by construction of deletion mutants around the structural gene (84,117). As for other genes (154) that are transcribed by RNA polymerase III, this approach has permitted the identification of an intragenic control region for VA RNAI transcription. An additional control region encompassing the 5′ flanking sequences of the VA RNAI gene also influences the transcription by changing the choice of site for initiation of transcription (305).

Although the VA RNAs were discovered in 1966 (251), a specific function has not yet conclusively been assigned to these RNAs. It was proposed that VA RNAs may serve as adapters in the splicing reaction by binding to the 5' and 3' borders of the exons destined to be joined together, thereby facilitating the cleavage and ligation reaction (193,207). The hypothesis was experimentally tested by Mathews (193), who showed that the VA RNAs bind, probably by forming classic base pairs, to unfractionated late viral mRNA. Furthermore, VA RNAI can hybridize to nitrocellulose filters carrying a cDNA clone containing the tripartite leader plus the fiber-specific y leader. However, it is not obvious from the sequence how VA RNA can interact with the tripartite leader through base pairing.

Small nuclear RNAs found in eukaryotic organisms as RNA–protein complexes, so-called snRNPs (171,172,331), have also been implicated in the splicing reaction by the same mechanism as proposed for the VA RNAs (172,193,207,257). Indirect evidence for the involvement of snRNPs in the processing of early adenovirus E1A mRNAs and certain late mRNA species has been reported (170,348). These studies add strength to the hypothesis that low-molecular-weight RNAs may function as adapter molecules during the splicing reaction event.

REPLICATION OF ADENOVIRUS DNA

The basic mechanism of adenovirus DNA replication is fairly well understood today. Several investigators (70,154,169,219,234,298,312) have shown that intermediates in adenovirus DNA replication are distinguished by their single-stranded character. This, together with the observation that the origin and the termini for replication are located at the molecular ends (15,126,166,271,299,308,332,344), led to the proposition of a model for adenovirus DNA replication that has been confirmed in its basic concepts (Fig. 3). The model suggests that replication starts at either end by so-called strand-displacement synthesis. Owing to the asynchrony in replication, one of the two strands is displaced during the first round of replication (Fig. 3). Because the adenovirus DNA carries inverted terminal repetitions (92,346), the liberated single strand presumably will form a circle, which is maintained through base pairing between the two ends, thus generating a panhandlelike a structure. The replication of the displaced single strand is presumed to initiate in the panhandle structure, which because of the inverted terminal duplication has a structure identical to the termini of double-stranded adenovirus DNA. The second strand is then completed by so-called complementary strand synthesis (Fig. 3).

An interesting property of the adenovirus genome is the existence of a protein covalently attached to the 5' ends of the DNA, as was originally discovered by Robinson et al. (255). Adenovirus DNA, isolated without protease treatment, contains one molecule of a 55K protein attached to each end, which makes the double-stranded DNA appear circular, presumably because of noncovalent interactions between the two terminal proteins (48,252,255,256). The protein is linked to the DNA via a serine residue (52) and can be liberated by treatment with weak base (33,294,307). The gene for the terminal protein has recently been identified by DNA sequence analysis (10,97,287), and its entire amino acid sequence has thereby been deduced. The site of linkage to the DNA has been identified and found to be

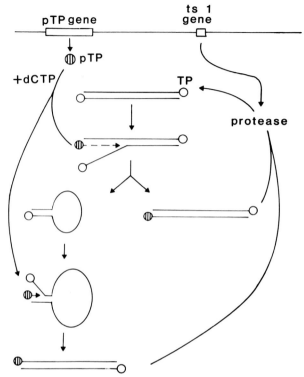

FIG. 3. A model for replication of adenovirus DNA. The precursor for the terminal protein, encoded by the viral DNA between map positions 29.5 and 23.5, binds dCTP and forms an initiation complex. Replication proceeds via a strand-displacement mechanism, producing a free single strand that will form a circular structure because of the inverted terminal repetition. The duplex part of the circular molecule forms a panhandlelike structure that is identical with the ends of the original duplex DNA. This structure presumably will be recognized by the initiation complex, and replication of the second strand will proceed by so-called complementary strand synthesis. A protease, presumably of viral origin, as defined by the ts1 mutation, cleaves the precursor for the terminal protein into a 55K protein. (Adapted from Stillman et al., ref. 294.)

located near the C-terminal end of the protein. The terminal protein is synthesized as a precursor with an approximate molecular weight of 80K (38,111,294), which through the action of a virus-specific protease is trimmed to an estimated size of 55K. The latter conclusion is based on the finding that a temperature-sensitive mutant of ad2 (ts1) that fails to cleave the precursors for the capsid proteins VI, VII, and VIII (26) also fails to cleave the precursor for the terminal protein. The cleavage of the protein appears to take place after initiation of DNA synthesis has occurred, and probably when the DNA has already entered the capsid.

A major breakthrough in research on adenovirus DNA replication is the development of soluble extracts that can replicate adenovirus DNA *in vitro* (14,36,-71,127,134,141,142,292,347). Extracts from infected cells can utilize exogenously added virus DNA (containing the terminal protein) as a template for replication. The presumed requirement for the terminal protein on the template has been found to be artifactual, because protein-free molecules also serve as templates, provided that no amino acids are left covalently attached to the template DNA (303). The availability of *in vitro* systems makes it possible to analyze the different steps in replication, to define the origin of replication, and furthermore to identify enzymes and other components that are necessary for adenovirus DNA replication.

Particular attention has been focused on the mechanism by which adenovirus DNA replication initiates. Adenovirus DNA does not seem to form either covalently closed circles (60) or concatenates during replication. Neither does replication seem to be primed through hairpin formation (293). Hence, if an RNA primer is required for initiation, there is no simple way to complete the replication of the linear double-stranded adenovirus genome without leaving a gap after the primer has been removed. In order to circumvent this problem, it has been proposed that the terminal protein serves as a primer for DNA replication by covalently binding the first nucleotide (a C residue for mammalian adenovirus) and then offering the 3' hydroxyl to the DNA polymerase (252,256) (Fig. 3). Experimental support for this model has been obtained recently. By the use of *in vitro* systems it has been shown that the precursor for the terminal protein can form a covalent complex with dCTP in the presence of adenovirus DNA, either completely free or carrying an intact molecule of terminal protein (71,183,303). In the second step the complex probably binds to the origin sequence, located at or near the two termini, and serves as a primer for the elongation process. The precise sequence at the termini that constitutes the origin remains to be defined. However, because DNAs from different adenovirus serotypes are interchangeable in the *in vitro* system, the origin sequence must be shared, at least among the different human adenoviruses. Several investigators (11,54,281,296,307) have performed comparative sequence studies of terminal repetitions from different adenoviruses in the hope of finding a unique and highly conserved sequence. The results show that a sequence located between nucleotides 9 and 14 is conserved in all inverted terminal repetitions that have been analyzed, thus being a candidate recognition sequence. In contrast, the first eight nucleotides in the sequences of different adenovirus termini show an unexpected degree of variation. It was recently shown (303) that adenovirus termini that are inserted and propagated in bacterial plasmids can, after excision from the plasmid, serve as origins in the *in vitro* system. It should thus be possible in the near future to create specific mutations in the terminal repetition and in this way define precisely the sequence required for initiation.

Our current knowledge about the enzymes and factors involved in replication of adenovirus DNA is very limited. The best characterized component is the 72K DNA binding protein (DBP) (148,184,258,316), which is encoded by the early region E2A (44,179). One function of this protein is defined by the mutation in the temperature-sensitive mutant H5ts125 (72,319). The protein binds strongly to single-stranded DNA (16,148,319) and also to the ends of double-stranded linear DNA (83,269). Its role in replication is not yet precisely defined in biochemical terms. However, it seems likely that the protein binds to the single-stranded tails that are exposed during displacement synthesis, perhaps thereby protecting them from nuclease action.

The 72K DBP seems to be a multifunctional protein, because several different properties have been attributed to it. Temperature-shift experiments indicate, for instance, that the DBP is involved in both initiation and elongation (127,318,320), although it has not yet been possible to demonstrate the former role *in vitro*. At least one of the functions linked to the DBP can be complemented by the *A* gene of SV40, because coinfection with SV40 compensates for the defect in the ts125 mutant (247). It is also clear that the DBP regulates its own expression (31,32) and also the expression of other early proteins (17,212), as will be described later.

Some other results suggest that the DBP influences the host range of the virus. It has been known for a long time that human adenoviruses replicate inefficiently in monkey cells (249), probably because mRNAs for the fiber protein are spliced incorrectly (151,152). Several investigators have studied the basis for the host-range restriction, and it has been found that mutants can be obtained that will grow efficiently in both human cells and monkey cells (149). These mutants have been mapped by marker rescue experiments (153) and by DNA sequence studies (156). The results show, unexpectedly, that the mutations map in the gene for the DBP, albeit in another part of the gene than the ts125 mutation.

Nicolas et al. (214) have reported that revertants of the ts125 mutant also exhibit certain remarkable host-range properties, again suggesting that the DBP is a multifunctional protein influencing the replication of the virus in a rather complex manner.

Host-range mutants that map in region E1A *(vide infra)* are also defective in DNA replication, although it is not yet known how this mutation affects viral DNA replication (122,163). Because region E1A is required for expression of the other early genes, it is conceivable that the effect on DNA replication is indirect, caused by defective expression of the E2 region encoding the DBP.

A particularly interesting group of DNA negative mutants are those that compose the complementation group N (ts36, ts149). Galos et al. (90) have mapped these mutants between coordinates 18.5 and 21 by marker rescue. This part of the genome has recently been sequenced (10,97), and the results show that the l strand in this region has the capacity to encode a hypothetical polypeptide with a molecular weight of approximately 120K, which most likely corresponds to the N gene product.

With regard to the DNA polymerase that replicates adenovirus DNA, the results are to some extent conflicting (71,187,279,317,321). By the use of inhibitors that selectively influence different host DNA polymerases it has been concluded that the replication of adenovirus DNA is carried out by an enzyme with properties that place it intermediate between the known host enzymes. These findings could be interpreted in several ways: A novel polymerase encoded by the virus or a modified host polymerase could be responsible for the observed properties of DNA polymerase in infected cells. Alternatively, several host polymerases could cooperate in the replication process. The product of the N gene is a possible candidate for being involved in viral DNA replication, either as a factor that modifies the host DNA polymerase or as a DNA polymerase itself.

REGULATION OF EARLY ADENOVIRUS GENE EXPRESSION

The production of adenovirus mRNAs during lytic infection is regulated by a complicated set of events in which both viral and cellular proteins are involved. It is clear that the cellular RNA polymerase II transcribes all adenovirus genes except the VA RNA genes (246,334), although the different promoters are regulated by viral gene products. This section will deal with three stages where regulation of gene expression has been demonstrated: (a) regulation of transcription from the early promoters, (b) regulation of viral mRNA stability, (c) control mechanisms for translation of viral mRNA.

During the infectious cycle the five early transcription units are expressed with different kinetics (211,230). Region E1A is the first to be expressed, and transcripts from this region can be detected 45 min after infection. The maximum rate of transcription from the E1A promoter is thereafter maintained for at least 6 hr. Transcription from regions E3 and E4 begins around 1.5 hr post infection and reaches a maximum rate around 3 hr post infection, followed by a decline. Region E2 is the last early transcription unit to be activated, and RNA synthesis begins around 3 hr post infection and reaches its maximum rate around 7 hr post infection (211). The transcription rate from the E1B promoter appears to be constant throughout the infection (343).

Taking advantage of infection of HeLa cells with host-range mutants (25) *(vide infra)* or deletion mutants (140) that have lesions in region E1A it has been possible to show that one or more products encoded by region E1A are necessary for efficient accumulation of cytoplasmic mRNA from early regions E1B, E2, E3, and E4. The failure to accumulate early viral mRNA in cells infected with E1A mutants is most likely due to a decreased level of transcription from the appropriate promoters (208). The mechanism of action of the E1A products on transcription per se seems to be quantitative rather than qualitative, because mRNA from these transcription units accumulates, although at a low rate, when infection with the E1A mutants is carried out at high multiplicities (140,208). The virus produced under these conditions is still of mutant genotype when assayed for its ability to form plaques on HeLa cells, thus demonstrating that wild-type genomes are not created by recombination between the mutant genome and the resident viral genome in the cells used to propagate the mutant virus. Taken together, these results suggest that there is no absolute requirement for the viral gene product from region E1A for activation of other early transcription units. This conclusion is also supported by the fact that all early and late promoters, with the exception of the IVa_2 promoter, are active when transcribed *in vitro* using cell extracts from uninfected cells (78,191,196,330).

Infection of HeLa cells (pretreated with protein synthesis inhibitors) with host-range mutants or deletion mutants with lesions in region E1A allows for the production of mRNAs from the other early regions (144,181,208). These results have led to the proposition that a cellular protein acts as a negative effector by inhibiting RNA transcription from early regions 2, 3, and 4 (144,208,230,231). The function of the E1A gene products is, according to the hypothesis, to inactivate this cellular protein, thereby allowing the activation of the other early regions. Treatment of cells before infection with protein synthesis inhibitors would thus reduce the concentration of this inhibitory protein, assuming that it has a short half-life. Therefore, even in the absence of a functional E1A gene product, transcription from all the early viral transcription units will occur to some extent.

Quantitative analysis of the effects of protein synthesis inhibitors on activation of the early transcription units (144,208,231) has shown that the most dramatic increase in the rate of transcription occurs for region E4. It is not clear why the early transcription units differ with regard to responses to protein synthesis inhibitors. One possible explanation that also would support the foregoing proposed model is that the various early promoters are more or less sensitive to the proposed cellular protein. The E2 and E3 promoters would then be much more sensitive to the cellular protein than the E4 promoter. As the E1A products start to inactivate the inhibitory protein, the least sensitive promoter (E4) will be activated first, and the most sensitive promoter will be activated last, thus providing a rational explanation why, for example, the E2 promoter is activated much later than the others during a lytic infection.

Addition of protein synthesis inhibitors 1 to 2 hr post infection with wild-type virus results in enhanced accumulation of early viral RNA (67,124,181,230). This enhancement is the result of increased stability of the mRNA (342), indicating that regulation of adenovirus gene expression also encompasses steps at the posttranscriptional level. Recent results obtained with a temperature-sensitive mutant (H5ts125) that has a defect in the 72K DBP demonstrate that the 72K DBP destabilizes early viral mRNAs, including that for the 72K DBP (17), resulting in autoregulation of its own expression (31,32). The actual mechanism by which the 72K DBP enhances the turnover of viral mRNA is unknown, because the protein itself does not seem to possess RNase activity (17). The turnover of viral mRNA is also regulated by factors other than the DBP. For instance, the change in abundance of the E1B 22S and 13S mRNAs seen at late times after infection (289,343) requires the synthesis of truly late proteins (17). Therefore, it seems that several regulatory elements are required for balanced accumulation of cytoplasmic mRNAs.

Adenovirus mRNAs are preferentially translated *in vivo* late after infection (40). Cellular transcription continues at late times, although cellular mRNA sequences do not seem to enter the cytoplasm (20), suggesting that processing or transport of cellular mRNA is restricted during adenovirus infection. Although decay of the existing cellular mRNAs alone could explain the preferential translation of viral mRNA, indirect evidence using protein synthesis inhibitors implies a control mechanism for early viral mRNA translation (230). These results have been interpreted to mean that a viral product, probably a protein from region E1A or region E1B, acts by facilitating translation of the early mRNAs. The identity of the early viral gene product in question and the mechanism by which it acts in enhancing translation remain to be established.

THE SWITCH BETWEEN EARLY AND LATE GENE EXPRESSION

During the late phase, the major late promoter at coordinate 16.5 controls most of the transcriptional activity. However, it is now clear that the major late promoter is also functional at early times after infection (45,86,146,181), although its activity is enhanced by gene products from region E1A (208) in the same manner as the early transcription units. The start site for transcription is the same at both early and late times of infection (280), although the structure of the mRNAs produced changes considerably. At late times, about 20 differently spliced mRNAs, falling into five 3' coterminal groups (L1–L5), are produced (Figs. 2 and 4). The primary transcript extends from coordinate 16.5 to the right-hand end of the genome near map coordinate 99 (85). At early times after infection, in contrast, the nuclear RNA terminates near the middle of the genome (6,213,280) and produces only two cytoplasmic mRNA species from region L1 (6,45) (Fig. 4). Thus, the transcription from the major late promoter is regulated by pretermination of transcription at early times of infection preventing the expression of promoter-distal cotermination groups L2 to L5 (Fig. 4). The major event responsible for the transition from early to late transcription (therefore enabling the expression of L2–L5 messengers) appears to be the DNA replication event, because unreplicated DNA, when introduced into cells in the late phase, still fails to express the late genes (306).

In addition to demonstrating the control of late gene expression by termination of transcription, studies of L1 mRNA synthesis have shown that the switch also involves virus-induced changes in the splicing machinery (6,213). The L1 nuclear

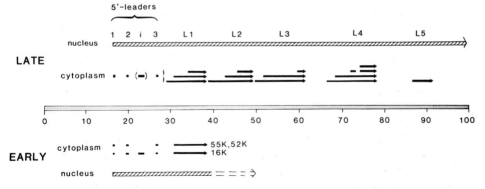

FIG. 4. Primary transcripts and mRNAs expressed from the major late promoter at early and late times of infection. Early after infection, the nuclear transcripts terminate around map position 50. They are spliced to form two mRNAs from region L1 encoding a 55K/52K polypeptide and a 16K polypeptide. The latter is presumably coded within the i leader segment. Late after infection, the primary transcript covers approximately 28,000 base pairs. The mRNAs are generated by splicing together the three segments that constitute the tripartite leader. The tripartite leader is joined to the different mRNA bodies. Several of these share poly(A) addition sites. In this way, the five coterminal families L1, L2, L3, L4, and L5 are formed.

RNA precursor is the same colinear RNA molecule at both early and late times, extending from the promoter site at coordinate 16.5 to the poly(A) addition site at coordinate 38.5 (Fig. 4). At early times, two L1 mRNA species accumulate preferentially (6,45), one of which encodes two structurally related polypeptides with molecular weights of 52K and 55K (6,45,205). The latter mRNA carries the normal tripartite leader, whereas the other species has a quadripartite leader with an extra 440-nucleotides-long leader segment derived from coordinates 22.0 to 23.2, designated the i leader. The i leader is spliced between the second and third leader segments (Fig. 4) (6,45), and its presence results in the translation of a 16K polypeptide (6,181,325). At late times, at least three L1 mRNAs are generated by splicing of the same nuclear precursor RNA (Fig. 4); in addition to the mRNA for the 55K/52K polypeptide, the mRNA for virion polypeptide IIIa and yet another mRNA with an unknown coding potential are produced (6,45). Analysis of pulse-labeled cytoplasmic and nuclear RNA has demonstrated that alterations in the splice pattern, rather than decreased mRNA stability or delayed transport from the nucleus, is the underlying cause of the observed change in expression of L1 mRNAs (213).

Our knowledge of the mechanism that causes differential splicing is very limited, although it seems clear that viral products are involved in this process. A promising approach for studying the details of the RNA processing mechanism may be via the temperature-sensitive mutant ad2ts206 (143), which appears to be defective for both DNA replication and RNA processing. Furthermore, the recent development of cell-free extracts that are able to process RNA precursors into functional mRNAs *in vitro* gives promise for rapid progress in this important area of research (101,333).

EARLY ADENOVIRUS PROTEINS

The proteins that are encoded by the early regions have been studied by several methods. One of these involves *in vitro* translation of mRNA isolated from adenovirus-infected cells that have been grown in the presence of protein synthesis inhibitors, such as cycloheximide. When the drug is added 1 to 2 hr after infection, accumulation of viral mRNA is enhanced considerably, and most of the early viral polypeptides can easily be detected above a background of host cell proteins (50,67,124,265). In addition, early viral polypeptides have been identified by *in vitro* translation of mRNA selected on DNA fragments representing the four early regions (120,123,179,181). Finally, the use of specific antisera from tumor-bearing animals has made it possible to identify many early adenovirus polypeptides (95,174,175,260,274,345). Particular attention has been focused on proteins expressed from region E1, because this region is of importance in transformation. The E1 polypeptides will be discussed later.

The main products of region E2 are the 72K DNA binding protein DBP (E2A) and the terminal protein (E2B) (Fig. 2). Both polypeptides are discussed in detail in the section dealing with DNA replication.

Region E3 is nonessential for viral replication in tissue culture cells, because it has been deleted in many of the replication-competent adenovirus/SV40 hybrids

(13,177) and also because viable deletion mutants have been isolated that lack sequences in this region. Two main proteins of molecular weights 19K and 14K have been assigned to region E3 (135,179,224,225,228,259). The best characterized is the glycosylated 19K protein that is found on the surfaces of infected and transformed cells, provided the latter contain the E3 region. A hydrophobic stretch of amino acids near the carboxy-terminal end appears to be inserted into the plasma membrane, whereas the amino-terminal part of the 19K protein is exposed on the cell surface (229). Recent studies have indicated that the 19K glycoprotein interacts with the major transplantation antigens both in ad2-transformed rat and hamster cells and in productively infected HeLa cells (158,227,284). The 19K polypeptide may therefore be involved in the so-called Zinkernagel-Doherty phenomenon (353), and the 19K protein may, in addition, be related to the tumor-specific transplantation antigen (TSTA) (285), which is known to be present on the surfaces of transformed cells. However, because the E3 region is absent in several transformed cell lines, the precise role of the 19K glycoprotein in transformation, tumorigenicity, and tumor immunity is still unclear. Three slightly different mRNAs encode the 19K glycoprotein (229), the difference being that they use three alternative poly(A) addition sites and thus vary in length at their 3' ends.

A 14K polypeptide, encoded by region E3, is preferentially found in the cytoplasm of infected cells. It has been purified to homogeneity, but no function has yet been assigned to this polypeptide (224).

Eight polypeptides with molecular weights ranging between 11K and 35K have been attributed to region E4 (28,114,123,179,197). However, tryptic peptide analysis reveals that at least six of these have sequences in common (197). The structural relationships between the polypeptides and the mRNAs of region E4 and their functions are at present unknown. Deletion mutants of ad2 have recently been isolated that lack sequences from region E4. Some of these are defective for the expression of certain late proteins (39).

GENERAL PROPERTIES OF ADENOVIRUS TRANSFORMATION

It was reported in 1962 that ad12 induces tumors in newborn rats and hamsters (130,310). Since then, it has been established that almost all human serotypes, including the nononcogenic ones, can induce transformation *in vitro* (201,202). Most of our information regarding the properties of adenoviruses as tumor viruses has been obtained from studies of *in vitro* transformation. As is the case with the papovaviruses, the adenoviruses appear preferentially to transform cells that are nonpermissive for replication. The most likely explanation of this observation is that virus replication leads to cell lysis, and nonpermissivity is hence a prerequisite for the transformed cell to survive. Support for this hypothesis comes from the fact that permissive cells nevertheless can be transformed by the use of virus that has been inactivated with ultraviolet (UV) light (178), by the use of mutants that are defective for replication (99,338,339), or by the use of viral DNA which has been fragmented to eliminate infectivity (103,105). For most transformation experiments, rat and hamster cells have been used. Transformation of mouse cells appears to be very inefficient, although it has been reported in a few cases (248,268). Also, transformation of permissive human cells has been achieved after transfection using fragmented adenovirus DNA, thereby preventing replication of the viral genome (105). Adenovirus transformation is a very inefficient process, usually requiring 10^4 to 10^6 infectious units to give rise to one transformation event. The role of the adenoviruses as tumor viruses in nature is therefore questionable. Extensive efforts to search for adenovirus-related nucleic acids or gene products in human tumors have thus far yielded negative results (96,109,176,200,262).

It is now a well-established fact that adenovirus-transformed cells contain viral DNA, viral mRNA, and viral proteins. In all cases, only a limited portion of the genome is expressed as mRNA, usually sequences in the early regions (79,80). When present in the transformed cell, the early promoters appear to be active, although there are exceptions to this rule. Cellular promoters usually are not used to transcribe integrated viral sequences, although sometimes aberrant transcripts are generated as a result of sequence rearrangement at the site of integration (267). The major late promoter usually is silent in transformed cells, although there have been some reports that late RNA and even late proteins are synthesized in certain adenovirus tumors (61,132,133).

TRANSFORMING GENES

It was shown a long time ago that the genes required for transformation are inactivated more slowly by ultraviolet irradiation than those required for replication, indicating that only a part of the adenovirus genome is required for transformation. In 1974, Sharp et al. (278) showed that the adenovirus-transformed rat cell line 8617 contains only about 50% of the ad2 genome, and shortly thereafter Gallimore et al. (89) described other ad2-transformed cell lines that also contain only parts of the ad2 genome, some as little as 14%. However, all cell lines possessed the left-hand end of the viral DNA, thus suggesting that the genes required for maintenance of transformation reside in this part of the genome.

The finding of Graham and Van der Eb in 1974 (102) that cells can be transformed by naked DNA, using the now well-known calcium phosphate technique, represented a breakthrough in research focusing on adenovirus transformation, because that made it possible to introduce specific restriction enzyme fragments into cells and thus to assay their transforming capacity. By means of this experimental approach it was shown that transformation can indeed be achieved by fragments containing the left-hand end of ad5 DNA, representing as little as 8% of the viral genome (103,104,314). Subsequently it was shown that even smaller fragments can transform cells, the minimum size being represented by the 4.5% *Hpa*I-E fragment of ad5 DNA (128). However, transformation with the *Hpa*I-E fragment of ad5 DNA is considerably less efficient than transformation with larger fragments, and *Hpa*I-E-transformed cells differ from those transformed by larger fragments in being fibroblastic, rather than having an epithelial morphology, and furthermore they grow to a lower saturation density. Thus, many of the phenotypic properties of transformed cells apparently are absent in cells transformed by the leftmost 4.5% of the adenovirus genome. The *Hpa*I-E-transformed cells are therefore considered "immortalized" because of their unlimited life-span, as opposed to "transformed" cells obtained by complete virus or larger fragments (315). Closer examination of cells transformed by the *Hind*III-G fragment (0–8 map units) has revealed that the T antigens are abnormally distributed in these cells (314,315). The information obtained by transfection of cells with different adenovirus fragments suggests that adenovirus transformation is a two-step process. Complete transformation is achieved by fragments including the entire E1 region. Fragments including region E1A alone result in immortalization, whereas fragments including region E1A plus the 5'-terminal part of region E1B give rise to transformed cells with a slightly altered phenotype.

Again, similar results have been obtained using DNA fragments from serotypes representing the weakly (55) and highly (198,282,283) oncogenic subgroups. In this respect, it is noteworthy that DNA from the highly oncogenic serotype 12 appears to transform rat cells in tissue culture with a lower frequency, as compared with DNA from the nononcogenic serotypes (A. J. Van der Eb, *personal communication*). With ad3 and ad7 DNA it has been shown that a 4% fragment located at the left-hand end gives rise to foci after transfection, although it has not been possible to establish cell lines from these foci (55). Therefore, the term "immortalization" seems inappropriate for these cells.

The results described here show that region E1 alone is sufficient for initiation and maintenance of transformation. Genetic studies (339,340) using group N mutants have suggested that these mutants are defective with regard to transformation, although the mutation has been mapped outside the E1 region *(vide infra)*. These results are difficult to reconcile with those described earlier, but they could be due to a different mechanism of integration when DNA is introduced through transfection, as opposed to the normal virus infection pathway. For instance, it is conceivable that DNA replication is required for integration when DNA enters the cell as a virus particle, and group N mutants are known to have a defect in the replication function.

mRNAs FROM THE TRANSFORMING REGION

Transcription Units

As described in detail in a previous section, promoter mapping studies have revealed that the early regions E1A, E1B, E2, E3, and E4 possess their own promoters. A third independent promoter has been defined in region E1B: that responsible for the expression of the unspliced mRNA coding for polypeptide IX (341). The E1A region is located between map coordinates 1.4 and 4.5, and region E1B is between coordinates 4.8 and 11.2. The transcription unit for polypeptide IX overlaps completely with region E1B and is located between coordinates 9.9 and 11.2 (Figs. 2 and 5).

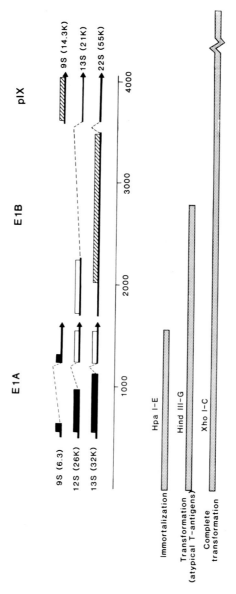

FIG. 5. Proposed structures of mRNAs from the transforming region of nononcogenic adenoviruses. The structures of the three spliced mRNAs from region E1A and the two spliced mRNAs from region E1B are indicated. The structure of the 9S mRNA from region E1A has been taken from data obtained with the weakly oncogenic ad7. Different parts of the mRNAs are translated from different reading frames as indicated. Polypeptide IX is an unspliced mRNA. The lower part of the figure shows the locations of fragments that give rise to cell transformation and cell immortalization.

mRNAs from Region E1A of Subgroup C Adenoviruses

S1 endonuclease mapping (24), electron microscopy (44,146), DNA sequencing (97,321), and molecular cloning (220,221) have been used as tools to define the mRNAs from the transforming region of subgroup C adenoviruses. The general conclusion drawn from these studies is that three mRNAs of 9S, 12S, and 13S are transcribed from a single promoter located in region E1A. All three species appear to have common 5′ as well as 3′ ends, and they differ by the size of the intervening sequence, which is excised during mRNA maturation (Fig. 5). In all likelihood they are processed from a common precursor, which thus can be spliced in three alternative fashions to generate the different mRNAs. The three mRNAs appear with different kinetics during the infectious cycle; the 9S mRNA, in contrast to the 12S and 13S mRNAs, is almost exclusively synthesized late after infection (289,342,343). The common cap site for the E1A mRNAs in ad5 is located 499 nucleotides from the left-hand end (18) and is, as expected, preceded by the so-called TATA box (100,321). The common poly(A) addition site for E1A mRNAs that is located at nucleotide 1,632 on the ad5 genome (220) is preceded by the hexanucleotide AAUAAA, which is known to precede the poly(A) addition site in most eukaryotic mRNAs. The precise positions of the splices in the 13S and 12S mRNAs have been determined by sequencing cDNA copies of the two mRNAs (220). The splicing events that generate the 12S and 13S mRNAs occur within the coding region of the mRNAs and result in the deletion of a markedly AT-rich region that contains many stop codons. In this respect, the splice has the same function as the splice in the mRNA for the large T antigen of SV40 (250). Also, as with the SV40 large T antigen mRNA, the 5′ and 3′ parts of both mRNAs will be translated from different reading frames (77,250) (Fig. 5). Thus the coding capacity of region E1A is used in the most efficient way possible. The polypeptides that are specified by the 13S and 12S mRNAs in ad5 will be 288 and 242 amino acids long, with molecular weights of 32,000 and 26,000, respectively, assuming that the AUG closest to the capped 5′ end is used for initiation of translation. The polypeptides will have identical amino- and carboxy-terminal ends, the only difference between them being a deletion of 46 internal amino acids from the polypeptide specified by the shorter mRNA (Fig. 5). The precise structure of the 9S mRNA from region E1A from subgroup C adenoviruses is not known, although the structure of the corresponding mRNA has been established in ad7 (57). The hypothetical product that is translated from the 9S mRNA in ad7 presumably initiates with the same AUG triplet but terminates in a different reading frame than the one used to translate the 12S and 13S mRNAs (Fig. 5), giving the protein product a predicted molecular weight of 6.3K (57). Because the 9S mRNA primarily accumulates late after infection (45,342), it is believed not to play a significant role in transformation.

mRNAs from Region E1B of Subgroup C Adenoviruses

Early after infection, two major mRNAs of 13S and 22S are transcribed from region E1B (44,243). As is the case for the E1A mRNAs, the early E1B mRNAs are completely overlapping and have common 5' and 3' ends. As a consequence, the 13S and 22S mRNAs of ad5 are likely to be formed by differential splicing of a single RNA precursor, and from looking at their structure it is apparent that each matures by the removal of a single intron. A promoterlike sequence is, as expected, located a short distance upstream from the cap site (18,321). The structure of the spliced 13S and 22S mRNAs is shown in Fig. 5, which also depicts the open translational reading frames predicted from the DNA sequence of region E1B in ad5 (275,321). The DNA sequence that covers the 13S and 22S mRNAs contains two large open translational reading frames (27). Both of these can be used in their entirety in the 22 mRNA, because both terminate before the small splice present in this mRNA (Fig. 5). Thus, the 22S mRNA is theoretically polycistronic, encoding a 55K polypeptide as well as a 21K polypeptide, provided both reading frames are used for translation. Experimental evidence indicates that both a small polypeptide and a large polypeptide can be translated from the 22S mRNA (27; A. J. Van der Eb, *personal communication*). The open translational reading frame that encodes a 21K polypeptide can also be utilized in its entirety in the 13S mRNA (Fig. 5). During the course of adenovirus infection there is a drastic change in the relative abundance of the 13S and 22S messengers (289,343). Early after infection, little 13S mRNA is present, as opposed to late after infection, when this mRNA becomes abundant.

The 13S and 22S mRNAs are unique, because different AUGs appear to be used for translation of the two mRNA species (27), even though they have identical 5' ends; in the 22S mRNA either the first or the second AUG appears to be selected for translation, whereas in the 13S mRNA the first AUG seems to be chosen. Theoretically it is possible that translation also begins at the second AUG in the 13S mRNA, in which case it would encode a 10K polypeptide by using sequences on both sides of the splice.

In addition to the 22S and 13S mRNAs that have been defined by S1 nuclease analysis, electron microscopy, and analysis of cDNA clones, Esche et al. (74) have detected the existence of an additional mRNA by *in vitro* translation of size-fractionated mRNA that is slightly larger than the 13S mRNA. The structure of this mRNA is not yet known, although it seems to encode a polypeptide of slightly larger size than that encoded by the 13S mRNA.

mRNA for Polypeptide IX

The polypeptide IX mRNA differs in several respects from other adenovirus mRNAs; it is the only adenovirus mRNA thus far characterized that is known with certainty to mature without splicing (9), and it also differs from most other adenovirus mRNAs in its temporal regulation (223). Small amounts of polypeptide IX mRNA are synthesized early after infection, even in the presence of inhibitors of DNA replication, whereas late after infection the polypeptide IX mRNA becomes one of the most abundant mRNA species in the infected cell (223,289). Sequence analyses of the E1B regions of ad2 and ad5, together with structural studies of the polypeptide IX mRNA, have shown that the cap site for the polypeptide IX mRNA is located in the intervening sequence, which is common to the 22S and 13S mRNAs of region E1B (9,97,321) (Fig. 5). The nucleotide sequence in ad2 and ad5 reveals, furthermore, the presence of a promoterlike sequence approximately 30 nucleotides upstream from the cap site (321), suggesting that this mRNA is regulated by a separate promoter, as is expected from its kinetics of appearance. The polypeptide IX mRNA overlaps with the 13S and 22S mRNAs and shares its poly(A) addition site with the other E1B mRNAs (9) (Fig. 5).

Polypeptide IX is a virion polypeptide and is believed to be located between the hexons in the adenovirus icosahedron, thereby holding the capsomers together (76,190). The fact that polypeptide IX is controlled by a different promoter than the other structural proteins may suggest that it has additional functions besides being a structural polypeptide. The observation that deletion mutant dl 313, which lacks the gene for polypeptide IX, is still viable, although the virions are less heat-stable than wild-type virions, may suggest that polypeptide IX is dispensable for virus replication (46). However, it should be pointed out that the mutant is prop-agated in cells that already contain integrated viral sequences. Therefore, the in-tegrated gene for polypeptide IX may produce the protein in sufficient amounts to carry out a hypothetical catalytic function, although the protein is not produced in quantities large enough for assembly into virions.

Because the gene for polypeptide IX is located outside of the minimum region required for transformation, there is no reason to suspect that polypeptide IX is involved in adenovirus transformation.

COMPARISON OF THE TRANSFORMING REGIONS OF HIGHLY AND WEAKLY ONCOGENIC AND NONONCOGENIC ADENOVIRUSES

Most structural information about adenovirus transforming genes has been derived from the human types 2 and 5, both of which belong to the nononcogenic subgroup C. An interesting question that is yet to be answered is what accounts for the differences in oncogenic properties between different adenoviruses. It was recog-nized a long time ago that the T antigens from adenoviruses belonging to different subgroups fail to cross-react (202) and that the transforming regions of adenoviruses belonging to different oncogenic subgroups share little or no sequence homology (107,112,189). During recent years, DNA sequence information has been collected from the transforming regions of adenoviruses belonging to different subgroups, and thus a direct comparison is today possible (27,56,296,321; K. Fujinaga, *per-sonal communication*). The cDNA copies of mRNAs from regions E1A and E1B of the highly oncogenic serotype 12 have also been cloned, thus allowing direct comparison between the mRNAs produced from the transforming region (222,326). The results show (27,222,322,326), contrary to expectations based on previous results, that the transforming regions of highly and weakly oncogenic and nonon-cogenic adenoviruses are very similar. The major open translational reading frames identified in ad2 and ad5 are also present in the weakly oncogenic ad7 and the highly oncogenic ad12 (Fig. 6). For region E1A it has furthermore been shown that 12S and 13S mRNAs with very similar structures are produced in cells infected with ad5 and ad12 (222) (Fig. 7). The amino acid compositions of the predicted proteins from region E1A of different subgroup members are very similar, suggesting that they all probably serve the same functions (27,322). In accord with this it has been demonstrated that ad12 can complement mutants of ad5 with defects in the transforming region (263).

For region E1A the overall DNA sequence homology between any pair of serotypes representing subgroups A, B, or C is approximately 50% (322), and from direct sequence comparison it is not possible to establish a closer relationship between any two subgroups. However, analyses of the structures at donor and

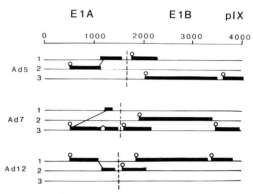

FIG. 6. The major open translational reading frames in regions E1A and E1B of adenoviruses, representing three different oncogenic subgroups. The location of the first ATG in each reading frame is shown. The frame shifts that result from the E1A splices are also illustrated. (Adapted from Dijkema, ref. 53.)

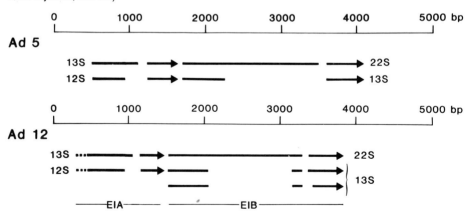

FIG. 7. A comparison of mRNAs from regions E1A and E1B of the nononcogenic ad5 and the highly oncogenic ad12. The principal structures of the different spliced mRNAs, as deduced from cDNA clones, are shown. (Adapted from Virtanen et al., ref. 325.)

acceptor sites for splicing suggest that subgroups A and B are more closely related to each other than to the nononcogenic serotypes (222,326).

For region E1B, serotypes 5, 7, and 12 have many features in common (27,53,97,296,321). In all cases there exist large (22S) and small (13S) mRNAs that in two separate but overlapping reading frames can give rise to large (54–55K) and small (19–21K) polypeptides (Figs. 6 and 7). In addition, the gene for poly-peptide IX can be identified in human adenoviruses representing all oncogenic subgroups. The structure of the 22S mRNA appears to be the same for the non-oncogenic ad5 and the highly oncogenic ad12 (326). However, the structures of the 13S mRNAs from region E1B differ significantly between oncogenic and non-oncogenic serotypes (Fig. 7). In cells infected with ad12 there exists no equivalent to the 13S mRNA with a single large splice (326). Instead, two different mRNAs have been found, both of which contain two intervening sequences. Both intervening sequences are located after the termination codon, which ends the reading frame that encodes the 19K polypeptide and hence will not cause any obvious change in the coding properties of the 13S mRNA. The difference between the two types of 13S mRNA present in ad12-infected cells is that two slightly different acceptor sites are used to splice out one of the introns, thus giving rise to two mRNAs with different 3' noncoding regions (326). This observation therefore leads to the inter-esting question whether or not the unique structure of the 13S mRNAs can account for the oncogenic properties of ad12. The two alternative splices in the 13S mRNAs of ad12 are both located in the 3' noncoding part of the mRNA, which is very unusual. So far, no splices have been encountered in the 3' noncoding region of cellular mRNAs; the only known example besides the E1B mRNAs of adenoviruses is the splice present in the mRNA for the small T antigen of SV40 (76,250). The biological function of the 3' noncoding region of eukaryotic mRNAs is poorly understood. It is conceivable that sequences present in this part of mRNAs influence the transport or the stability of the mRNAs. Provided that the difference between oncogenic and nononcogenic viruses is quantitative rather than qualitative, the unique 3' noncoding parts of the ad12 mRNAs could play a decisive role in de-termining the oncogenic potential of the virus.

ADENOVIRUS T ANTIGENS

By definition, tumor antigens (T antigens) are proteins that are immunoprecip-itated with sera from tumor-bearing animals (131). Because different transformed cells contain different quantities of adenovirus DNA, the T antigens will not be the same in all cell lines and tumors. For instance, sera from certain tumor-bearing animals contain antibodies against the 72K DBP, because this protein is expressed in some, but not all, tumors (95,173). Therefore, by definition, the 72K protein could be regarded as a T antigen. Likewise, proteins from the E3 and E4 regions are precipitable with certain tumor sera. However, in our opinion it is inappropriate to include among the T antigens polypeptides that are encoded by parts of the viral genome other than those required for transformation, and therefore only proteins encoded by the E1 region will be considered in this section. T antigens can be identified by several different methods: (a) A commonly used procedure involves selection of mRNA by hybridization to restriction endonuclease fragments representing the transforming regions and subsequent translation of this mRNA *in vitro*. (b) An alternative method is to analyze isotope-labeled polypeptides from lytically infected or transformed cells, followed by immunoprecipitation using sera either from tumor-bearing animals or from animals that have been immunized with transformed cells.

These two methods do not necessarily give identical results, for several reasons: First, some polypeptides are poor immunogens and hence will elicit a weak immune response. Second, many polypeptides suffer different kinds of posttranslational modifications *in vivo* that do not happen *in vitro*. Also, different *in vitro* systems translate different mRNA species with widely different efficiencies, and in addition polypeptide fragments are sometimes generated by proteolytic degradation. Another particularly disturbing complication encountered is that many investigators use different marker proteins for their studies and therefore arrive at different molecular weight estimates for otherwise identical proteins. As a consequence, the literature on adenovirus T antigens describes a vast number of candidate polypeptides, many of which are related in one way or another. In this chapter we shall consider primarily those that can with certainty be correlated to specific mRNAs from the transforming region.

T Antigens Encoded by Region E1A

The 12S and 13S mRNAs from region E1A appear to give rise to several related polypeptides ranging in size between 35K and 53K (74,120,123,136,137,179,182, 188). Four discrete bands having estimated molecular weights of 35K, 41K, 47K, and 53K[3] usually can be identified after one-dimensional SDS polyacrylamide gel electrophoresis. By *in vitro* translation of size-fractionated RNA it has been shown that the 13S mRNA encodes the 41K and 53K polypeptides, whereas the 12S mRNA yields the 35K and 47K polypeptides (74,120,253). After two-dimensional gel electrophoresis these components can be resolved into additional species (123). The results are interpreted to mean that each early mRNA from region E1A can give rise to two or more polypeptides, presumably by posttranslational modification, the nature of which is not yet understood. Tryptic peptide analysis and amino acid radio-sequence analysis have shown that all polypeptides encoded by the 12S and 13S mRNAs are related, as would be expected from the structure of the mRNAs (110,114,119,123,173,286). The molecular weights of the E1A polypeptides as predicted from the DNA sequence are 33K and 26K (220,321). There is thus considerable discrepancy between the predicted and estimated molecular weights; this could be accounted for in part by the comparatively high proline content in both polypeptides.

---

[3]The estimated molecular weights of the E1A polypeptides have varied in different studies because different size markers have been used.

The protein product that is translated from the 9S mRNA of region E1A has been reported to be a 28K polypeptide (74,290). However, the estimated molecular weight exceeds by far the predicted molecular weight (57) (6.3K and ad7), and further work will be necessary to resolve this discrepancy.

In addition to the polypeptides mentioned earlier, many other polypeptides have been ascribed to region E1A. Of particular interest is a polypeptide with a molecular weight of 10K/11K that is efficiently precipitated with sera from certain tumor-bearing animals and that is absent from cells infected with host-range mutants belonging to class I (164,261). Recent results indicate that the 10K polypeptide may be translated from an mRNA encoded by the viral l strand in region E1 (145). The exact structure of the mRNA for the 10K polypeptide is at present not known.

T Antigens Encoded by Region E1B

The polypeptides encoded by the 12S and 13S mRNAs of region E1A are weak immunogens and hence are difficult to detect by immunoprecipitation. The major polypeptides from region E1B, in contrast, are more easily detectable by immunoprecipitation (using sera from immunized animals) and thus should be regarded as the major adenovirus T antigens. One of these has an estimated molecular weight of 21K[4] and appears to be the major translation product of the 13S mRNA from region E1B, whereas the major translation product of the 22S mRNA appears to be a 55K polypeptide (74,120,137,188). The 21K and 55K polypeptides are translated from different but overlapping reading frames in region E1B (27) and are therefore totally unrelated, as has been verified by tryptic peptide analysis (27,114,119). However, as mentioned in a previous section, the 22S mRNA is polycistronic, and it has been shown *in vitro* that the 22S mRNA can be translated to yield both the 21K and 55K polypeptides (27,188; A. J. Van der Eb, *personal communication*). It appears, however, that the 55K polypeptide is the main translation product of the 22S mRNA, because at early times after infection, when little 13S mRNA is present, the 55K polypeptide is the most abundant E1B protein. Another prominent polypeptide with an estimated molecular weight of 18K has been assigned to region E1B (110,114,315). This polypeptide has, in contrast to the 21K polypeptide, many of its tryptic peptides in common with the 55K polypeptide.

The T antigens described earlier are the major proteins produced in cells infected or transformed by subgroup C adenoviruses. Several studies have been carried out using cells transformed by highly and weakly oncogenic adenoviruses, and the results appear to be similar (1,73,136,272). However, in many cases large numbers of additional polypeptides have been identified, but the relationship between these and the E1 mRNAs remains to be established.

---

[4]The estimated molecular weights for the E1B polypeptides differ considerably in different reports, presumably because of the use of different size markers. For convenience, we use the values that are predicted from the DNA sequence.

Roles of Different T Antigens in Adenovirus Transformation

Region E1A is sufficient for immortalization of cells, and thus the products of the 12S and 13S mRNAs are likely to be responsible for this property. Genetic experiments have shown that the product of the 13S mRNA is probably responsible for the regulation of early gene expression and for the first step in adenovirus transformation (25,140).

The phenotypic properties that are connected with transformation appear to be associated with the E1B region, most likely with the product of the 13S mRNA, the 21K polypeptide. This conclusion rests on the observation that cells transformed by the *Hin*dIII-G fragment (0–8.0 map units) of ad5 express the transformed pheno- type. Fragment *Hin*dIII-G includes the entire coding region for the 21K protein, but only the amino-terminal end of the 55K polypeptide (Fig. 5). Provided that a suitable poly(A) addition site is found within the flanking host sequences after integration, the 21K protein would be expected to be synthesized in *Hin*dIII-G transformants, in contrast to the 55K protein. Analyses of T antigens in *Hin*dIII- G-transformed cells show, as expected, that a 21K protein is present, but not the 55K protein (137,315). From these observations it can be concluded that the 21K polypeptide is likely to account for the major transforming properties of adenovi- ruses. Because a product from region E1A is necessary to activate the other early regions of the adenovirus genome, including the E1B region, the main role of region E1A in transformation could be to activate region E1B. However, a certain cor- relation has been obtained between the presence of the 55K sequences and tumor- igenicity in the case of ad12 (M. Perricaudet and A. J. Van der Eb, *personal communication*). It is thus conceivable that the oncogenic potential of the virus is influenced by the 55K polypeptide.

POSSIBLE FUNCTIONS OF ADENOVIRUS T ANTIGENS

Although a wealth of information has been collected concerning the structures of adenovirus transforming genes and their mRNAs, our knowledge of the functions of the transforming proteins is still very incomplete. As discussed earlier, a product from region E1A regulates the expression of the other early genes, probably by blocking an inhibitory protein of cellular origin. It seems logical that the inhibitory protein also suppresses some cellular genes. Therefore, the transforming protein of region E1A could derepress a group of cellular genes, thereby affecting the growth properties of the cells in such a way that they become immortalized.

The function of the E1B polypeptides is less clearly established. Following the original observation of Collett and Erikson (47) that the transforming genes of avian sarcoma viruses are associated with protein kinase activity, it was reported that a virus-induced protein kinase also can be detected in adenovirus-infected and -transformed cells (29,165). This kinase activity was demonstrated by immuno- precipitation, using sera from a tumor-bearing animal, and as in the case of the *src* protein, the adenovirus-induced kinase phosphorylates the heavy chain of IgG pres- ent in the immunoprecipitate. However, it can also phosphorylate exogenous acceptor proteins such as histones. From its kinetics of appearance, the adenovirus-induced kinase appears to be an early protein, most likely encoded by region E1 (29). The latter conclusion is based on the fact that the tumor serum that was used for detection was prepared after immunization with cells expressing only the E1 region. However, it has not yet been established which of the E1 proteins is associated with the kinase activity, although studies using host-range mutants suggest that the kinase activity is low or absent in cells infected with mutants carrying lesions in the E1B region (29). The kinases that are induced by the nononcogenic serotype 5 and the highly oncogenic serotype 12 are immunologically different, as would be expected, because the T antigens of adenoviruses from different subgroups fail to cross-react (29). Unlike the product of the *src* gene, the adenovirus protein kinase does not seem to phosphorylate tyrosine residues, but rather threonine and serine residues (29). The 21K polypeptide from region E1B of ad2 has been purified to homogeneity, and the results indicate that it is membrane-bound (233). It is not yet known if the purified protein contains any kinase activity.

Sarnow et al. (268) have shown that the large E1B protein (55K) in transformed cells is complexed with a cellular 54K polypeptide. It had previously been established that SV40-transformed cells contain increased levels of a 54K polypeptide and that the 54K polypeptide is complexed with the SV40 large T antigen (162,185). It has been shown more recently that in EBV-transformed cells a 54K polypeptide is complexed with the so-called EBNA antigen. Also, cells transformed by chemical carcinogens appear to contain increased levels of a 54K protein (51). Using monoclonal antibodies, Sarnow et al. (268) demonstrated that the 54K polypeptides associated with the SV40 large T antigen and the 55K protein from the E1B region of adenovirus are identical. Although this finding gives no direct clue as to the function of the T antigens, it nevertheless suggests that several different agents may transform cells by a common mechanism.

INTEGRATION OF ADENOVIRUS DNA IN THE GENOMES OF TRANSFORMED CELLS

It is now well established that adenovirus-transformed cells contain integrated viral genomes and not episomal copies of the viral DNA. The structure of the integrated genome has been studied by several methods, including reassociation kinetics, Southern's blotting method, and molecular cloning. The most surprising conclusion that can be drawn from these studies is that cells transformed by subgroup C adenoviruses usually contain viral genomes with large deletions. Following the original observation that the ad2-transformed rat cell line 8617 contains only half of the ad2 genome (278), integration of fragments of adenovirus DNA has been shown to be the rule rather than the exception (82,89,138,266,267,327,336). There is no simple way to explain why only partial genomes are integrated, although this may be related to the fact that hamster and rat cells are semipermissive for replication of subgroup C adenoviruses (88). Because adenovirus replication leads to cell lysis, there is probably a strong selection pressure to prevent viral replication by deleting functional parts of the genome. There is as yet no way to discriminate between the two main alternatives for how these deleted genomes are created: Either transformation is caused by integration of a defective viral genome, or selected areas of the integrated DNA are eliminated after the original integration event.

Some cell lines do not follow the general pattern of integration, but instead contain sequences representing the complete viral DNA. Transformation at the nonpermissive temperature with the H5ts125 mutant, which is defective for viral DNA replication, results in a higher frequency of transformation than with wild-type ad5, and analysis of the integrated genomes in the resulting transformants has shown that multiple copies of the complete viral DNA usually are present (62,99,199). Integration of complete viral genomes occurs also after transformation with host-range mutants belonging to complementation class I (264). Although defective for transformation in a strict sense, these mutants induce transient transformation of baby rat kidney cells (106), and it has been seen that the transformed cells, which can be established as cell lines starting with polyclonal cultures, often contain complete copies of the transforming virus (264). Finally, cells transformed by the highly oncogenic sero-type 12 contain multiple copies representing the complete viral DNA (59,61,113,133,291,301). The explanation for the presence of integrated intact ad12 genomes is presumably that the target hamster and rat cells are entirely nonpermissive for replication of ad12, unlike ad2 and ad5.

Studies of the integrated viral genomes by the Southern blotting technique have revealed in most cases very complicated patterns of integration (266,324,327). Different cell lines transformed by live or UV-inactivated subgroup C virus contain widely different amounts of viral DNA sequences, ranging from about 15% to the complete viral genome (89,138,274,327). The results have also demonstrated that different parts of the viral genome are present in different molar amounts, suggesting that integration is accompanied by amplification and rearrangement of the viral sequences. Sequences from the left-hand end often are amplified, suggesting that there may be a selective advantage of having multiple copies of the transforming region (89,327). Other common findings are that the central parts of the viral genome often are deleted and that the right- and left-hand parts are juxtaposed (266,327). All transformed cell lines thus far analyzed contain sequences from the left-hand end, again emphasizing the importance of this region for viral transformation. By means of restriction enzyme mapping of the sequences that flank the viral inserts it has been found that there is no preferred site of integration in the genome of the host cell (327). However, it should be emphasized that all cell lines that have been analyzed have been propagated for several generations in tissue culture prior to analysis. Although it is unlikely, it cannot be completely excluded that integration originally took place in a unique position, with deletions and rearrangements subsequently occurring at the site of integration.

For the highly oncogenic ad12, a different pattern of integration is usually found. Large numbers of ad12-transformed cell lines and ad12-induced tumors from animals have been analyzed [for a review, see Doerfler (59)], and the conclusion drawn is that most ad12 cell lines and tumors contain several complete copies of the ad12 genome (133,198,291). Studies using Southern's blotting technique have shown that limited numbers of integration sites do exist, because in each cell line fewer unique fragments are found that are joined to flanking sequences than are copies of viral DNA. The most likely explanation for this observation is that viral integration first occurs at one or a few sites and that selective amplification of the integrated genome, together with some flanking sequences, generates tandemly integrated copies separated by cellular sequences (291). Furthermore, for integrated ad12 genomes, rearrangement of the viral sequences leading to noncolinearity has also been reported (68).

An interesting question is whether or not integration is caused by recombination events involving homologous sequences. The answer to this question requires the isolation of integrated viral genomes by molecular cloning and subsequent DNA sequence studies of junctions between cellular and viral sequences. Several such junctions have been studied from cell lines transformed by ad2, ad5, and ad12, and the general conclusion from these studies is that the flanking sequences usually are joined to the viral DNA within the terminal repetition, although exceptions to this rule have been found (63,267,336). Computer-assisted analysis of the flanking sequences has revealed that no homology exists between host and viral DNA sequences at the site of integration. However, Deuring et al. (63) have recently reported that a patchlike homology between host and viral sequences can be found at the site of integration in some cell lines. The biological significance of this observation remains to be established. As pointed out earlier, it should be emphasized that deletions, amplifications, and rearrangements probably take place after the original integration events, and the significance of the lack of sequence homology cannot be properly evaluated until cellular sites of integration have been analyzed at the molecular level before and after integration.

Revertants of ad12-transformed cells have been studied with regard to the structure of the integrated viral genomes. The results show that revertants exhibit different integration patterns; in some cell lines all copies of viral DNA are lost, whereas in others selected parts are preserved (68,69,114). The revertants do not seem to express T antigen, not even those that retain viral DNA sequences from the transforming region (69,116). In this respect, it is interesting that the viral DNA sequences become methylated in the revertants (69).

METHYLATION OF INTEGRATED VIRAL SEQUENCES

Recently a great deal of attention has been focused on DNA methylation, because an inverse correlation between the degree of DNA methylation and the level of gene activity has been established in some eukaryotic systems (300); for a review, see Doerfler (58). The adenovirus DNA is undermethylated, inside the virus particle and also during replication, and it contains considerably fewer methylated bases than the DNA of its host (118). The mechanism by which the viral DNA escapes the action of the host methyltransferases is not known, although it may in some way or other be related to the general shutoff of host gene functions during viral replication. In contrast, the integrated DNA becomes methylated, and because only certain regions are expressed in most transformed cell lines, different parts of the integrated viral genome exhibit different levels of methylation. A particularly interesting correlation between methylation and gene activity has been established for the ad2-hamster-transformed cell lines HE1, HE2, and HE3 (323). All these cell lines contain the gene for the DBP from region E2A (138,324). However, only the HE1 cell line expresses the DBP, and analysis of the methylation pattern has shown that the E2 region in HE1 cells is undermethylated, whereas the corresponding regions in cell lines HE2 and HE3 are methylated. Other studies, including tumor cells from animals, have shown less striking correlations between methylation and inactive regions in the integrated genomes, suggesting that the relationship between gene activity and methylation could be complex (157).

GENETICS OF ADENOVIRUS TRANSFORMATION

It has been surprisingly difficult to isolate temperature-sensitive mutants with lesions in the early regions, and not a single one in a large collection of ad5 mutants maps in the E1 region. Therefore, more sophisticated tools have been employed for construction of mutants that carry defects in the transforming region. The 293 cell line, originally isolated by Graham et al. (105), has been of considerable importance for genetic studies of the transforming region. The 293 cell line was established by transformation of human embryonic kidney (HEK) cells with fragmented ad5 DNA. Although the HEK cell is permissive for replication of adenovirus, fragmentation prevents the lytic response, and a stable transformed cell line was established after a large number of passages (105). This cell line has been used extensively in many laboratories for genetic experiments. The 293 cells contain sequences from the left-hand end of the ad5 genome, and mRNAs and proteins are expressed from both the E1A and E1B regions (2,105,274). The cell line can, because of the integrated viral genome, complement a superinfecting virus with lesions in the E1 region. An array of deletion mutants has been constructed lacking various amounts of sequences in the E1 region (139). The mutants were selected because of their host-range properties; they grow efficiently on 293 cells but fail to replicate in HeLa cells. The most interesting result that has come from studies of mutants with deletions in region E1A (such as dl 312 and dl 314) is that they fail to express mRNAs and proteins not only from the E1A region but also from the other early regions (140). The conclusion from these results is that a product from region E1A serves as positive regulator of the expression of the other early regions.

Transformation assays, as expected, show that mutants that have deletions in region E1A or E1B have defective transformation capacity (270).

Another set of mutants having a host-range phenotype has been selected after mutagenesis of wild-type ad5 and subsequent screening for plaques that grow on 293 cells but not on HeLa cells (122). In this way a large collection of so-called host-range (hr) mutants has been isolated on the basis of complementation analysis. They can be subdivided into two groups: class I and class II hr mutants. By means of marker rescue procedures, class I mutants have been mapped in region E1A, whereas class II mutants map in region E1B, between coordinates 6.0 and 11.1 (87,91). The class I hr mutants have a phenotype very similar to that of the deletion mutants with defects in the E1A region; they express mRNAs from the E1A region, but not from the other early transcription units (25).

The hr mutants are, as expected, defective for transformation (106). Those belonging to class II do not transform cells at all, or with a drastically reduced frequency, as compared with wild-type virus, and an analysis of productively infected cells with class II mutants indicates the E1B polypeptides are not properly expressed after infection with class II mutants (163,164,261). This again reinforces the idea that one or both of the E1B proteins are of crucial importance for transformation. The class I mutants have a different phenotype with regard to transformation, being unable to transform rat embryo or rat embryo brain cells. However, they are able to cause a semiabortive transformation of baby rat kidney cells (106). Transformation of baby rat kidney cells with hr-I virus gives rise to transient transformation with a higher frequency than wild-type virus, but it is difficult or impossible to establish transformed cell lines from the foci that result. Analysis of the genotype of polyclonally derived transformed cells indicates that they contain integrated viral genomes, in some cases copies of the complete genome, and the results furthermore show that the 21K and 55K proteins are expressed (264). Taken together, these observations may suggest that class I mutants are defective in maintenance of transformation, whereas class II mutants fail to initiate transformation.

Sequence studies of the hr-I genome belonging to the complementation class I have been particularly informative (253). It has been observed that the mutant genome contains a series of point mutations that introduce a termination codon in the reading frame that is utilized for translation of the 12S and 13S mRNAs (74,253). Because the termination codon is located between the donor sites that are used for splicing of the 12S and 13S mRNAs, the mutation will alter only the product of the 13S mRNA, giving rise to a truncated polypeptide. This has been experimentally verified by *in vitro* translation of mRNA from mutant-infected cells (74). Because the hr-I mutant is defective for transformation and expression of mRNAs from the other early regions, these findings suggest that the region that is unique to the 13S mRNA, encoding 46 amino acids, is of critical importance both for the regulatory function and for transformation (253).

During recent years, more sophisticated methods have become available to allow the introduction of specific point mutations in strategic regions of viral genomes (206,273,295). Such methods presumably will be of critical importance for more detailed functional analysis of the transforming region, because large deletions give less informative results often altering several different mRNAs because of the overlapping nature of the mRNAs in region E1A and region E1B. Recently, mutations have been introduced into the splice site that generates the 12S mRNA of region E1A without affecting the coding properties of the 13S mRNA (206). Results of experiments using this mutant have shown that although the 12S mRNA is not expressed, the mutant is nondefective for replication. This finding again emphasizes the importance of the sequence that is unique to the 13S mRNA. McKinnon et al. (204) have used another interesting technique to introduce specific mutations: By propagation of a cloned fragment containing the transforming region in a bacterial host, they were able to isolate mutant clones that carried a transposable element introduced into different positions of the transforming region. Results obtained by this procedure show that insertion of the transposable element Tn5 into the E1A region or into the N-terminal part of early region E1B eliminates the transforming properties of the DNA, confirming the significance of early regions E1A and part of region E1B for transformation.

The design of additional mutants in the E1 region will be of critical importance in the future for further dissection of the transforming functions. It will also be necessary to construct mutants with defects in other areas of the genome in order to understand better the details of viral gene regulation and expression. For this purpose it will be important to establish cell lines that are equivalent to the 293 cells but that express other regions of the adenovirus genome. In this respect, it is a promising possibility that adenovirus DNA can be introduced in a functional form into cells by the use of cotransfection procedures with the thymidine kinase gene from herpes simplex virus (115,153).

Mutations outside the transforming region can also influence the frequency of virion-mediated transformation. The group N mutants that map between coordinates 18.0 and 22.5 are defective for transformation (339). This defect may be caused by the fact that DNA replication is necessary when the viral genome is introduced as virions, whereas this is not the case when the DNA is introduced via transfection.

CONCLUDING REMARKS

In this chapter we have attempted to give a comprehensive survey of our current knowledge regarding the molecular biology of adenovirus transformation. It is obvious that considerable work remains to be done in order to answer the fundamental questions regarding the mechanisms by which the adenoviruses cause cell transformation. Thus, the adenovirus system promises fertile ground for further and more sophisticated experimentation. The information that will come from work on the simple adenoviruses will certainly be of primary importance for our comprehension of the complex and intricate manner in which eukaryotic DNA is regulated and expressed.

ACKNOWLEDGMENTS

We thank Drs. Doerfler, Levine, Graham, Roberts, Van Ormondt, Van der Eb, Persson, and Philipson for preprints of unpublished work. We would also like to express our gratitude to Drs. Philipson, Therwath, and Virtanen for valuable comments on the manuscript. Marianne Gustafson, Ingegärd Schiller, and Christina Pellettieri provided excellent and patient secretarial help. Studies from the authors' laboratory were supported by grants from the Swedish Cancer Society, The Swedish Medical Research Council, and the Swedish Board for Technical Development.

REFERENCES

1. Achten, S., and Doerfler, W. (1982): Virus-specific proteins in adenovirus type 12-transformed and tumor cells as detected by immunoprecipitation. *J. Gen. Virol.*, 59:357–366.
2. Aiello, L., Guilfoyle, R., Huebner, K., and Weinmann, R. (1979): Adenovirus 5 DNA sequences present and RNA sequences transcribed in transformed human embryo kidney cells (HEK-Ad5 or 293). *Virology*, 94:460–469.
3. Akusjärvi, G., and Pettersson, U. (1979): Sequence analysis of adenovirus DNA: Complete nucleotide sequence of the spliced 5′ noncoding region of adenovirus 2 hexon messenger RNA. *Cell*, 16:841–850.
4. Akusjärvi, G., and Pettersson, U. (1979): The genomic sequences encoding the common tripartite leader of late adenovirus messenger RNA. *J. Mol. Biol.*, 134:143–158.
5. Akusjärvi, G., Mathews, M. B., Anderson, P., Vennström, B., and Pettersson, U. (1980): Structure of genes for virus-associated RNA$_I$ and RNA$_{II}$ of adenovirus type 2. *Proc. Natl. Acad. Sci. USA*, 77:2424–2428.
6. Akusjärvi, G., and Persson, H. (1981): Controls of RNA splicing and termination in the major late adenovirus transcription unit. *Nature*, 292:420–426.
7. Akusjärvi, G., and Persson, H. (1981): Gene and mRNA for precursor polypeptide VI from adenovirus type 2. *J. Virol.*, 38:469–482.
8. Akusjärvi, G., Zabielski, J., Perricaudet, M., and Pettersson, U. (1981): The sequence of the 3′-non-coding region of the hexon mRNA discloses a novel adenovirus gene. *Nucleic Acids Res.*, 9:1–17.
9. Aleström, P., Akusjärvi, G., Perricaudet, M., Mathews, M. B., Klessig, D. F., and Petterson, U. (1980): The gene for polypeptide IX of adenovirus type 2 and its unspliced messenger RNA. *Cell*, 19:671–681.
10. Aleström, P., Akusjärvi, G., Pettersson, M., and Pettersson, U. (1982): DNA sequence analysis of the region encoding the terminal protein and the hypothetical N-gene product of adenovirus type 2. *J. Biol. Chem.*, 257:13492–13498.
11. Aleström, P., Stenlund, A., Li, P., and Pettersson, U. (1982): A common sequence in the inverted terminal repetitions of human and avian adenoviruses. *Gene*, 18:193–197.
12. Anderson, C. W., Baum, P. R., and Gesteland, R. F. (1973): Processing of adenovirus 2-induced proteins. *J. Virol.*, 12:241–252.
13. Anderson, C. W., Lewis, J. B., Baum, P. R., and Gesteland, R. F. (1976): Simian virus 40-specific polypeptide in ad2$^+$ ND1- and ad2$^+$ ND4-infected cells. *J. Virol.*, 18:686–692.
14. Arens, M., Yamashita, T., Padmanabahn, R., Tsuro, T., and Green, M. (1977): Adenovirus DNA replication: Characterizations of the enzyme components of a soluble replication system. *J. Biol. Chem.*, 252:7947–7954.
15. Ariga, H., and Shimojo, H. (1977): Initiation and termination sites of adenovirus 12 DNA replication. *Virology*, 78:415–424.
16. Axelrod, N. (1978): Phosphoproteins of adenovirus 2. *Virology*, 87:366–383.
17. Babich, A., and Nevins, J. R. (1981): The stability of early adenovirus mRNA is controlled by the viral 72K DNA binding protein. *Cell*, 26:371–379.
18. Baker, C. C., and Ziff, E. B. (1980): Biogenesis, structures and sites encoding the 5′-termini of adenovirus-2 mRNAs. *Cold Spring Harbor Symp. Quant. Biol.*, 44:415–428.
19. Bellett, A. J. D., and Younghusband, H. B. (1972): Replication of the DNA of chick embryo lethal orphan virus. *J. Mol. Biol.*, 72:691–709.
20. Beltz, G. A., and Flint, S. J. (1979): Inhibition of HeLa cell protein synthesis during adenovirus infection. Restriction of cellular messenger RNA sequences to the nucleus. *J. Mol. Biol.*, 131:353–373.
21. Berget, A. M., and Sharp, P. A. (1979): Structure of late adenovirus 2 heterogeneous nuclear RNA. *J. Mol. Biol.*, 129:547–565.
22. Berget, S. M., Moore, C., and Sharp, P. A. (1977): Spliced segments at the 5′ terminus of adenovirus 2 late mRNA. *Proc. Natl. Acad. Sci. USA*, 74:3171–3175.

23. Berk, A. J., and Sharp, P. A. (1977): Ultraviolet mapping of the adenovirus 2 early promoters. *Cell*, 12:45–55.
24. Berk, A. J., and Sharp, P. A. (1978): Structure of adenovirus 2 early mRNAs. *Cell*, 14:695–711.
25. Berk, A. J., Lee, F., Harrison, T., Williams, J., and Sharp, P. A. (1979): Pre-early adenovirus 5 gene product regulates synthesis of early viral messenger RNAs. *Cell*, 17:1935–1944.
26. Bhatti, A. R., and Weber, J. (1979): Protease of adenovirus type 2. *J. Biol. Chem.*, 254:12265–12268.
27. Bos, J. L., Polder, L. J., Bernards, R., Schrier, P. I., Van den Elsen, P. J., Van der Eb, A. J., and Van Ormondt, H. (1981): The 2.2kb E1b mRNA of human ad12 and ad5 codes for two tumor antigens starting at different AUG triplets. *Cell*, 27:121–131.
28. Brackman, K. H., Green, M., Wold, W. S. M., Cartas, M., Matsuo, T., and Hashimoto, S. (1980): Identification and peptide mapping of human adenovirus type 2-induced early polypeptides isolated by two-dimensional gel electrophoresis. *J. Biol. Chem.*, 255:6772–6779.
29. Branton, P. E., Lassam, N. J., Downey, J. F., Yee, S.-P., Graham, F. L., Mak, S., and Bayley, S. T. (1981): Protein kinase activity immunoprecipitated from adenovirus-infected cells by sera from tumor-bearing hamsters. *J. Virol.*, 37:601–608.
30. Breatnach, R., and Chambon, P. (1981): Organization and expression of eucaryotic split genes coding for proteins. *Annu. Rev. Biochem.*, 50:349–383.
31. Carter, T. H., and Blanton, R. A. (1978): Possible role of the 72,000-dalton DNA-binding protein in regulation of adenovirus type 5 early gene expression. *J. Virol.*, 25:664–674.
32. Carter, T. H., and Blanton, R. A. (1978): Autoregulation of adenovirus type 5 early gene expression. II. Effect of temperature-sensitive early mutations on virus RNA accumulation. *J. Virol.*, 28:450–456.
33. Carusi, E. A. (1977): Evidence for blocked termini in human adenovirus DNA. *Virology*, 76:380–394.
34. Celma, M. L., Pan, J., and Weissman, S. M. (1977): Studies of low molecular weight RNA from cells infected with adenovirus 2. I. The sequence at the 3' end of VA-RNAI. *J. Biol. Chem.*, 252:9032–9043.
35. Celma, M. L., Pan, J., and Weissman, S. M. (1977): Studies of low molecular weight RNA from cells infected with adenovirus 2. II. Heterogeneity at the 5' end of VA-RNAI. *J. Biol. Chem.*, 252:9043–9046.
36. Challberg, M. D., and Kelly, T. J., Jr. (1979): Adenovirus DNA replication *in vitro*. *Proc. Natl. Acad. Sci. USA*, 76:655–659.
37. Challberg, M. D., Desiderio, S. V., and Kelly, T. J., Jr. (1980): Adenovirus DNA replication in vitro: Characterization of a protein covalently linked to nascent DNA strands. *Proc. Natl. Acad. Sci. USA*, 77:5105–5109.
38. Challberg, M. D., and Kelly, T. J., Jr. (1981): Processing of the adenovirus terminal protein. *J. Virol.*, 38:272–277.
39. Challberg, S. S., and Ketner, G. (1981): Deletion mutants of adenovirus 2: Isolation and initial characterization of virus carrying mutations near the right end of the viral genome. *Virology*, 114:196–209.
40. Cherney, C. S., and Wilhelm, J. M. (1979): Differential translation in normal and adenovirus type 5-infected human cells and cell-free systems. *J. Virol.*, 30:533–542.
41. Chow, L. T., and Broker, T. R. (1978): The spliced structures of adenovirus 2 fiber message and other late mRNAs. *Cell*, 15:497–510.
42. Chow, L. T., Gelinas, R. E., Broker, T. R., and Roberts, R. J. (1977): An amazing sequence arrangement at the 5' ends of adenovirus 2 messenger RNA. *Cell*, 12:1–8.
43. Chow, L. T., Roberts, J. M., Lewis, J. B., and Broker, T. R. (1977): A map of cytoplasmic RNA transcripts from lytic adenovirus type 2, determined by electron microscopy of RNA:DNA hybrids. *Cell*, 11:819–836.
44. Chow, L. T., Broker, T. R., and Lewis, J. B. (1979): Complex splicing patterns of RNAs from the early regions of adenovirus-2. *J. Mol. Biol.*, 134:265–303.
45. Chow, L. T., Lewis, J. B., and Broker, T. R. (1980): RNA transcription and splicing at early and intermediate times after adenovirus 2 infection. *Cold Spring Harbor Symp. Quant. Biol.*, 44:401–414.
46. Colby, W. W., and Shenk, T. (1981): Adenovirus type 5 virions can be assembled in vivo in the absence of delectable polypeptide IX. *J. Virol.*, 39:977–980.

47. Collett, M. S., and Erikson, R. L. (1978): Protein kinase activity associated with the avian sarcoma virus src gene product. *Proc. Natl. Acad. Sci. USA*, 75:2021–2024.

48. Coombs, D. H., Robinson, A. J., Boduar, J. W., Jones, C. J., and Pearson, G. D. (1978): Detection of covalent DNA-protein complexes: The adenovirus DNA-terminal protein complex and HeLa DNA-protein complexes. *Cold Spring Harbor Symp. Quant. Biol.*, 43:741–753.

49. Corden, J., Engelking, H. M., and Pearson, G. D. (1976): Chromatin-like organization of the adenovirus chromosome. *Proc. Natl. Acad. Sci. USA*, 73:401–404.

50. Craig, E. A., and Raskas, H. J. (1974): Effect of cycloheximide on RNA metabolism early in productive infection with adenovirus 2. *J. Virol.*, 14:26–32.

51. De Leo, A. B., Jay, G., Apella, E., Dubois, G. C., Law, L. W., and Old, L. J. (1979): Detection of a transformation related antigen in chemically induced sarcomas and other transformed cells of the mouse. *Proc. Natl. Acad. Sci. USA*, 76:2420–2424.

52. Desideiro, S. V., and Kelly, T. J., Jr. (1981): Structure of the linkage between adenovirus DNA and the 55.000 molecular weight terminal protein. *J. Mol. Biol.*, 145:319–337.

53. Dijkema, R. (1981): Thesis, University of Leiden, Holland. The structure and organization of the transforming region of weakly oncogenic human adenovirus type 7.

54. Dijkema, R., and Dekker, B. M. M. (1979): The inverted terminal repetition of the DNA of weakly oncogenic adenovirus type 7. *Gene*, 8:7–15.

55. Dijkema, R., Dekker, B. M. M., Van der Feltz, M. J. M., and Van der Eb, A. J. (1979): Transformation of primary rat kidney cells by fragments of weakly oncogenic adenoviruses. *J. Virol.*, 32:943–950.

56. Dijkema, R., Dekker, B. M. M., and Van Ormondt, H. (1980): The nucleotide sequence of the transforming BglII-H fragment of adenovirus type 7 DNA. *Gene*, 9:141–156.

57. Dijkema, R., Dekker, B. M. M., Van Ormondt, H., de Waard, A., Maat, J., and Boyer, H. W. (1980): Gene organization of the transforming region of weakly oncogenic adenovirus type 7: The E1A region. *Gene*, 12:287–299.

58. Doerfler, W. (1981): DNA methylation—a regulatory signal in eukaryotic gene expression. *J. Gen. Virol.*, 57:1–20.

59. Doerfler, W. (1982): Uptake, fixation and expression of foreign DNA in mammalian cells: The organization of integrated adenovirus DNA sequences. *Curr. Top. Microbiol. Immunol.*, 101:127–194.

60. Doerfler, W., Lundholm, U., Rensing, U., and Philipson, L. (1973): Intracellular forms of adenovirus deoxyribonucleic acid. II. Isolation in dye-buoyant density gradients of a deoxyribonucleic acid–ribonucleic acid complex from KB cells infected with adenovirus type 2. *J. Virol.*, 12:793–807.

61. Doerfler, W., Stabel, S., Ibelgaufts, H., Sutter, D., Neumann, R., Groneberg, J., Scheidtmann, K. H., Deuring, R., and Winterhoff, U. (1980): Selectivity in integration sites of adenoviral DNA. *Cold Spring Harbor Symp. Quant. Biol.*, 44:551–564.

62. Dorsch-Häsler, K., Fisher, P., Weinstein, B., and Ginsberg, H. (1980): Patterns of viral DNA integration in cells transformed by wild type or DNA-binding protein mutants of adenovirus type 5 and effect of chemical carcinogenesis on integration. *J. Virol.*, 34:305–314.

63. Duering, R., Winterhoff, U., Tamanoi, F., Stabel, S., and Doerfler, W. (1981): Site of linkage between adenovirus type 12 and cell DNAs in hamster tumor line CLAC3. *Nature*, 293:81–84.

64. Dunn, A. R., and Hassell, J. A. (1977): A novel method to map transcripts: Evidence for homology between an adenovirus mRNA and discrete multiple regions of the viral genome. *Cell*, 12:23–36.

65. Dunn, A. R., Mathews, M. B., Chow, L. T., Sambrook, J., and Keller, W. (1978): A supplementary adenoviral leader sequence and its role in messenger translation. *Cell*, 15:511–526.

66. Edvardsson, B., Everitt, E., Jörnvall, H., and Philipson, L. (1976): Intermediates in adenovirus assembly. *J. Virol.*, 19:533–547.

67. Eggerding, F., and Raskas, H. J. (1978): Effect of protein synthesis inhibitors on viral mRNAs synthesized early in adenovirus type 2 infection. *J. Virol.*, 25:453–458.

68. Eick, D., and Doerfler, W. (1982): Integrated adenovirus type 12 DNA in the transformed hamster cell line T637: Sequence arrangement at the termini of viral DNA and mode of amplification. *J. Virol.*, 42:317–321.

69. Eick, D., Stabel, S., and Doerfler, W. (1980): Revertants of adenovirus type 12 transformed hamster cell line T637 as tools in the analysis of integration patterns. *J. Virol.*, 36:41–49.

70. Ellens, D. J., Sussenbach, J. S., and Jansz, H. S. (1974): Studies on the mechanism of replication of adenovirus DNA. III. Electron microscopy of replicating DNA. *Virology*, 61:427–442.

71. Enomoto, T., Lichy, J. H., Ikeda, J. E., and Hurwitz, J. (1981): Adenovirus DNA replication in

vitro. Purification of the terminal protein in a functional form. *Proc. Natl. Acad. Sci. USA*, 78:6779–6783.

72. Ensinger, M. J., and Ginsberg, H. S. (1972): Selection and preliminary characterization of temperature-sensitive mutants of type 5 adenovirus. *J. Virol.*, 10:328–339.

73. Esche, H., Schilling, R., and Doerfler, W. (1979): In vitro translation of adenovirus type 12-specific mRNA isolated from infected and transformed cells. *J. Virol.*, 30:21–31.

74. Esche, H., Mathews, M. B., and Lewis, J. B. (1980): Proteins and messenger RNAs of the transforming region of wild-type and mutant adenoviruses. *J. Mol. Biol.*, 142:399–417.

75. Evans, R. M., Fraser, N., Ziff, E., Weber, J., Wilson, M., and Darnell, J. E. (1977): The initiator site for RNA transcription in ad2 DNA. *Cell*, 12:733–739.

76. Everitt, E., Sundquist, B., Pettersson, U., and Philipson, L. (1973): Structural proteins of adenoviruses. X. Isolation and topography of low molecular weight antigens from the virion of adenovirus type 2. *Virology*, 52:130–147.

77. Fiers, W., Contreras, R., Haegeman, G., Rogiers, R., Van de Voorde, A., Van Heuverswyn, H., Van Herreweghe, J., Volckaert, G., and Ysebaert, M. (1978): Complete nucleotide sequence of SV40 DNA. *Nature*, 273:113–120.

78. Fire, A., Baker, C. C., Manley, J. L., Ziff, E. B., and Sharp, P. A. (1982): In vitro transcription of adenovirus. *J. Virol.*, 40:703–719.

79. Flint, S. J. (1980): Molecular biology of adenoviruses. In: *Viral Oncology*, edited by G. Klein, Raven Press, New York.

80. Flint, S. J., and Sharp, P. A. (1976): Adenovirus transcription. V. Quantitation of viral RNA sequences in adenovirus 2 infected and transformed cells. *J. Mol. Biol.*, 106:749–771.

81. Flint, S. J., Gallimore, P. H., and Sharp, P. A. (1975): Comparison of viral RNA sequences in adenovirus 2 transformed and lytically-infected cells. *J. Mol. Biol.*, 96:47–68.

82. Flint, S. J., Sambrook, J., Williams, J., and Sharp, P. A. (1976): Viral nucleic acid sequences in transformed cells. IV. A study of the sequences of adenovirus 5 DNA and RNA in four lines of adenovirus 5 transformed rodent cells using specific fragments of the viral genome. *Virology*, 72:456–470.

83. Fowlkes, D. M., Lord, S. T., Linné, T., Pettersson, U., and Philipson, L. (1979): Interaction between the adenovirus DNA-binding protein and double-stranded DNA. *J. Mol. Biol.*, 132:163–180.

84. Fowlkes, D. M., and Shenk, T. (1980): Transcriptional control regions of the adenovirus VAI RNA gene. *Cell*, 22:405–413.

85. Fraser, N. W., Nevins, J. R., Ziff, E., and Darnell, J. E. (1979): The major late adenovirus type-2 transcription unit: Termination is down stream from the last poly(A) site. *J. Mol. Biol.*, 129:643–656.

86. Fraser, N., Sehgal, P., and Darnell, J. E. (1979): Multiple discrete sites for premature RNA chain termination late in Ad2 infection: Enhancement by 5,6-dichloro-1-β-D-ribofuranosylbenzimidazole. *Proc. Natl. Acad. Sci. USA*, 76:2571–2575.

87. Frost, E., and Williams, J. (1978): Mapping temperature-sensitive and host-range mutations of adenovirus type 5 by marker rescue. *Virology*, 91:39–50.

88. Gallimore, P. H. (1974): Interactions of adenovirus type 2 with rat embryo cells: Permissiveness, transformation and *in vitro* characterization of adenovirus 2 transformed rat embryo cells. *J. Gen. Virol.*, 25:263–273.

89. Gallimore, P. H., Sharp, P. A., and Sambrook, J. (1974): Viral DNA in transformed cells. II. A study of the sequences of adenovirus 2 DNA in nine lines of transformed rat cells using specific fragments of the viral genome. *J. Mol. Biol.*, 89:49–72.

90. Galos, R. S., Williams, J., Binger, M. H., and Flint, S. J. (1979): Location of additional early gene sequences in the adenovirus chromosome. *Cell*, 17:945–956.

91. Galos, R. S., Williams, J., Shenk, T., and Jones, N. (1980): Physical location of host-range mutations of adenovirus type 5: Deletion and marker rescue mapping. *Virology*, 104:510–513.

92. Garon, C. F., Berry, K. W., and Rose, J. A. (1972): A unique form of terminal redundancy in adenovirus DNA molecules. *Proc. Natl. Acad. Sci. USA*, 69:2391–2395.

93. Garon, C. F., Berry, K., Hierholzer, J. C., and Rose, J. (1973): Mapping of base sequence heterologies between genomes from different adenovirus serotypes. *Virology*, 54:414–426.

94. Gelinas, R. E., and Roberts, R. J. (1977): One predominant 5′-undecanucleotide in adenovirus 2 late messenger RNAs. *Cell*, 11:533–544.

95. Gilead, Z., Jeng, Y., Wold, W. S. M., Sugawara, H., Rho, M., Harter, M. L., and Green, M.

(1976): Immunological identification of two adenovirus 2-induced early proteins possibly involved in cell transformation. *Nature*, 264:263–266.

96. Gilden, R. V., Kern, J., Lee, Y. K., Rapp, F., Melnick, J. L., Riggs, J. L., Lennette, E. H., Zbar, B., Rapp, H. J., Turner, H. C., and Huebner, R. J. (1970): Serologic surveys of human cancer patients for antibody to adenovirus T antigens. *Am. J. Epidemiol.*, 91:500–509.

97. Gingeras, T. R., Sciaky, D., Gelinas, R. E., Bing-Dang, J., Yen, C., Kelly, M., Bullock, P., Parsons, B., O'Neill, K., and Roberts, R. J. (1982): Nucleotide sequences from the adenovirus-2 genome. *J. Biol. Chem.*, 257:13475–13491.

98. Ginsberg, H. S. (1979): Adenovirus structural proteins. *Comprehensive Virology*, 13:409–457.

99. Ginsberg, H. S., Ensinger, M. J., Kaufman, R. S., Mayer, A. J., and Lundholm, U. (1974): Cell transformation: A study of regulation with types 5 and 12 adenovirus temperature sensitive mutants. *Cold Spring Harbor Symp. Quant. Biol.*, 39:419–426.

100. Goldberg, D. (1979): Thesis. Stanford University.

101. Goldenberg, C. J., and Raskas, H. J. (1981): In vitro splicing of purified precursor RNAs specified by early region 2 of the adenovirus 2 genome. *Proc. Natl. Acad. Sci. USA*, 78:5430–5434.

102. Graham, F. L., and Van der Eb, A. J. (1973): A new technique for the assay of infectivity of human adenovirus DNA. *Virology*, 52:456–467.

103. Graham, F. L., Abrahams, P. J., Mulder, C., Heijneker, H. L., Warnaar, S. O., de Vries, F. A. J., Fiers, W., and Van der Eb, A. J. (1974): Studies on *in vitro* transformation by DNA and DNA fragments of human adenoviruses and simian virus 40. *Cold Spring Harbor Symp. Quant. Biol.*, 39:637–750.

104. Graham, F. L., Van der Eb, A. J., and Heijneker, H. L. (1974): Size and location of the transforming region in human adenovirus type 5 DNA. *Nature*, 251:687–691.

105. Graham, F. L., Smiley, J., Russell, W. C., and Nairu, R. (1977): Characterization of a human cell line transformed by DNA from human adenovirus type 5. *J. Gen. Virol.*, 36:59–72.

106. Graham, F. L., Harrison, T., and Williams, J. (1978): Defective transforming capacity of adenovirus type-5 host-range mutants. *Virology*, 86:10–21.

107. Green, M. (1970): Oncogenic viruses. *Annu. Rev. Biochem.*, 39:701–756.

108. Green, M., Pina, M., Kimes, R. C., Wensink, P. C., MacHattie, L. A., and Thomas, C. A., Jr. (1967): Adenovirus DNA: I. Molecular weight and conformation. *Proc. Natl. Acad. Sci. USA*, 57:1302–1309.

109. Green, M., and Mackey, J. K. (1977): Are oncogenic human adenoviruses associated with human cancer? Analysis of human tumors for adenovirus transforming gene sequences. In: *Origins of Human Cancer*, edited by H. H. Hiatt, J. D. Watson, and J. A. Winsten, pp. 1013–1026. Cold Spring Harbor Laboratory, Cold Spring Harbor, N.Y.

110. Green, M., Wold, W. S. M., Brackman, K. H., and Cartas, M. A. (1979): Identification of families of overlapping polypeptides coded by early region 1 of human adenovirus type 2. *Virology*, 97:275–286.

111. Green, M., Symington, J. Brackman, K. H., Cartas, M. A., Thornton, H., and Young, L. (1981): Immunological and chemical identification of intracellular forms of adenovirus type 2 terminal protein. *J. Virol.*, 40:541–550.

112. Green, M., Mackey, J. K., Wold, W. S. M., and Rigden, P. (1979): Thirty-one human adenovirus serotypes (Ad1-Ad31) form five groups (A-E) based upon DNA genome homologies. *Virology*, 93:481–492.

113. Green, M. R., Chinnadurai, G., Mackey, J. K., and Green, M. (1976): A unique pattern of integrated viral genes in hamster cells transformed by highly oncogenic human adenovirus 12. *Cell*, 7:419–428.

114. Green, M., Wold, W. S. M., Brackmann, K., and Cartas, M. A. (1980): Studies of early proteins and transformation proteins of human adenoviruses. *Cold Spring Harbor Symp. Quant. Biol.*, 44:457–470.

115. Grodzicker, T., and Klessig, D. F. (1980): Expression of unselected adenovirus genes in human cells co-transformed with the HSV-1 tk gene and adenovirus 2 DNA. *Cell*, 21:453–463.

116. Groneberg, J., and Doerfler, W. (1979): Revertants of adenovirus type 12 transformed hamster cells have lost part of the viral genomes. *Int. J. Cancer*, 24:67–74.

117. Guilfoyle, R., and Weinmann, R. (1981): Control region for adenovirus VA RNA transcription. *Proc. Natl. Acad. Sci. USA*, 78:3378–3382.

118. Günthert, U., Schweiger, M., Stupp, M., and Doerfler, W. (1976): DNA methylation in adenovirus, adenovirus transformed cells, and host cells. *Proc. Natl. Acad. Sci. USA*, 73:3923–3927.

119. Halbert, D. N., and Raskas, H. J. (1982): Tryptic and chymotryptic methionine peptide analysis of the *in vitro* translation products specified by the transforming region of adenovirus type 2. *Virology*, 116:406–418.
120. Halbert, D. N., Spector, D. J., and Raskas, H. J. (1979): In vitro translation products specified by the transforming region of adenovirus type 2. *J. Virol.*, 31:621–629.
121. Hammarsköld, M.-L., and Winberg, G. (1980): Encapsidation of adenovirus 16 DNA is directed by a small DNA sequence at the left end of the genome. *Cell*, 20:787–795.
122. Harrison, T., Graham, F., and Williams, J. (1977): Host range mutants of adenovirus type 5 defective for growth in HeLa cells. *Virology*, 77:319–329.
123. Harter, M. L., and Lewis, J. B. (1978): Adenovirus type 2 early proteins synthesized in vitro and in vivo: Identification in infected cells of the 38,000- to 50,000-molecular-weight protein encoded by the left end of the adenovirus type 2 genome. *J. Virol.*, 26:736–749.
124. Harter, M. L., Shanmugam, G., Wold, W. S. M., and Green, M. (1976): Detection of adenovirus type 2-induced early polypeptides using cycloheximide pretreatment to enhance viral protein synthesis. *J. Virol.*, 19:232–242.
125. Hashimoto, S., and Green, M. (1980): Adenovirus 2 early messenger RNA-genome mapping of 5'-terminal RNase T1 oligonucleotides and heterogeneity of 5'-termini. *J. Biol. Chem.*, 255:6780–6788.
126. Horwitz, M. S. (1976): Bidirectional replication of adenovirus type 2 DNA. *J. Virol.*, 18:307–315.
127. Horwitz, M. S. (1978): Temperature-sensitive replication of H5ts125 adenovirus DNA in vitro. *Proc. Natl. Acad. Sci. USA*, 75:4291–4295.
128. Houweling, A., Van den Elsen, P. J., and Van der Eb, A. J. (1980): Partial transformation of primary rat cells by the leftmost 4.5% fragment of adenovirus 5 DNA. *Virology*, 105:537–550.
129. Huebner, R. J. (1967): Adenovirus-directed tumor and T-antigens. In: *Perspectives in Virology, Vol. 5*, edited by M. Pollard, pp. 147–167. Academic Press, New York.
130. Huebner, R. J., Rowe, W. P., and Lane, W. T. (1962): Oncogenic effects in hamsters of human adenovirus type 12 and 18. *Proc. Natl. Acad. Sci. USA*, 48:2051–2058.
131. Huebner, R. J., Rowe, W. P., Turner, H. C., and Lane, W. T. (1963): Specific adenovirus complement-fixing antigens in virus-free hamster and rat tumors. *Proc. Natl. Acad. Sci. USA*, 50:379–389.
132. Huebner, R. J., Pereira, H. G., Allison, A. C., Hollinshead, A. C., and Turner, H. C. (1964): Production of type-specific C antigen in virus-free hamster tumor cells induced by adenovirus type 12. *Proc. Natl. Acad. Sci. USA*, 51:432–439.
133. Ibelgaufts, H., Doerfler, W., Scheidtmann, K. H., and Wechsler, W. (1980): Adenovirus type 12 induced rat tumor cells of neuroepithelial origin: Persistence and expression of the viral genome. *J. Virol.*, 33:423–427.
134. Ikeda, J.-E., Enomoto, T., and Hurwitz, J. (1981): Replication of adenovirus DNA-protein complex with purified proteins. *Proc. Natl. Acad. Sci. USA*, 78:884–888.
135. Jeng, T. H., Wold, W. S. M., Sugawara, K., and Green, M. (1978): Evidence for an adenovirus type 2-coded early glycoprotein. *J. Virol.*, 28:314–323.
136. Jochemsen, H. (1981): Thesis, Studies on the transforming genes and their products of human adenovirus types 12 and 5. University of Leiden, Holland.
137. Jochemsen, H., Hertoghs, J. J. L., Lupker, J. H., Davis, A., and Van der Eb, A. J. (1981): In vitro synthesis of adenovirus type 5 T antigens. II. Translation of virus-specific RNA from cells transformed by fragments of adenovirus type 5 DNA. *J. Virol.*, 37:530–534.
138. Johansson, K., Persson, H., Lewis, A. M., Pettersson, U., Tibbetts, C., and Philipson, L. (1978): Viral DNA sequences and gene products in hamster cells transformed by adenovirus type 2. *J. Virol.*, 27:628–639.
139. Jones, N., and Shenk, T. (1979): Isolation of adenovirus type 5 host range deletion mutants defective for transformation of rat embryo cells. *Cell*, 17:683–689.
140. Jones, N., and Shenk, T. (1979): An adenovirus type 5 early gene functions regulates expression of other early viral genes. *Proc. Natl. Acad. Sci. USA*, 76:3665–3669.
141. Kaplan, L. M., Kleinman, R. E., and Horwitz, M. S. (1977): Replication of adenovirus type 2 DNA *in vitro*. *Proc. Natl. Acad. Sci. USA*, 74:4425.
142. Kaplan, L. M., Hiroyoshi, A., Hurwitz, J., and Horwitz, M. (1979): Complementation of the temperature-sensitive defect in H5ts125 adenovirus DNA replication in vitro. *Proc. Natl. Acad. Sci. USA*, 76:5534–5538.

143. Kathman, P., Schick, J., Winnacker, E.-L., and Doerfler, W. (1976): Isolation and characterization of temperature-sensitive mutants of adenovirus type 2. *J. Virol.*, 19:43–53.

144. Katze, M. G., Persson, H., and Philipson, L. (1981): Control of adenovirus early gene expression: A post-transcriptional control mediated by region E1A products. *Mol. Cell. Biol.*, 1:807–813.

145. Katze, M. G., Persson, H., and Philipson, L. (1982): A leftward reading transcript from the transforming region of adenovirus DNA encodes a low molecular weight polypeptide *Embo.*, 1:783–790.

146. Kitchingman, G. R., and Westphal, H. (1980): The structure of adenovirus 2 early nuclear and cytoplasmic RNAs. *J. Mol. Biol.*, 137:23–48.

147. Kitchingman, G., Lai, S. P., and Westphal, H. (1977): Loop structures in hybrids of early RNA and the separated strands of adenovirus DNA. *Proc. Natl. Acad. Sci. USA*, 74:4392–4395.

148. Klein, H., Maltzman, W., and Levine, A. J. (1979): Structure-function relationships of the adenovirus DNA-binding protein. *J. Biol. Chem.*, 254:11051–11060.

149. Klessig, D. F. (1977): Isolation of a variant of human adenovirus serotype 2 that multiplies efficiently on monkey cells. *J. Virol.*, 21:1243–1246.

150. Klessig, D. F. (1977): Two adenovirus mRNAs have a common 5' terminal leader sequence encoded at least 10 kb upstream from their main coding regions. *Cell*, 12:9–21.

151. Klessig, D. F., and Chow, L. T. (1980): Incomplete splicing and deficient accumulation of the fiber messenger RNA in monkey cells infected by human adenovirus type 2. *J. Mol. Biol.*, 139:221–242.

152. Klessig, D. F., and Anderson, C. W. (1975): Block to multiplication of adenovirus serotype 2 in monkey cells. *J. Virol.*, 16:1650–1668.

153. Klessig, D. F., and Grodzicker, T. (1979): Mutations that allow human ad2 and ad5 to express late genes in monkey cells map in the viral gene encoding the 72K DNA binding protein. *Cell*, 17:957–966.

154. Korn, L. J. (1982): Transcription of *Xenopus* 5S ribosomal RNA genes. *Nature*, 295:101–105.

155. Kozak, M. (1978): How do eucaryotic ribosomes select initiation regions in messenger RNA? *Cell*, 15:1109–1123.

156. Kruijer, W., Van Schaik, F. M. A., and Sussenbach, J. S. (1981): Structure and organization of the gene coding for the DNA binding protein of adenovirus type 5. *Nucleic Acids Res.*, 9:4439–4457.

157. Kuhlman, I., and Doerfler, W. (1982): Shift in extent and pattern of DNA methylation upon explanation and subcultivation of adenovirus type 12 induced hamster tumor cells. *Virology*, 118:169–180.

158. Kvist, S., Östberg, L., Persson, H., Philipson, L., and Pettersson, P. A. (1978): Molecular association between transplantation antigens and a cell surface antigen in an adenovirus-transformed cell line. *Proc. Natl. Acad. Sci. USA*, 75:5674–5678.

159. Lacy, S., Sr., and Green, M. (1964): Biochemical studies on adenovirus multiplication. VII. Homology between DNA's of tumorigenic and nontumorigenic human adenoviruses. *Proc. Natl. Acad. Sci. USA*, 52:1053–1059.

160. Lacy, S., Sr., and Green, M. (1965): Genetic relatedness of tumorigenic human adenovirus type 7,12,18. *Science*, 150:1296–1298.

161. Lacy, S., Sr., and Green, M. (1967): The mechanism of viral carcinogenesis by DNA mammalian viruses: DNA-DNA homology relationship among the "weakly" oncogenic human adenoviruses. *J. Gen. Virol.*, 1:413–418.

162. Lane, D., and Crawford, L. V. (1979): T-antigen is bound to a host protein in SV40 transformed cells. *Nature*, 278:261–263.

163. Lassam, N. J., Bayley, S. T., and Graham, F. L. (1978): Synthesis of DNA, late polypeptides, and infectious virus by host-range mutants of adenovirus 5 in nonpermissive cells. *Virology*, 87:463–467.

164. Lassam, N. J., Bayley, S. T., and Graham, F. L. (1979): Tumor antigens of human ad5 in transformed cells and in cells infected with transformation-defective host range mutants. *Cell*, 18:781–791.

165. Lassam, N. J., Bayley, S. T., Graham, F. L., and Branton, P. E. (1979): Immunoprecipitation of protein kinase activity from adenovirus 5-infected cells using antiserum directed against tumour antigens. *Nature*, 277:241–243.

166. Lavelle, G., Patch, C., Khoury, G., and Rose, J. (1975): Isolation and partial characterization of single stranded adenoviral DNA produced during synthesis of adenovirus type 2 DNA. *J. Virol.*, 16:775–782.

167. Laver, W. G. (1970): Isolation of an arginine-rich protein from particles of adenovirus type 2. *Virology*, 41:15–24.
168. Laver, W. G., Younghusband, H. B., and Wrigley, N. G. (1971): Purification and properties of chick embryo lethal orphan virus (an avian adenovirus). *Virology*, 45:598–614.
169. Lechner, R. L., and Kelly, T. J., Jr. (1977): The structure of replicating adenovirus 2 DNA molecules. *Cell*, 12:1007–1020.
170. Lenk, R. P., Maizel, J. V., and Crouch, R. J. (1982): Expression of two late adenovirus genes is altered by introducing antibodies against ribonucleoprotein into living HeLa cells. *Eur. J. Biochem.*, 121:475–482.
171. Lerner, M. R., and Steitz, J. A. (1979): Antibodies to small nuclear RNAs complexed with proteins are produced by patients with systemic lupus erythematosus. *Proc. Natl. Acad. Sci. USA*, 76:5495–5499.
172. Lerner, M. R., Boyle, J. A., Mount, S. M., Wolin, S. L., and Steitz, J. A. (1979): Are snRNPs involved in splicing? *Nature*, 283:220–224.
173. Levinson, A., Levine, A. J., Anderson, S., Osborn, M., Rosenwirth, B., and Weber, K. (1976): The relationship between group C adenovirus tumor antigen and the adenovirus single-strand DNA binding protein. *Cell*, 7:575–584.
174. Levinson, A., and Levine, A. J. (1977): The isolation and identification of the adenovirus group C tumor antigens. *Virology*, 76:1–11.
175. Levinson, A. D., and Levine, A. J. (1977): The group C adenovirus tumor antigens: Infected and transformed cells and a peptide map analysis. *Cell*, 11:871–879.
176. Lewis, A. M., Jr., Wiese, W. H., and Rowe, W. P. (1967): The presence of antibodies in human serum to early (T) adenovirus antigens. *Proc. Natl. Acad. Sci. USA*, 57:622–629.
177. Lewis, A. M., Jr., Levin, M. J., Wiese, W. H., Crumpacker, C. S., and Henry, P. H. (1969): A non-defective (competent) adenovirus-SV40 hybrid isolated from the ad2-SV40 hybrid population. *Proc. Natl. Acad. Sci. USA*, 63:1128–1135.
178. Lewis, A. M., Jr., Rabson, A. S., and Levine, A. S. (1974): Studies of nondefective adenovirus 2-simian virus 40 hybrid viruses. Transformation of hamster kidney cells by adenovirus 2 and the nondefective hybrid viruses. *J. Virol.*, 13:1291–1301.
179. Lewis, J. B., Atkins, J. F., Baum, P. R., Solem, R., Gesteland, R. B., and Anderson, C. W. (1976): Location and identification of the genes for adenovirus type 2 early polypeptides. *Cell*, 7:141–151.
180. Lewis, J. B., Anderson, C. W., and Atkins, J. F. (1977): Further mapping of late adenovirus genes by cell-free translation of RNA selected by hybridization to specific DNA fragments. *Cell*, 12:37–44.
181. Lewis, J. B., and Mathews, M. B. (1980): Control of adenovirus early gene expression: A class of immediate early products. *Cell*, 21:303–313.
182. Lewis, J. B., Esche, H., Smart, J. E., Stillman, B. W., Harter, M. L., and Mathews, M. B. (1980): Organization and expression of the left third of the genome of adenovirus. *Cold Spring Harbor Symp. Quant. Biol.*, 44:493–508.
183. Lichy, J. H., Horwitz, M. S., and Hurwitz, J. (1981): Formation of a covalent complex between the 80.000-dalton adenovirus terminal protein and 5'-dCMP in vitro. *Proc. Natl. Acad. Sci. USA*, 78:2678–2682.
184. Linné, T., Jörnvall, H., and Philipson, L. (1977): Purification and characterization of the phosphorylated DNA-binding protein from adenovirus type 2 infected cells, *Eur. J. Biochem.*, 76:481–491.
185. Linzer, D. I. H., and Levine, H. J. (1979): Characterization of a 54K dalton cellular SV40 tumor antigen present in SV40 transformed cells and uninfected embryonal carcinoma cells. *Cell*, 17:43–52.
186. Lonberg-Holm, K., and Philipson, L. (1969): Early events of virus infection in an adenovirus system. *J. Virol.*, 4:323–338.
187. Longiaru, M., Ikeda, J. E., Jarkovsky, Z., Horwitz, S. B., and Horwitz, M. S. (1979): The effect of aphidicolin on adenovirus DNA synthesis. *Nucleic Acids Res.*, 6:3369–3386.
188. Lupker, J. H., Davis, A., Jochemsen, H., and Van der Eb, A. J. (1981): In vitro synthesis of adenovirus type 5 T antigens. I. Translation of early region 1-specific RNA from lytically infected cells. *J. Virol.*, 37:524–529.
189. Mackey, J., Wold, W., Rigden, P., and Green, M. (1979): Transforming region of group A, B,

and C adenoviruses: DNA homology studies with twenty-nine human adenovirus serotypes. *J. Virol.*, 29:1056–1064.

190. Maizel, J. V., Jr., White, D. O., and Scharff, M. D. (1968): The polypeptides of adenovirus. II. Soluble proteins, cores, top components and the structure of the virion. *Virology*, 36:115–125.

191. Manley, J. L., Fire, A., Cano, A., Sharp, P. A., and Gefter, M. L. (1980): DNA dependent transcription of adenovirus genes in a soluble whole-cell extract. *Proc. Natl. Acad. Sci. USA*, 77:3855–3859.

192. Mathews, M. B. (1975): Genes for VA-RNA in adenovirus 2. *Cell*, 6:223–229.

193. Mathews, M. B. (1980): Binding of adenovirus VA RNA to mRNA: A possible role in splicing? *Nature*, 285:575–577.

194. Mathews, M. B., and Pettersson, U. (1978): The low molecular weight RNAs of adenovirus 2-infected cells. *J. Mol. Biol.*, 119:293–328.

195. Mathews, M. B., and Grodzicker, T. (1981): Virus-associated RNAs of naturally occurring strains and variants of group C adenoviruses. *J. Virol.*, 38:849–862.

196. Mathis, D. J., Elkaim, R., Kedinger, C., Sassone-Corsi, P., and Chambon, P. (1981): Specific in vitro initiation of transcription on the adenovirus type 2 early and late EII transcription units. *Proc. Natl. Acad. Sci. USA*, 78:7383–7387.

197. Matsuo, T., Hashimoto, S., Wold, W. S. M., and Green, M. (1982): Identification of adenovirus type 2 early region E4 polypeptides by in vitro translation and tryptic peptide map analysis. *J. Virol.*, 41:334–339.

198. Mak, S., Mak, I., Smiley, J. R., and Graham, F. L. (1979): Tumorigenicity and viral gene expression in rat cells transformed by ad12 virions or by the EcoRI C fragment of ad12 DNA. *Virology*, 98:456–460.

199. Mayer, A. J., and Ginsberg, H. S. (1977): Persistence of type 5 adenovirus DNA in cells transformed by a temperature sensitive mutant, H5ts125. *Proc. Natl. Acad. Sci. USA*, 74:785–788.

200. McAllister, R. M., Gilden, R. V., and Green, M. (1972): Adenoviruses in human cancer. *Lancet*, 1:831–833.

201. McAllister, R. M., Nicolson, M. O., Lewis, A. M., Jr., Macpherson, I., and Huebner, R. J. (1969): Transformation of rat embryo cells by adenovirus type 1. *J. Gen. Virol.*, 4:29–36.

202. McAllister, R. M., Nicolson, M. O., Reed, G., Kern, J., Gilden, V., and Huebner, R. J. (1969): Transformation of rodent cells by adenovirus 19 and other group D adenoviruses. *J. Natl. Cancer Inst.*, 43:917–923.

203. McGrogan, M., and Raskas, H. J. (1978): Two regions of the adenovirus 2 genome specify families of late polysomal RNAs containing common sequences. *Proc. Natl. Acad. Sci. USA*, 75:625–629.

204. McKinnon, R. D., Bacchetti, S., and Graham, F. L. (1982): Tn5 mutagenesis of the transforming genes of human adenovirus type 5. *Gene*, 19:33–42.

205. Miller, J. S., Ricciardi, R., Roberts, B. E., Paterson, B., and Mathews, M. B. (1980): Arrangement of messenger RNAs and protein coding sequences in the major late transcription unit of adenovirus 2. *J. Mol. Biol.*, 142:455–488.

206. Montell, C., Fisher, E. F., Caruthers, M. H., and Berk, A. J., (1982): Resolving the functions of overlapping viral genes by site-specific mutagenesis at a mRNA splice site. *Nature*, 295:380–384.

207. Murray, V., and Holliday, R. (1979): Mechanism for RNA splicing of gene transcripts. *F.E.B.S. Lett.*, 106:5–7.

208. Nevins, J. R. (1981): Mechanism of activation of early viral transcription by the adenovirus E1A gene products. *Cell*, 26:213–220.

209. Nevins, J. R., and Darnell, J. E. (1978): Groups of adenovirus type 2 mRNAs derived from a large primary transcript: Probable nuclear origin and possible common 3'-ends. *J. Virol.*, 25:811–823.

210. Nevins, J. R., and Darnell, J. E. (1978): Steps in the processing of ad2 mRNA: poly(A)⁺ nuclear sequences are conserved and poly(A) addition precedes splicing. *Cell*, 15:1477–1493.

211. Nevins, J. R., Ginsberg, H. S., Blanchard, J. M., Wilson, M. C., and Darnell, J. E. (1979): Regulation of the primary expression of early adenovirus transcription units. *J. Virol.*, 32:727–733.

212. Nevins, J. R., and Winkler, J. J. (1980): Regulation of early adenovirus transcription: A protein product of early region 2 specifically represses region 4 transcription. *Proc. Natl. Acad. Sci. USA*, 77:1893–1897.

213. Nevins, J. R., and Wilson, M. C. (1981): Regulation of adenovirus-2 gene expression at the level of transcriptional termination and RNA processing. *Nature*, 290:113–118.
214. Nicolas, J. C., Suarez, F., Levine, A. J., and Girard, M. (1981): Temperature-independent revertants of adenovirus H5 + s125 and Ht + s107 mutants in the DNA binding protein: Isolation of a new class of host range temperature conditional revertants. *Virology*, 108:521–524.
215. Norrby, E. (1968): Biological significance of structural adenovirus components. *Curr. Top. Microbiol. Immunol.*, 43:1–43.
216. Norrby, E., Bartha, A., Boulanger, P., Dreizin, R. S., Ginsberg, H. S., Kalter, S. S., Kawamura, H., Rowe, H. P., Russell, W. C., Schlesinger, R. W., and Wigand, R. (1976): Adenoviridae. *Intervirology*, 7:117.
217. Ortin, J., Scheidtmann, K. H., Greenberg, R., Westphal, H., and Doerfler, W. (1976): Transcription of the genome of adenovirus type 12. III. Maps of stable RNA from productively infected human cells and abortively infected human cells and abortively infected and transformed hamster cells. *J. Virol.*, 20:355–372.
218. Pan, J., Celma, M. L., and Weissman, S. M. (1977): Studies of low molecular weight RNA from cells infected with adenovirus 2. III. The sequence of the promoter for VA RNAI. *J. Biol. Chem.*, 252:9047–9054.
219. Pearson, G. D. (1975): Intermediates in adenovirus type 2 replication. *J. Virol.*, 16:17–26.
220. Perricaudet, M., Akusjärvi, G., Virtanen, A., and Pettersson, U. (1979): Structure of two spliced mRNAs from the transforming region of human subgroup C adenoviruses. *Nature*, 281:694–696.
221. Perricaudet, M., Le Moullec, J. P., and Pettersson, U. (1980): The predicted structure of two adenovirus T-antigens. *Proc. Natl. Acad. Sci. USA*, 77:3778–3782.
222. Perricaudet, M., Le Moullec, J.-M., Tiollais, P., and Pettersson, U. (1980): Structure of two adenovirus type 12 transforming polypeptides and their evolutionary implications. *Nature*, 288:174–176.
223. Persson, H., Pettersson, U., and Mathews, M. B. (1978): Synthesis of a structural adenovirus polypeptide in the absence of viral DNA replication. *Virology*, 90:67–79.
224. Persson, H., Öberg, B., and Philipson, L. (1978): Purification and characterization of an early protein (E14K) from adenovirus type 2-infected cells. *J. Virol.*, 28:119–139.
225. Persson, H., Signäs, C., and Philipson, L. (1979): Purification and characterization of an early glycoprotein from adenovirus type 2-infected cells. *J. Virol.*, 29:938–948.
226. Persson, H., Mathisen, B., Philipson, L., and Pettersson, U. (1979): A maturation protein in adenovirus morphogenesis. *Virology*, 93:198–208.
227. Persson, H., Kvist, S., Östberg, L., Peterson, P. A., and Philipson, L. (1979): The early adenovirus glycoprotein E3-19K and its association with transplantation antigens. *Cold Spring Harbor Symp. Quant. Biol.*, 44:509–517.
228. Persson, H., Jansson, M., and Philipson, L. (1980): Synthesis of and genomic site for an adenovirus type 2 early glycoprotein. *J. Mol. Biol.*, 136:375–394.
229. Persson, H., Jörnvall, H., and Zabielski, J. (1980): Multiple mRNA species for the precursor to an adenovirus-encoded glycoprotein: Identification and structure of the signal sequence. *Proc. Natl. Acad. Sci. USA*, 77:6349–6353.
230. Persson, H., Monstein, H.-J., Akusjärvi, G., and Philipson, L. (1981): Adenovirus early gene products may control viral mRNA accumulation and translation *in vivo*. *Cell*, 23:485–496.
231. Persson, H., Katze, M. G., and Philipson, L. (1981): Control of adenovirus early gene expression: Accumulation of viral mRNA after infection of transformed cells. *J. Virol.*, 40:358–366.
232. Persson, H., and Philipson, L. (1982): Regulation of adenovirus gene expression. *Curr. Top. Microbiol. Immunol.*, 97:157–203.
233. Persson, H., Katze, M. G., and Philipson, L. (1982): An adenovirus tumor antigen associated with membranes in vivo and in vitro. *J. Virol.*, 42:905–917.
234. Pettersson, U. (1973): Some unusual properties of replicating adenovirus type 2 DNA. *J. Mol. Biol.*, 81:521–527.
235. Pettersson, U., and Philipson, L. (1975): Location of sequences on the adenovirus genome coding for the 5.5S RNA. *Cell*, 6:1–4.
236. Pettersson, U., Tibbetts, C., and Philipson, L. (1976): Hybridization maps of early and late mRNA sequences on the adenovirus type 2 genome. *J. Mol. Biol.*, 101:479–502.
237. Pettersson, U., and Mathews, M. B. (1977): The gene and messenger RNA for adenovirus polypeptide IX. *Cell*, 12:741–750.

238. Philipson, L. (1979): Adenovirus proteins and their messenger RNAs. *Adv. Virus Res.*,25:357–405.
239. Philipson, L., Lonberg-Holm, K., and Pettersson, U. (1968): Virus receptor interaction in an adenovirus system. *J. Virol.*, 2:1064–1075.
240. Philipson, L., Pettersson, U., Lindberg, U., Tibbetts, C., Vennström, B., and Persson, T. (1974): RNA synthesis and processing in adenovirus infected cells. *Cold Spring Harbor Symp. Quant. Biol.*, 39:447–456.
241. Pina, M., and Green, M. (1965): Biochemical studies on adenovirus multiplication. IX. Chemical and base composition analysis of 28 human adenoviruses. *Proc. Natl. Acad. Sci. USA*, 54:547–551.
242. Pina, M., and Green, M. (1968): Base composition of the DNA of oncogenic simian adenovirus SA7 and homology with human adenovirus DNAs. *Virology*, 36:321–323.
243. Pincus, S., Robertson, W., and Rekosh, D. M. K. (1981): Characterization of the effect of aphidicholin on adenovirus DNA replication: Evidence in support of a protein primer model of initiation. *Nucleic Acids Res.*, 9:4919–4938.
244. Prage, L., and Pettersson, U. (1971): Structural proteins of adenoviruses. VII. Purification and properties of an arginine-rich core protein from adenovirus type 2 and type 3. *Virology*, 45:364–373.
245. Prage, L., Pettersson, U., and Philipson, L. (1968): Internal basic proteins in adenovirus. *Virology*, 36:508–511.
246. Price, R., and Penman, S. (1972): Transcription of the adenovirus genome by an amanitine-sensitive ribonucleic acid polymerase in HeLa cells. *J. Virol.*, 9:621–626.
247. Rabek, J. P., Zakian, V. A., and Levine, A. J. (1981): The SV40 A gene product suppresses the adenovirus H5+ts125 defect in DNA replication. *Virology*, 109:290–302.
248. Rabson, A. S., O'Conor, G. T., Berezesky, I. K., and Paul, F. J. (1964): Tumors produced by adenovirus 12 in mastomys and mice. *J. Natl. Cancer Inst.*, 32:77–87.
249. Rabson, A. S., O'Conor, G. T., Berezesky, I. K., and Paul, J. F. (1964): Enhancement of adenovirus growth in African Green monkey kidney cell cultures by SV40. *Proc. Soc. Exp. Biol. Med.*, 116:187–190.
250. Reddy, V. B., Ghosh, P. K., Lebowith, P., Piatak, M., and Weissman, S. M. (1979): Simian virus 40 early mRNAs. I. Genomic localization of 3' and 5' termini and two major splices in mRNA from transformed and lytically infected cells. *J. Virol.*, 30:279–296.
251. Reich, P. R., Forget, B. G., Weissman, S. H., and Rose, J. A. (1966): RNA of low molecular weight in KB cells infected with adenovirus type 2. *J. Mol. Biol.*, 17:428–439.
252. Rekosh, D. M. K., Russell, W. C., Bellett, A. J. D., and Robinson, A. J. (1977): Identification of a protein linked to the ends of adenovirus DNA. *Cell*, 11:283–295.
253. Riccardi, R. P., Jones, R. L., Cepko, C. L., Sharp, P. A., and Roberts, B. E. (1981): Expression of early adenovirus genes requires a viral encoded acidic polypeptide. *Proc. Natl. Acad. Sci. USA*, 78:6121–6125.
254. Robin, J., Bourgoux-Ramoizy, D., and Bourgaux, P. (1973): Single-stranded regions in replicating DNA of adenovirus type 2. *J. Gen. Virol.*, 20:233–237.
255. Robinson, A. J., Younghusband, H. B., and Bellett, A. J. D. (1973): A circular DNA-protein complex from adenoviruses. *Virology*, 56:54–69.
256. Robinson, A. J., and Bellett, A. J. D. (1974): A circular DNA-protein complex from adenoviruses and its possible role in DNA replication. *Cold Spring Harbor Symp. Quant. Biol.*, 39:523–531.
257. Rogers, J., and Wall, R. (1980): A mechanism for RNA splicing. *Proc. Natl. Acad. Sci. USA*, 77:1877–1879.
258. Rosenwirth, B., Shiroki, K., Levine, A. J., and Shimojo, H. (1975): Isolation and characterization of adenovirus type 12 DNA binding proteins. *Virology*, 67:14–23.
259. Ross, S., and Levine, A. J. (1979): The genomic map position of the adenovirus type 2 glycoprotein. *Virology*, 99:427–430.
260. Ross, S. R., Flint, S. J., and Levine, A. J. (1980): Identification of the adenovirus early proteins and their genomic map positions. *Virology*, 100:419–432.
261. Ross, S. R., Levine, A. J., Galos, R. S., Williams, J., and Shenk, T. (1980): Early viral proteins in HeLa cells infected with adenovirus type 5 host range mutants. *Virology*, 103:475–492.
262. Rowe, W. P., and Lewis, A. M., Jr. (1968): Serologic surveys for viral antibodies in cancer patients. *Cancer Res.*, 28:19–20.

263. Rowe, D. T., and Graham, F. L. (1981): Complementation of adenovirus type 5 host range mutants by adenovirus type 12 in coinfected HeLa and BHK-21 cells. *J. Virol.*, 38:191–197.

264. Ruben, M., Bacchetti, S., and Graham, F. L. (1982): Integration and expression of viral DNA in cells transformed by host-range mutants of adenovirus type 5. *J. Virol.*, 41:674–685.

265. Saborio, J. L., and Öberg, B. (1976): *In vivo* and *in vitro* synthesis of adenovirus type 2 early proteins. *J. Virol.*, 17:865–875.

266. Sambrook, J., Botchan, M., Gallimore, P., Ozanne, B., Pettersson, U., Williams, J., and Sharp, P. A. (1975): Viral DNA sequences in cells transformed by simian virus 40, adenovirus type 2 and adenovirus type 5. *Cold Spring Harbor Symp. Quant. Biol.*, 39:615–632.

267. Sambrook, J., Greene, R., Stringer, J., Mitchison, J., Hu, S. L., and Botchan, M. (1980): Analysis of the sites of integration of viral DNA sequences in rat cells transformed by adenovirus 2 or SV40. *Cold Spring Harbor Symp. Quant. Biol.*, 44:569–584.

268. Sarnow, P., Ho, Y. S., Williams, J., and Levine, A. J. (1982): Adenovirus E1B-58kd tumor antigen and SV40 large tumor antigen are physically associated with the same 54kd cellular protein in transformed cells. *Cell*, 28:387–394.

269. Schechter, N. M., Davies, W., and Anderson, C. W. (1980): Adenovirus coded DNA binding protein. Isolation physical properties and effects of proteolytic degradation. *Biochemistry*, 19:2802–2810.

270. Schenk, T., Jones, N., Colby, W., and Fowlkes, D. (1979): Functional analysis of adenovirus type 5 host range deletion mutants defective for transformation of rat embryo cells. *Cold Spring Harbor Symp. Quant. Biol.*, 44:367–375.

271. Schilling, R., Weingärtner, B., and Winnacker, E. L. (1974): Adenovirus type 2 replication. *Cold Spring Harbor Symp. Quant. Biol.*, 39:523–531.

272. Schirm, S., and Doerfler, W. (1981): Expression of viral DNA in adenovirus type 12-transformed cells, in tumor cells, and in revertants. *J. Virol.*, 39:694–702.

273. Scolnick, D. (1981): An adenovirus mutant defective in splicing RNA from early region 1A. *Nature*, 291:508–510.

274. Schrier, P. I., Van den Elsen, P. J., Hertoghs, J. J. L., and Van der Eb, A. J. (1979): Characterization of tumor antigens in cells transformed by fragments of adenovirus type 5 DNA *Virology*, 99:372–385.

275. Sehgal, P. B., Fraser, N. W., and Darnell, J. E. (1979): Early Ad-2 transcription units: Only promoter-proximal RNA continues to be made in the presence of DRB. *Virology*, 94:185–191.

276. Sergeant, A., Tigges, M. A., and Raskas, H. J. (1979): Nucleosome like structural subunits of intranuclear parental adenovirus type 2 DNA. *J. Virol.*, 29:888–898.

277. Sharp, P. A., Gallimore, P. H., and Flint, S. J., (1974): Mapping of adenovirus 2 RNA sequences in lytically infected cells and transformed cell lines. *Cold Spring Harbor Symp. Quant. Biol.*, 39:457–474.

278. Sharp, P. A., Pettersson, U., and Sambrook, J. (1974): Viral DNA in transformed cells. I. A study of the sequences of adenovirus 2 DNA in a line of transformed rat cells using specific fragments of the viral genome. *J. Mol. Biol.*, 86:709–726.

279. Shaw, C. H., Rekosh, D. M. K., and Russell, W. C. (1980): Catalysis of adenovirus DNA synthesis *in vitro* by DNA polymerase. *J. Gen. Virol.*, 48:231–236.

280. Shaw, A. R., and Ziff, E. B. (1980): Transcripts from the adenovirus-2 major late promoter yield a single family of a coterminal mRNAs during early infection and five families at late times. *Cell*, 22:905–916.

281. Shinagawa, M., and Padmanabhan, R. (1980): Comparative sequence analysis of the inverted terminal repetitions from different adenovirus. *Proc. Natl. Acad. Sci. USA*, 77:3831–3835.

282. Shiroki, K., Shimojo, H., Sawada, Y., Uemizu, Y., and Fujinaga, K. (1979): Incomplete transformation of rat cells by a small fragment of adenovirus 12 DNA. *Virology*, 95:127–136.

283. Shiroki, K., Segawa, K., Saito, I., Shimojo, H., and Fujinaga, K. (1979): Products of the adenovirus-12 transforming genes and their functions. *Cold Spring Harbor Symp. Quant. Biol.*, 44:533–540.

284. Signäs, C., Katze, M. G., Persson, H., and Philipson, L. (1982): An adenovirus glycoprotein is tightly bound to class I transplantation antigens. *Nature*, 299:175–178.

285. Sjögren, H. O., Minowada, J., and Ankerst, J. (1967): Specific transplantation antigens of mouse sarcoma induced by adenovirus type 12. *J. Exp. Med.*, 125:689–701.

286. Smart, J. E., Lewis, J. B., Mathews, M. B., Harter, M. L., and Anderson, C. W. (1981): Ad-

enovirus type 2 early proteins. Assignment of the early region 1A proteins synthesized *in vivo* and *in vitro* to specific mRNAs. *Virology*, 112:703–713.

287. Smart, J. E., and Stillman, B. W. (1982): Adenovirus terminal protein precursor: Partial amino acid sequence and the site of covalent linkage to virus DNA. *J. Biol. Chem.*, 257:13499–13506.
288. Smiley, J. R., and Mak, S. (1978): Transcription map for adenovirus type 12 DNA. *J. Virol.*, 28:227–239.
289. Spector, D. J., McGrogan, M., and Raskas, H. J. (1978): Regulation of the appearance of cytoplasmic RNAs from region 1 of the adenovirus genome. *J. Mol. Biol.*, 126:395–414.
290. Spector, D. J., Crossland, L. D., Halbert, D. N., and Raskas, H. J. (1980): A 28K polypeptide is the translation product of 9S RNA encoded by region 1A of adenovirus 2. *Virology*, 102:218–221.
291. Stabel, S., Doerfler, W., and Friis, R. R. (1980): Integration sites of adenovirus type 12 DNA in transformed hamster cells and hamster tumor cells. *J. Virol.*, 36:22–40.
292. Stillman, B. W. (1981): Adenovirus DNA replication *in vitro*: A protein linked to the 5'-end of nascent DNA strands. *J. Virol.*, 37:139–147.
293. Stillman, B. W., and Bellet, A. J. D. (1977): Replication of linear adenovirus DNA is not hairpin-primed. *Nature*, 269:723–725.
294. Stillman, B. W., Lewis, J. B., Chow, L. T., Mathews, M. B., and Smart, J. E. (1981): Identification of the gene and mRNA for the adenovirus terminal protein precursor. *Cell*, 23:497–508.
295. Stow, N. B. (1981): Cloning of a DNA fragment from the left-hand terminus of the adenovirus type 2 genome and its use in site-directed mutagenesis. *J. Virol.*, 37:171–280.
296. Sugisaki, H., Sugimoto, K., Takanami, M., Shiroki, K., Saito, I., Shimojo, H., Sawada, Y., Uemizu, Y., Uesugi, S.-I., and Fujinaga, K. (1980): Structure and gene organization in the transforming HindIII-G fragment of ad12. *Cell*, 20:777–786.
297. Sundquist, B., Everitt, E., Philipson, L., and Höglund, S. (1973): Assembly of adenoviruses. *J. Virol.*, 11:449–459.
298. Sussenbach, J. S., Van der Vliet, P. C., Ellens, D. J., and Jansz, H. S. (1972): Linear intermediates in the replication of adenovirus DNA. *Nature [New Biol.]*, 239:47–49.
299. Sussenbach, J. S., and Kuijk, M. G. (1977): Studies on the mechanism of replication of adenovirus DNA. V. The location of termini of replication. *Virology*, 77:149–157.
300. Sutter, D., and Doerfler, W. (1980): Methylation of integrated adenovirus type 12 DNA sequences in transformed cells is inversely correlated with viral gene expression. *Proc. Natl. Acad. Sci. USA*, 77:253–256.
301. Sutter, D., Westphal, M., and Doerfler, W. (1978): Patterns of integration of viral DNA sequences in the genomes of adenovirus type 12 transformed hamster cells. *Cell*, 14:569–585.
302. Söderlund, H., Pettersson, U., Vennström, B., Philipson, L., and Mathews, M. B. (1976): A new species of virus-coded low molecular weight RNA from cells infected with adenovirus type 2. *Cell*, 7:585–593.
303. Tamanoi, F., and Stillman, B. W. (1982): Function of adenovirus terminal protein in the initiation of DNA replication. *Proc. Natl. Acad. Sci. USA*, 79:2221–2225.
304. Tate, V., and Philipson, L. (1979): Parental adenovirus DNA accumulation in nucleosome-like structures in infected cells. *Nucleic Acids Res.*, 6:2769–2785.
305. Thimmappaya, B., Jones, N., and Shenk, T. (1979): A mutation which alters initiation of transcription by RNA polymerase III on the Ad5 chromosome. *Cell*, 18:947–954.
306. Thomas, G. P., and Mathews, M. B. (1981): DNA replication and the early to late transition in adenovirus infection. *Cell*, 22:523–532.
307. Tolun, A., Aleström, P., and Pettersson, U. (1979): Sequence of inverted terminal repetitions from different adenoviruses: Demonstration of conserved sequences and homology between SA7 termini and SV40 DNA. *Cell*, 17:705–713.
308. Tolun, A., and Pettersson, U. (1975): Termination sites for adenovirus type 2 DNA replication. *J. Virol.*, 16:759–766.
309. Tooze, J. (1980): *The Molecular Biology of Tumor Viruses*, ed. 2. Cold Spring Harbor Laboratory, Cold Spring Harbor, N.Y.
310. Trentin, J. J., Yabe, Y., and Taylor, G. (1962): The quest for human cancer viruses. *Science*, 137:835–841.
311. Uhlén, M., Svensson, C., Josephson, S., Aleström, P., Chattapadhyaya, J. B., Pettersson, U., and Philipson, L. (1982): Leader arrangement in the adenovirus fiber mRNA. *E.M.B.O. Journal*, 1:249–254.

312. Van der Eb, A. J. (1973): Intermediates in type 5 adenovirus DNA replication. *Virology*, 51:11–23.
313. Van der Eb, A. J., Van Kesteren, L. W., and Van Bruggen, E. F. J. (1969): Structural properties of adenovirus DNAs. *Biochim. Biophys. Acta*, 182:530–541.
314. Van der Eb, A. J., Mulder, C., Graham, F. L., and Houwelling, A. (1977): Transformation with specific fragments of adenovirus DNAs. I. Isolation of specific fragment with transforming activity of adenovirus 2 and 5 DNA. *Gene*, 2:115–132.
315. Van der Eb, A. J., Van Ormondt, H., Schrier, P. I., Lupker, J. H., Jochemsen, H., Van den Elsen, P. J., de Leys, R. J., Maat, J., Van Beveren, C. P., Dijkema, R., and de Waard, A. (1979): Structure and function of the transforming genes of human adenoviruses and SV40. *Cold Spring Harbor Symp. Quant. Biol.*, 44:383–399.
316. Van der Vliet, P. C., and Levine, A. J. (1973): DNA-binding proteins specific for cells infected by adenovirus. *Nature*, 246:170–174.
317. Van der Vliet, P. C., and Kwant, M. M. (1978): Role of DNA polymerase in adenovirus DNA replication. *Nature*, 276:532–534.
318. Van der Vliet, P. C., and Sussenbach, J. S. (1975): An adenovirus type 5 gene function required for initiation of viral DNA replication. *Virology*, 64:415–426.
319. Van der Vliet, P. C., Levine, A. J., Ensinger, M. S., and Ginsberg, H. S. (1975): Thermolabile DNA binding proteins from cells infected with a temperature-sensitive mutant of adenovirus defective in viral DNA synthesis. *J. Virol.*, 15:348–354.
320. Van der Vliet, P. C., Zandberg, J., and Jansz, H. S. (1977): Evidence for a function of the adenovirus DNA-binding protein in initiation of DNA synthesis as well as in elongation of nascent DNA chains. *Virology*, 80:98–110.
321. Van Ormondt, H., Maat, J., and Van Beveren, C. P. (1980): The nucleotide sequence of the transforming region E1 of adenovirus type 5 DNA. *Gene*, 11:299–309.
322. Van Ormondt, H., Maat, J., and Dijkema, R. (1980): Comparison of nucleotide sequences of the early E1a regions for subgroups A,B and C of human adenoviruses. *Gene*, 12:63–76.
323. Vardimon, L., Neuman, R., Kuhlman, I., Sutter, D., and Doerfler, W. (1980): DNA methylation and viral gene expression in adenovirus-transformed and -infected cells. *Nucleic Acids Res.*, 8:2461–2473.
324. Vardimon, L., and Doerfler, W. (1981): Patterns of integration of viral DNA in adenovirus type 2-transformed hamster cells. *J. Mol. Biol.*, 147:227–246.
325. Virtanen, A., Aleström, P., Persson, H., Katze, M., and Pettersson, U. (1982): A adenovirus agnogene. *Nucleic Acids Res.*, 10:2539–2548.
326. Virtanen, A., Pettersson, U., Le Moullec, J. M., Tiollais, P., and Perricaudet, M. (1982): Different mRNAs from the transforming region (E1B) of highly- and non-oncogenic human adenoviruses. *Nature*, 295:705–707.
327. Visser, L., Maarschalkerweerd, M. W., Rozijn, T. H., Wasenaar, A. D. C., Reemst, A. M. C. B., and Sussenbach, J. S. (1979): Viral DNA sequences in adenovirus transformed cells. *Cold Spring Harbor Symp. Quant. Biol.*, 44:541–550.
328. Von Acken, U., Simon, D., Grunert, F., Döring, H. P., and Kröger, H. (1979): Methylation of viral DNA in vivo and in vitro. *Virology*, 99:152–157.
329. Wadell, G., Hammarskjöld, M.-L., Winberg, G., Varsanyi, T. W., and Sundell, G. (1980): Genetic variability of adenoviruses. *Ann. N.Y. Acad. Sci.*, 354:16–42.
330. Weil, P. A., Luse, D. S., Segal, J., and Roeder, R. G. (1979): Selective and accurate initiation of transcription at the Ad2 major late promoter in a soluble system dependent on purified RNA polymerase II and DNA. *Cell*, 18:469–484.
331. Weinberg, R. A., and Pennman, S. (1968): Small molecular weight monodisperse nuclear RNA. *J. Mol. Biol.*, 38:289–304.
332. Weingärtner, B., Winnacker, E. L., Tolun, A., and Pettersson, U. (1976): Two complementary-strand specific termination sites for adenovirus DNA replication. *Cell*, 7:557–566.
333. Weingärtner, B., and Keller, W. (1981): Transcription and processing of adenoviral RNA by extracts from HeLa cells. *Proc. Natl. Acad. Sci. USA*, 78:4092–4096.
334. Weinmann, R., Raskas, H. J., and Roeder, R. G. (1974): Role of DNA dependent RNA polymerases II and III in transcription of the adenovirus genome late in productive infection. *Proc. Natl. Acad. Sci. USA*, 71:3436–3438.
335. Weinmann, R., Raskas, H. J., and Roeder, R. G. (1976): Low molecular weight viral RNAs transcribed by RNA polymerase III during ad2-infection. *Cell*, 7:557–566.

336. Westin, G., Visser, L., Zabieski, J., Van Manfeld, A. D. M., Rozijn, T., and Pettersson, U. (1982): Sequence organization of a viral DNA insertion present in the Ad5 transformed hamster line BHK 268-231. *Gene*, 17:263–270.

337. Wigand, R., Bartha, A., Dreizin, R. S., Esche, H., Ginsberg, H. S., Green, M., Hierholzer, J. C., Kalter, S. S., McFerran, J. B., Pettersson, U., Russell, W. C., and Wadell, G. (1982): Adenoviridae, second report. *Intervirology*, 18:169–176.

338. Williams, J. F. (1973): Oncogenic transformation of hamster embryo cells *in vitro* by adenovirus type 5. *Nature*, 243:162–163.

339. Williams, J. F., Young, C. S. H., and Austin, P. E. (1975): Genetic analysis of human adenovirus type 5 in permissive and nonpermissive cells. *Cold Spring Harbor Symp. Quant. Biol.*, 39:427–437.

340. Williams, J., Galos, R. S., Binger, M. H., and Flint, S. J. (1979): Location of additional early regions within the left quarter of the adenovirus genome. *Cold Spring Harbor Symp. Quant. Biol.*, 44:353–365.

341. Wilson, M., Fraser, N., and Darnell, J. (1979): Mapping of RNA initiation sites by high doses of UV irradiation. Evidence for three independent promoters within the left 11% of the Ad-2 genome. *Virology*, 94:175–184.

342. Wilson, M. C., Nevins, J. R., Blanchard, J. M., Ginsberg, H. S., and Darnell, J. E., Jr. (1979): The metabolism of mRNA from the transforming region of adenovirus type 2. *Cold Spring Harbor Symp. Quant. Biol.*, 44:447–455.

343. Wilson, M. C., and Darnell, J. E., Jr. (1981): Control of mRNA concentration by differential cytoplasmic half-life: Adenovirus mRNAs from transcription units 1A and 1B. *J. Mol. Biol.*, 148:231–251.

344. Winnacker, E. L. (1975): Origins and termini of adenovirus type 2 DNA replication. *Cold Spring Harbor Symp. Quant. Biol.*, 39:547–550.

345. Wold, W. S. M., and Green, M. (1979): Adenovirus type 2 early polypeptides immunoprecipitated by antisera to five lines of adenovirus-transformed rat cells. *J. Virol.*, 30:297–310.

346. Wolfson, J., and Dressler, D. (1972): Adenovirus-2-DNA contains an inverted terminal repetition. *Proc. Natl. Acad. Sci. USA*, 69:3054–3057.

347. Yamashita, T., Arens, M., and Green, M. (1977): Adenovirus DNA replication: Isolation of a soluble replication system and analysis of the *in vitro* DNA product. *J. Biol. Chem.*, 252:7940–7946.

348. Yang, V. W., Lerner, M., Steitz, J. A., and Flint, S. J. (1981): A small, nuclear ribonucleoprotein is required for splicing of adenoviral early RNA sequences. *Proc. Natl. Acad. Sci. USA*, 78:1371–1375.

349. Zain, S., Sambrook, J., Roberts, R. J., Keller, W., Fried, M., and Dunn, A. R. (1979): Nucleotide sequence analysis of the leader segments in a cloned copy of adenovirus 2 fiber mRNA. *Cell*, 16:851–861.

350. Zeevi, M., Nevins, J. R., and Darnell, J. E. (1981): Nuclear RNA is spliced in the absence of poly(A) addition. *Cell*, 26:39–46.

351. Ziff, E., and Fraser, N. (1978): Adenovirus type 2 late mRNA's: Structural evidence for 3'-coterminal species. *J. Virol.*, 25:897–906.

352. Ziff, E. B., and Evans, R. M. (1978): Coincidence of the promoter and capped 5' terminus of RNA from the adenovirus 2 major late transcription unit. *Cell*, 15:1463–1475.

353. Zinkernagel, R. M., and Doherty, P. C. (1974): Restriction of in vitro T cell-mediated cytotoxicity in lymphocytic choriomeningitis within a syngeneic or semiallogeneic system. *Nature*, 248:701–704.

Advances in Viral Oncology, Volume 3, edited by
George Klein. Raven Press, New York © 1983.

Epstein-Barr Virus Transformation and Replication

Elliott Kieff, Timothy Dambaugh, Mary Hummel, and Mark Heller

Division of Biological Sciences, The University of Chicago, Chicago, Illinois 60637

Epstein-Barr virus (EBV) was the fifth human herpesvirus to be discovered. Prior to its discovery, a great deal of research had been done with the other human herpesviruses: herpes simplex virus type 1 (HSV-1), herpes simplex virus type 2 (HSV-2), cytomegalovirus (CMV), and varicella-zoster virus (VZV). There was substantial knowledge of the biology and morphology of HSV, CMV, and VZV and of the biochemistry of HSV. Although morphologically indistinguishable from these other herpesviruses, EBV has little, if any, antigenic relatedness to them. EBV also differs from these and other viruses in its narrowly restricted host range *in vitro*. *In vitro*, EBV will infect only primate lymphocytes of the immunoglobulin-producing or B lymphocyte series (87,97,157,158). As a consequence of virus infection, the lymphocyte is stimulated to multiply. The infected cell continues to multiply indefinitely as long as it is provided with adequate nutrition.

Antibodies to EBV can be distinguished from antibodies directed against other herpesviruses, and this provides a useful marker of primary and latent human infection (86). The age of primary EBV infection varies among human populations. The clinical manifestations of primary infection are age-dependent. Infection in the first few years of life is common among lower socioeconomic groups. Clinical manifestations of early childhood infection are usually mild. In contrast, 50% of college students with primary EBV infection develop clinical manifestations of infectious mononucleosis (182). Primary EBV infection is the usual cause of infectious mononucleosis. Some children with Duncan's syndrome or other poorly characterized immune defects or those undergoing immunosuppression for organ transplantation develop prolonged primary infection syndromes (70,164,177). These syndromes are characterized by proliferation of multiple clones of virus-infected lymphoid cells and may result in death. In normal individuals, the proliferation of virus-infected, growth-stimulated cells is contained by suppressor and specifically immune T cells, by antibody, by natural killer cells and nonspecific resistance factors, including interferons (198). The containment of EBV-infected cells in normal individuals and the growth of these cells in some immunosuppressed individuals suggest that specific immunity to EBV-infected cells is important in natural restriction of infected cell proliferation. However, the relative role of specific immunity versus nonspecific immune factors such as lymphokines and interferons has not been assessed.

Following primary human infection, the virus persists indefinitely, latent in some B lymphocytes (141). Latent EBV infection is prevalent in every human population. Latently infected cells are capable of sustained growth in tissue culture and in the brains of nude mice, but they will not grow in subcutaneous tissues of nude mice. Uninfected B lymphocytes rapidly undergo senescence; they have a limited lifespan *in vitro* and will not grow in subcutaneous tissue or brains of nude mice. Virus shedding in nasopharyngeal secretions may continue for years after primary EBV infection and may recur with immunosuppression (130). Lymphomas develop in some immunosuppressed children who appear to have recovered from prolonged primary EBV infection.

EBV is historically associated with Burkitt's lymphoma, an unusual malignancy that is endemic in certain tropical regions of equatorial Africa (11,38). The virus was discovered in lymphoblast cultures of Burkitt's lymphoma. At the time of the discovery of EBV in Burkitt tumor cells, other viruses were known to cause malignancy after experimental infection of animals. Furthermore, some naturally occurring animal cancers were known to be transmitted by virus infection. Therefore, from the moment of the discovery of EBV in cultures of biopsied tumor cells, an important question has been whether or not EBV is the cause of African Burkitt lymphoma.

The EBV nuclear antigen, EBNA, and the complete viral genome are present in almost all African Burkitt tumor cells (119). EBNA and viral DNA are also present in all cells of the polyclonal and late uniclonal lymphomas that develop in immunosuppressed children. In normal people who have been infected with EBV, the virus is latent in a small fraction of the B lymphocyte clones. The latently infected cells express EBNA and a new surface antigen. The lymphoma cells that rarely emerge as late tumors in immunosuppressed or African children are uniclonal (45) and are able to grow in both the skin and brain in nude mice (141). The uniclonality of the tumor cells suggests that malignancy results from an unusual change in a single latently infected cell. Cells from Burkitt's lymphoma have reciprocal 8:14 chromosome translocations, or variant translocations of chromosome 8 to chromosome 2 or 22 (124). These chromosomal translocations are characteristic of malignant B lymphocytes regardless of whether the B cell malignancy is associated with EBV. Because the malignant change is regularly associated with the translocation of a part of chromosome 8, the translocated segment may be of pathophysiologic significance in the evolution of the malignancy. The other involved chromosome regions (14, 2, and 22) are those that contain immunoglobin genes (110). These genes would be expected to be active in transcription and in recombination in B lymphocytes. The translocated portion of chromosome 8 may be a key reason for control of cell growth, which then becomes activated as a consequence of the translocation. Latent virus infection is neither absolutely necessary nor sufficient for malignant degeneration, because most adult humans have B cells infected with EBV and never develop malignant B cells, and malignant B cells with the 8:14 translocation occur without EBV infection.

Because every cell in African Burkitt tumors and in the uniclonal malignancies of immunosuppressed children is infected with EBV, EBV infection probably antedates the malignant change. Infection may prime the cell for malignant transformation. Alternatively, EBV may be a passenger that infects every malignant B lymphocyte. The uniform presence of latent EBV genomes in all African Burkitt tumor cells is strong evidence that infection precedes malignant proliferation, especially when weighed against the observation that EBV infection of malignant B cells is an infrequent event in other clinical situations, even when the patient harbors latent virus.

If infection is neither necessary nor sufficient for malignant transformation of lymphocytes, what role may the virus play in development of malignancy? EBV causes lymphocytes to grow continuously. One hypothesis is that by promoting cell growth, the virus increases the likelihood of occurrence of spontaneous malignant transformation, a low-probability chance event. The frequent occurrence of EBV-associated Burkitt lymphoma in equatorial Africa would then be due to a geographically confined host immunologic response or a cocarcinogenic factor that further promotes the emergence of the malignant B cell. General suppression of host immunity seems to be an unlikely factor, because purposeful immunosuppression for organ transplantation or for antineoplastic chemotherapy rarely gives rise to tumors in latently infected adults or children. However, the recent discovery that newer immunosuppressive regimens which include cyclosporin A yield a high rate of EBV-associated polyclonal and uniclonal malignancies suggests that there may be a key cyclosporin A sensitive component of immunity to EBV-induced cell proliferation (70). A second hypothesis is that African EBV isolates differ from other EBV isolates and may decrease host immunoresponsiveness or may act as cocarcinogenic factors. For example, a change in a viral gene that specifies or modulates the expression of infected B cell surface neoantigens that are recognized by immune T cells could render the cell less subject to immune surveillance. Alternatively, African virus isolates could differ from other isolates in the function of the promoter for an important growth-transforming gene, in the presence of a nucleotide sequence that promotes recombination with cell DNA, or in a gene that regulates the extent of virus replication, so that after primary infection a larger number of cells would harbor the virus in a latent state. A prospective seroepidemiologic study in the Burkitt-lymphoma-endemic region has suggested that children with higher levels of antibody to EBV are more likely to develop malignancy (28). These data suggest that reactivated EBV infection, chronic progressive infection, or more severe primary infection antedates the development of malignancy.

If strain variation occurs, the prevalence of latent EBV infection in adult human populations would confine strains of EBV to the initial geographic niche. An important expectation of the strain-variation hypothesis is not met by epidemiologic observations. There is an immediate increase in the incidence of lymphoma among the progeny of tribes migrating into the Burkitt-lymphoma-endemic region (12).

Progeny should become infected with the mother's EBV, because the mother would be the closest infected contact. If virus strain variation is a factor in malignancy, the lymphoma incidence would be expected to change over many generations. Thus, the epidemiologic data suggest that other environmental factors interact with the latently infected host as a cocarcinogen.

Experimental infection of some species of nonhuman primates with EBV results in tumor formation (127). Although the tumor cells are B lymphocytes, they differ from EBV-infected human B lymphocytes in some cell surface characteristics. It is uncertain whether the animal model is more similar to primary human EBV infection with polyclonal lymphoid proliferation or to uniclonal malignant B cell proliferation associated with the 8:14 translocation. Analyses of cell surface markers and karyotype studies of a few animals suggest that some of the tumors may be polyclonal. Baboons and other Old World primates are naturally infected with agents that are biologically and genetically related to EBV (42,54,56). One baboon colony in the U.S.S.R. has a high incidence of malignant B cell lymphomas. The lymphomas occur among animals that are latently infected with the baboon EBV-related agent, HVPapio (170).

EBV has been associated with a second human malignancy, anaplastic nasopharyngeal carcinoma (111). Nasopharyngeal cancer (NPC) occurs infrequently in most populations, but it has a high incidence in southern China, where it is the most common cancer. Because of the large population of southern China, NPC is one of the most common malignancies afflicting humans. The cancer cells of NPC tumors are uniformly latently infected with EBV. Nothing is known about the karyotype or clonal origin of these tumors. The tumor cells will grow in the subcutaneous tissue of nude mice. Although other data suggest that EBV can infect epithelial cells, the presence of latent virus infection in nasopharyngeal tumor cells is the only definitive evidence that the host range of the virus in humans is broader than B lymphocytes. As in EBV-associated B cell malignancies, the role of the virus in malignant transformation is uncertain. The high incidence of NPC among southern Chinese, the intermediate incidence among first-generation overseas Chinese, and the low incidence in most other populations suggest both environmental and genetic factors. The uniform presence of virus DNA and EBNA in anaplastic nasopharyngeal carcinomas from patients worldwide suggests that EBV infection is a necessary condition for the evolution of this malignancy. Prospective field studies in southern China indicate that increased antibody response to EBV precedes malignant transformation (213). In the adult Chinese population, rising IgA titers to EBV antigens are a prognostic indicator of subsequent evolution of nasopharyngeal carcinoma.

Studies of EBV have been complicated by lack of an *in vitro* system that is permissive for virus replication. This deficiency has forestalled classic genetic studies and hinders biochemical analysis. The *in vitro* host range of the virus is limited to B lymphocytes. Viral infection conveys new growth ability to the lymphocytes, so that only virus-infected cells can be grown in culture as continuous cell lines. The cell lines that result are either latently infected or partially permissive of virus replication. Virus replication can be induced in some continuous cultures by the addition of phorbol esters, sodium butyrate, nucleoside analogues, or anti-IgM to the culture medium. Partially permissive infection has also been achieved by superinfection of a particular latently infected cell line (Raji) with virus produced by cultures of an unusual clone of Burkitt tumor cells, P3HR-1 (7). The P3HR-1 virus differs from all other EBV isolates in two characteristics. P3HR-1 virus can induce replication in Raji cells (either the superinfecting P3HR-1 or endogenous Raji EBV or both), and P3HR-1 virus can infect, but cannot induce growth transformation of, B lymphocytes (132,172).

In part, the restricted host range of EBV *in vitro* may be due to the difficulty of culturing other differentiated cells that may have receptors for the virus. Viral DNA that has been transfected into mouse or human placental cells is expressed and induces a single abortive or productive round of infection (133,208). The efficiency of the transfection process is low, so that transfection has not been useful for studies requiring virus replication.

STRUCTURAL COMPONENTS OF THE VIRUS

Morphology of the Virus

The few detailed studies of EBV have been made using thin sections of lymphoblastoid cell cultures in which small percentages of the cells have been productively infected or have been made using virus purified from such partially permissive cultures (Fig. 1) (29,30,33–36,39,41,94,148,157,158,191,204). The innermost component of the virus particle, the core, varies in appearance with the plane of sectioning. The core appears similar to the toroid of HSV (50) and therefore probably consists of DNA coiled around protein. The core is surrounded by the icosahedral capsid. Hexameric capsomers are commonly seen in negatively stained preparations of partially enveloped or maturing virus and in negatively stained preparations of virus treated with nonionic detergent. Petameric capsomers should also be present to permit puckering of the capsid. The capsid is enveloped by a trilaminar membrane with spikes on its outer surface. The space between the capsid shell and the envelope is filled with amorphous tegument.

Polypeptides of the Virus

Enveloped virus is generally purified from extracellular fluids of partially permissive cultures by velocity sedimentation in dextran gradients (29,30). Two isolates of viruses have been most extensively studied (29,30,138–140): virus produced by B95-8, a culture of a clone of marmoset lymphocytes infected with virus from a culture of lymphocytes from a patient with infectious mononucleosis (128,129), and virus produced by P3HR-1, a clone of the Jijoye Burkitt tumor cell line (89). At a level of purity of B95-8 virus at which at least 98% of the labeled protein is viral, 33 component polypeptides can be resolved in denaturing polyacrylamide gels (Fig. 2) (29,30). On the basis of experience with the more thoroughly studied

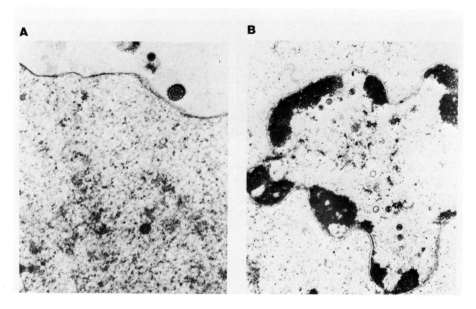

FIG. 1. Electron photomicrographs of thin sections of a productively infected Burkitt tumor cell growing in culture (×40,000). **A:** Enveloped extracellular virus located near the cytoplasmic membrane. **B:** The nucleus of the same cell with marginated chromatin, empty and full nucleocapsids.

polypeptides on HSV (189), some of the 33 EBV polypeptides are likely to share common polypeptide components and differ in molecular weight as a consequence of varying degrees of posttranslational modification, principally glycosylation or phosphorylation. Some of the minor components may be products of partial proteolysis of major components. Of the 33 polypeptides, 18 are more abundant than the others and differ in molar abundance among themselves by 20- to 30-fold. The apparent sizes of the most abundant polypeptides are 290, 160, 152, 90, 78, 47, 43, 33, and 28 × 10^3 daltons (d), based on their electrophoretic mobility in acrylamide gels under denaturing conditions. Nonionic detergents that strip the envelope from the nucleocapsid solubilize the 290, 152, 90, 43, and 33 × 10^3 d components, suggesting that these polypeptides are external to the capsid. On the basis of labeled glucosamine incorporation and periodic-acid-Schiff (PAS) staining, the 290 × 10^3-d polypeptide is the major glycoprotein; the 120–130, 70–90, and 43 × 10^3-d polypeptides label less heavily with glucosamine and stain less with PAS. Because these polypeptides are stripped from the virion with nonionic detergents and are glycosylated, they are also tentatively designated as envelope components. The 150 × 10^3-d polypeptide is the major nonglycosylated polypeptide removed from the virion by nonionic detergent. Because this abundant polypeptide is extracted from the virion, leaving the nucleocapsid apparently intact, it is likely to be the principal component of the tegument or of the core membrane. The 160, 78, 44–47, and 28 × 10^3-d polypeptides remain associated with the

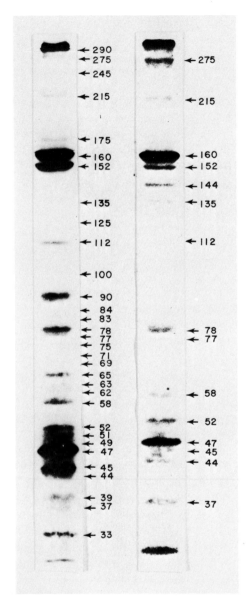

FIG. 2. Fluorograms of ^{35}S-labeled polypeptides of enveloped virus *(left)* and nucleocapsids *(right)* separated on sodium dodecyl sulfate polyacrylamide gels. The numbers indicate the estimated molecular weights. (Adapted from Dolyniuk et al., refs. 29 and 30.)

nucleocapsid through nonionic-detergent extraction and are the principal nucleocapsid components.

Antigenic Determinants of the Virus

Sera from infected patients have been used to identify the major antigenic polypeptides of the envelope and capsid (98,138–140,155,165,166,192,200,201). Most studies of the envelope or membrane antigens (MA) have prepared the antigens from nonionic-detergent extracts of cell cultures in which as many as 50% of the cells have been induced to express MA. In some studies the outer plasma membrane was specifically surface-labeled by iodination or borohydride reduction (139,140,166,192). In other studies, plasma membranes or virus were purified prior to nonionic-detergent extraction (200,201). The major surface-labeled antigens are 350, 220 and 85 $\times$ 10^3 d. The three antigens are heterogeneous in size, label with radioactive glucosamine, bind to ricin lectin, and elute with galactose. The three proteins have been designated gp350, gp220, and gp85, respectively. The 220–250 component is slightly more abundant than the 320–350 in extracts of P3HR-1 virus or P3HR-1 cells, whereas the 320–350 component is much more abundant than the 220–250 on the surface of B95-8 virus or B95-8 cells. Two sets of monoclonal antibodies recognize both the 220–250 and 320–350 components (90,202), indicating shared antigenicity through either common polypeptide or oligosaccharide components. These monoclonal antibodies also neutralize virus, confirming that the 220–350 $\times$ 10^3-d complex is on the outer surface of the virus. With the reactivity demonstrated by human sera to these antigens, it is likely that the 220–350 complex is an important neutralizing antigen in natural human infection. The 80–90 $\times$ 10^3-d glycoprotein complex may also be an important neutralizing antigen. Surface labeling indicates that it is also on the outer surface of the virus envelope. Convalescent human sera react with antigenic determinants of the 80–90 $\times$ 10^3-d complex.

Superinfection of latently infected Raji cells with the P3HR-1 virus induces the synthesis of gp350, gp220, and gp85 (139,140,166). A 70 $\times$ 10^3-d polypeptide appears on the cell surface within 2 hr of P3HR-1 superinfection and before the 80–90 $\times$ 10^3-d polypeptide can be detected. Over the ensuing 24 to 48 hr, the relative intensity of heterogeneously migrating polypeptide species in the size range 80–90 $\times$ 10^3 d increases suggesting that the 70 $\times$ 10^3-d protein is a precursor to the 80–90 $\times$ 10^3-d glycoprotein. In one study, the synthesis of the 70 and 80–90 $\times$ 10^3-d polypeptides was unaffected by the use of cytosine arabinoside to inhibit viral DNA synthesis. In other studies, the 80–90 $\times$ 10^3-d complex was reduced by treatment with phosphonoacetic acid, a better characterized inhibitor of EBV DNA synthesis.

The 43 $\times$ 10^3-d envelope polypeptide is labeled less heavily by surface iodination and is less evident in immunoprecipitates with human sera than gp350, gp220, and gp85 (98,139,140,166,192,200,201). A 130 $\times$ 10^3-d polypeptide has also been detected as a minor component in immunoprecipitates of glucosamine-labeled cell extracts. Trypsin treatment of infected cells before surface iodination exposes the 150 $\times$ 10^3-d polypeptide to iodination. The exposure of this protein after trypsin treatment suggests that it is probably a core protein rather than an outer-membrane or tegument protein.

The 160 $\times$ 10^3-d major nucleocapsid polypeptide is also the major capsid component precipitated by immune human sera (98,139,140). This polypeptide is probably an important component of the viral capsid antigen (VCA) complex detected by immunofluorescence in the nucleus and cytoplasm of permissively infected cells (85,125).

Little is known about the biochemistry of the antigenic determinants or structural polypeptides of the primate EBV-related viruses, herpesvirus pan (HVPan) and herpesvirus papio (HVPapio). Human and primate sera that have activity in homologous assays cross-react extensively in heterologous VCA, MA, and neutralization tests, suggesting that EBV, HVPan, and HVPapio have similar antigenic determinants on their capsids and envelopes (42,54,56,57).

Viral DNA

Comparative analysis of EBV DNAs is a particularly important issue in EBV research. Because of the nonpermissive outcome of EBV infection *in vitro*, more of the phenotypic properties of the genome are cryptic in culture than is the case with other herpesviruses. Comparison of the phenotypic properties of EBV isolates is therefore difficult and imprecise. Further, although seroepidemiologic studies indicate that infection with EBV is prevalent in all human populations, the virus has an unusual association with Burkitt lymphoma and nasopharyngeal cancer. Burkitt lymphoma is an endemic disease in equatorial Africa. EBV is also invariably found in every African Burkitt tumor cell (174), but elsewhere EBV is not a regular passenger in malignant B cells. EBV is almost invariably present in anaplastic nasopharyngeal cancer cells (113,210,216). This disease occurs worldwide in association with EBV (25,154). However, there is endemic clustering of cases in southern China (27). One hypothesis that could explain the restricted geography of Burkitt lymphoma and the high incidence of nasopharyngeal cancer in southern China is geographic strain variation among EBV isolates.

The DNA of the B95-8 isolate of EBV has been the prototype for detailed restriction endonuclease mapping, for cloning into *Escherichia coli* plasmids and into bacteriophage lambda, and for nucleotide sequencing (14,15,17,20,21,59–61,186). Comparative restriction endonuclease maps of eight other EBV isolates have been derived (10,77,78,167). DNA fragments from two other EBV isolates, AG876 and W91, have been partially cloned into plasmid vectors (17,167). AG876 is a culture of an African Burkitt lymphoma biopsy (156). W91 is a clone of marmoset cells infected with an African Burkitt lymphoma EBV isolate (131). Studies of these EBV DNAs have provided most of our current knowledge of the homoscadicity of EBV isolates.

General Features

EBV DNA is a linear, double-stranded molecule of approximately 170×10^3 nucleotide base pairs (bp) (73,161,162). The density of EBV DNA in neutral CsCl is 1.718 g·cm^{-3} (96,161,162,209). Assuming that the DNA consists entirely of unmodified bases, the overall base composition that corresponds to this density is 57% guanine plus cytosine (G + C) and 43% adenine plus thymine. Comparison of the restriction endonuclease fragments of virion DNA digested with the isoschizomers *Msp*I and *Hpa*II indicates that CG residues are not methylated (109). The DNA in most virus preparations from chronically infected cultures is extensively and randomly nicked by endonuclease (61). As with HSV, as many as 50% of the single strands of nascent virion DNA are intact, as shown by alkaline sucrose sedimentation (161,162).

The general structure of EBV DNA is shown in Fig. 3 (20,21). There is a terminal repeat (TR) at each end of the DNA (59,61,108). The TR is 500 bp long. The repetitions are tandem and direct and vary in number at each end. There are usually 4 to 8 copies per end, although some ends have as many as 12 copies. TR is in the same orientation at both ends of the DNA (61). There is no homology between TR and internal DNA. Although the functions of TR are not fully known, one recognized role is to facilitate circularization of EBV DNA following infection (120). Inside the infected cells, TRs at opposite ends of the DNA become covalently linked. The process is likely to be mediated by homologous recombination. The joined ends can be cloned from infected cells as a single DNA fragment (20,21). The repeats of TR could facilitate circularization by enabling base pairing between the ends or by binding a bivalent protein that could hold the two ends in close proximity. It is not known if a protein is involved in circularization of the EBV genome. The 5′ ends of virion DNA are susceptible to lambda-exonuclease digestion, indicating that there is no protein linked to the 5′ terminus (73).

Multiple direct tandem repeats of a 3,071-bp sequence, IR1 (15), separate the genome into two domains: a short unique region of 15,000 bp, US or U1, and a long, largely unique region of 150,000 bp, UL. Other direct repeats, IR2, IR3, and IR4 (18,79), further subdivide UL into the unique-sequence domains U2, U3, U4, and U5. IR2 and IR4 are tandem repeats of sequences of 124 and 103 bp, respectively. A sequence (DL) of approximately 2 kbp in the region of U3 adjacent to IR2 is partially homologous to a sequence (DR) of approximately 2.1 kbp in U5 that is adjacent to IR4 (18,167). IR3 designates a sequence of 708 bp that consists of direct repeats of three nucleotide triplets, GGG, GCA, and GGA (79). The triplets are organized into a hexanucleotide sequence GCAGGA (H) and two non-anucleotide sequences, GCAGGAGGA (N1) and GGGGCAGGA (N2). At a higher level of organization, H or NI sequences are interspersed between N2 sequences or tandem copies of N2.

The nucleotide sequence of IR1 is shown in Fig. 4 (15). The sequence is 67% guanine plus cytosine. There is a CCAAT sequence 39 nucleotides 5′ to a TATAAA, which could be a promoter for transcription. The longest open reading frame is 1,124 bp, which is 3′ to the promoter sequence. There are many potential splice donor and acceptor sequences through IR1, so that the structure of the processed RNA encoded by IR1 cannot be readily predicted. Within IR1 is a sequence similar to the papovavirus origin of DNA replication. The *ori*-like sequence is within a long 500-bp imperfect palindrome. This 500-bp palindrome is 3′ to the promoter and would be expected to have a profound effect on the secondary structure of an RNA transcribed from this region. Shorter dyad symmetries act as terminators of transcription of SV40 late RNA and may be attenuators of transcription or modu-

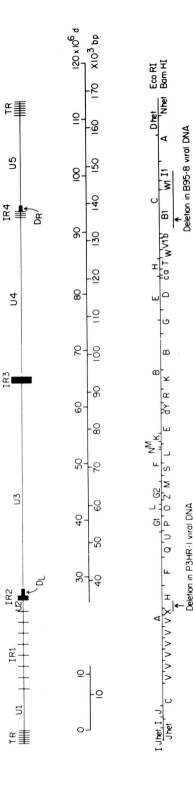

FIG. 3. The physical structure of the linear EBV DNA molecule is indicated by the first line. As described in the text, the EBV genome is divided into five domains of unique-sequence complexity (U1–U5) bounded by direct tandem copies of repeated DNA sequences located at the termini of the molecule (TR) and at internal sites within the molecule (IR1–IR4). DL and DR represent partially homologous unique sequences of approximately 2 kbp that lie adjacent to IR2 and IR4, respectively. The discontinuity in the map coordinates in the IR1 region reflects variation in the average number of copies of IR1 among different EBV isolates. The locations of BamHI and EcoRI restriction enzyme sites in EBV DNA are shown in the third line. The locations of DNA sequences that are deleted from P3HR-1 EBV and B95-8 EBV are indicated by the horizontal bars. The deletion within P3HR-1 EBV DNA is described in the text.

```
         10         20         30         40         50         60         70
GATCCCCCA  CCGGCCCTTC TCTCTGTCCC CCTGCTCCTC TCCAACCTTC GCTCCACCCT AGACCCCAGC

         80         90        100        110        120        130        140
TTCTGGCCTC CCCGGGTCCA CAAGGCCAGC CGGAGGGACC CCGGCGAGTCG GGGGCAGTCG CCTTCCCTCT

        150        160        170        180        190        200        210
CCCTGGCCT  CTCCTTCCCG CCTCCCACCC GAGCCCCTTC AGCTTGCCTC CCCACCGGGT CCATCAGGCC

        220        230        240        250        260        270        280
GGGCGGAGGG ACCCCGGCGG CCCGGTGTCA GTCTCTGCCTG CAGCCGCCCA GTCTCTGCCT CCAGGCAAGG

        290        300        310        320        330        340        350
GCGCCAGCTT TTCTCCCCC  AGCCTGAGGC CCAGTCTGTC TGTAAAGTCC AGCCTCCCAC

        360        370        380        390        400        410        420
GCCGTCCAC  GGCTCCGGGG CCCAGCCTCG TCCACCCCTC CCCACGGTGG ACAGCCCCTC TGTCCACCCG

        430        440        450        460        470        480        490
GGCCATCCCC GCCCCCCTGT GTCCACCCCA GTCCGTCCA  GGGGGGACTT TATGTGACCC TTGGGCCTGG

        500        510        520        530        540        550        560
CTCCCATAG  ACTCCCATGT AAGCCTGCCT CGAGTAGGTG CCTTCAGAGC CCCTTTTGCC CCCCTGGCGG

        570        580        590        600        610        620        630
CCAGCCCGA  CCCCGGGGCG CCCCCAAACT TTGTCCAGAT GTCCAGGGGT CCCCGAGGGT GAGGCCCAGC

        640        650        660        670        680        690        700
CCCCTCCCGC CCCTGTCCAC TGCCCCGGTC CCCCCAGAAG CCCCCAAAAG TAGAGGCTCA GGCCATGCGC

        710        720        730        740        750        760        770
GCCCGTCAC  CAGGCCTGCC AAAGAGCCAG ATCTAAGGCC GGGAGAGGCA GCCCCAAAGC GGGTGCAGTA


       1550       1560       1570       1580       1590       1600       1610
GCCAAGAACC CAGACGAGTC CGTAGAAGGG TCCTCGTCCA GCAAGAAGAG GAGGTGGTAA GCGGTTCACC

       1620       1630       1640       1650       1660       1670       1680
TTCAGGGGTA AGTAACCTGA CCTCTCCAGG GCTCACATAA AGGGAGGCTT AGT[TATA]CATG CTTCTTGCTT

       1690       1700       1710       1720       1730       1740       1750
TTCACAGGAA CCTGGGGGCT AGTCTGGGTG GGATTAGGCT GCCTCAAGTT GCATCAGCCA GGGCTTCATG

       1760       1770       1780       1790       1800       1810       1820
CCCTCCTCAG TTCCCTAGTC CCCGGGCTTC AGGCCCCCTC CGTCCCCGTC CTCCAGAGAC CCGGGCTTCA

       1830       1840       1850       1860       1870       1880       1890
GGGCCTGCCT CTCCTGTTAC CCTTTTAGAA CCACAGCCTG GACACATGTG CCAGACGCCT TGGCCTCTAA

       1900       1910       1920       1930       1940       1950       1960
GGGCCTCGGG TCCCCGTGGA CCCCGGCCTC AGCAACCCTG CTGCTCCCCT CCTGCCACCC CAGCCTCCCC

       1970       1980       1990       2000       2010       2020       2030
CCCTCCCGT  CCCCCTTCGC TCCTGATCCT CCCCGGTCC  CCAGTAGGGC CGCTGCCCC  CCTGCACCCA

       2040       2050       2060       2070       2080       2090       2100
GTACCTGCCC CTCTTGGCCA CGCACCCCGG GCCAGCGCAC CTTAGACCCG GCCAAGCCCC ATCCCTGAAG

       2110       2120       2130       2140       2150       2160       2170
ACCCAGCGGC CATTCTCTCT GGTAACGAGC AGAGAAGAAG TAGAGGCCCG CGGCCATTGG GCCCAGATTG

       2180       2190       2200       2210       2220       2230       2240
AGAGACCAGT CCAGGGGCCC GAGGTTGGAG CCAGCGGGCA CCGGAGGTTC CAGCACCCCG TCCCTGCGGG

       2250       2260       2270       2280       2290       2300       2310
GGGCAGAGAC AGGCAGGGCC CCCCGGCAGC TGGCCCCGAG GAGGCGCCCG GAGTGGGGGC GGTGGGCTGG
```

FIG. 4. Nucleotide sequence of IR1 in EBV DNA. The entire *Bam*HI V fragment (IR1) of B95-8 virus has been sequenced by the chemical degradation method (15). It has 3,071 base pairs (bp) and is composed of 66.8% guanosine (G) and cytosine (C) and therefore 33.2% thymidine (T) and adenosine (A). Promoter sequences for transcription (CCAAT, TATAAA, and TATA) are detected at 1,098 bp, 1,137 bp, and 1,663 bp, respectively. A cluster of dyad symmetries is located between 2,205 bp and 2,715 bp that shares common features with the Alu family sequences and eukaryotic transposable elements. Within this cluster is a 19-bp sequence that is homologous to the papovaviruses *ori*. The promoter sequences are boxed, and the potential origin of DNA replication is underlined.

```
 780       790        800        810        820        830        840
ACAGTAATC TCTGGTAGTG ATTTGGACCC GAAATCTGAC ACTTTAGAGC TCTGGAGGAC TTTAAAACTC

 850       860        870        880        890        900        910
TAAAATCAA AACTTTAGAG GCGAATGGGC GCCATTTGT CCCCACGCGC GCATAATGGC GGACCTAGGC

 920       930        940        950        960        970        980
CTAAAACCCC CAGGAAGCGG GTCTATGGTT GGCTGCGCTG CTGCTATCTT TAGAGGGGAA AAGAGGAATA

 990       1000       1010       1020       1030       1040       1050
AGCCCCAGA CAGGGGAGTG GGCTTGTTTG TGACTTCAGG GCCCAAGGGG GTTCGCGTTG

 1060      1070       1080       1090       1100       1110       1120
CTAGGCCACC TTTCTCAGTCC AGCGCGTTTA CGTAAGGCAG ACAGCAGC[CA A]TGTCAGTT CTAGGGAGGG

 1130      1140       1150       1160       1170       1180       1190
GGACCACTGC CCCTG[TATA AAG]GGTCCT GCAGCTATTT CTGGTCGCAT CAGAGCGCCA GGAGTCCACA

 1200      1210       1220       1230       1240       1250       1260
CAAATGTAAG AGGGGGTCTT CTACCTTCCC CTAGCCCTCC GCCCCCTCCA AGGACTCGGG CCCAGTTTCT

 1270      1280       1290       1300       1310       1320       1330
AACTTTTCCC CTTCCCTCCC TCGTCTTTGCC CTGCGCCCGG GGCCACCTTC ATCACCGTCG CTGACTCCGC

 1340      1350       1360       1370       1380       1390       1400
CATCCAAGCC TAGGGGAGAC CGAAGTGAAG GCCCTGGACC AACCCGGCCC GGGCCCCCCG GTATCGGGCC

 1410      1420       1430       1440       1450       1460       1470
AGAGGTAAGT GGACTTTAAT TTTTTCTGCT AAGCCCAACA CTCCACACA CCCAGGCACA CACTACACAC

 1480      1490       1500       1510       1520       1530       1540
ACCCACCGT CTCAGGTCC CCTCGGACAG CTCCTAAGAA GGCACCGGTC GCCCAGTTCCT ACCCAGAGGGG

 2320      2330       2340       2350       2360       2370       2380
GCTGCCGAG CCCGGGTCTG GGAGGCTCGG GGTGGCGAGC CTGCTGTCTC AGGAGGGGCC TGGCTCCGCC

 2390      2400       2410       2420       2430       2440       2450
GGGTGGCCCT GGGTAAGTC AGGGTCGGCC TAGGCCCGGG GAAGTGGAGG GGGATCGCCC

 2460      2470       2480       2490       2500       2510       2520
GGGTCTTCGT TGGCAGAGTC CGGGCGATCC TCTGAGACCC TCCGGGCCCG GACTGTCGCC CTCAGCCCCC

 2530      2540       2550       2560       2570       2580       2590
CAGACAGACC CCAGGGTCTC CAGGCAGGGT CCGGCATCTT CAGGGGCAGC AGGCTCACCA CCACAGGCCC

 2600      2610       2620       2630       2640       2650       2660
CCCAGACCCG GGTCTCGGCC AGCCGAGCCG ACCGGCCCGC TCCTGGCGGC TCCTCGGGGC CAGCCGCCGG

 2670      2680       2690       2700       2710       2720       2730
GGTTGGTTCT GCCCCTCTCT CTGTCCTTCA GAGGAACCAG GGACCTCGGG CACCCCAG(AG) CCCCTCGGGC

 2740      2750       2760       2770       2780       2790       2800
CCGCCTCCAG GCGCCCTCCT GGTCTCCGCT CCCCTCTGAG CCCGTTAAA CCCAAAGAAT GTCTGAGGGG

 2810      2820       2830       2840       2850       2860       2870
AGCCACCTTC GGGCCCAGC CCCAGAGTC CAGAGGTCAG GGGCACCTCA CCGGGTCCCA

 2880      2890       2900       2910       2920       2930       2940
GGCCAGCGAG AGGGACCCCG CGAGCCCAGG CGGCCCCAGA GGCGGGTTCC TCGCCCCTTC CCCGGGCTTC

 2950      2960       2970       2980       2990       3000       3010
AGAGCCCAGG ATGTCCCCA GAAGGGACCC TAGGCGTCCC CTTCCTCCCC CTCCAGGCCC GAGCCTCTCC

 3020      3030       3040       3050       3060       3070
CTCGCGGAGA GGGGCGCTCTT TGGGCCTCA AGTCCAGCCC CACCGAGACC CGAGTGGCCC  G
```

lators of processing or translocation. Relative to the U1-IR1 juncture, the last copy of IR1 is a partial repeat that consists of only the beginning 1,850 nucleotides.

There are 11 to 14 tandem direct repeats of IR2 in the DL region of EBV DNA and 30 tandem direct repeats of IR4 in DR. IR2 and IR4 are similar sequences (Fig. 5) (18) that evolved from a common progenitor sequence. IR2 and IR4 are 84% guanine and cytosine and have limited homology to the HSV-1 inverted terminal "a" sequence.

IR3 is a simple array that consists of three tandem direct repeat units, GCAGGA, GCAGGAGGA, and GGGGCAGGA. The length of the overall array varies among EBV isolates. The array has a high degree of homology to a family of interspersed repeat sequences in cell DNA (80). Cytological hybridization shows that IR3 is homologous to at least one region on each human chromosome except the Y chromosome.

Range of Variability among EBV DNAs

The restriction endonuclease fragments and the linkage maps of nine EBV DNAs vary sufficiently to specifically identify each of the DNAs (10,21,46,59,77,78,167). Although four DNAs from Africans with Burkitt lymphoma, three from Americans with infectious mononucleosis, one from an Australian with myeloblastic leukemia, and one from a patient with nasopharyngeal cancer have been analyzed, no features have been identified that correlate with a specific geographic or pathological origin. Some of the analyses have been pursued at the level of mapping nearly a hundred restriction endonuclease sites. Most of the variations observed among the DNAs could be the consequence of mutations at existing or potential restriction endonuclease sites, because there is no discernible change in the order or size of the surrounding DNA sequences (21,77,78). Similar kinds of differences have been observed with passage of the B95-8 virus in cord-blood cells (21,107,167). The DNA of each isolate has a distinctive arrangement of restriction endonuclease sites. Spread of EBV could therefore be traced, should the need arise.

Although it is clear from these studies that the isolates do not segregate into discernible subtypes, it is premature to conclude that sufficient variability could not exist to account for the differences in the epidemiology of the diseases associated with EBV infection. The level of resolution of most of the comparative restriction endonuclease studies of different EBV isolates is of the order of several hundred nucleotides. This level of investigation is barely adequate to detect the extensive variability in the U2 region described below. Therefore, the analyses that have been done neither support nor rigorously exclude the hypothesis that biologically significant strain differences exist. As functions of the viral genome that could participate in malignant transformation become better defined, the hypothesis will require continued testing. Relatively minor changes in nucleotide sequence could have profound effects on expression of one or several genes of pathophysiological significance.

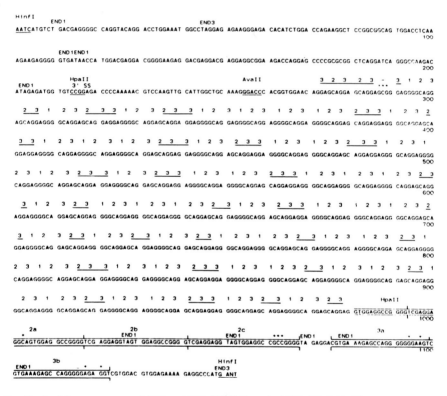

FIG. 5. Nucleotide sequences of IR2 and IR4 **(A)** (18) and of IR3 **(B)** (79). The sequences are in the polarity 5′ to 3′ in the orientation of the map shown in Fig. 3. **A:** The recognition sites for HaeII and SstI enzymes, which cut once within IR2 and IR4, respectively, are indicated in boxes. IR2 and IR4 each contain different 7-bp dyad symmetries indicated by a vertical arrow at the axis of the symmetry. The single solid line indicates the positions of a perfect direct repeat of 11 bp in IR2. The double line indicates the position of a 9-bp perfect tandem direct repeat in IR4 and the same 9-bp tandem direct repeat in IR2. The triangle marks the position of a missing T residue in the second 9-bp repeat in IR2. The dash lines indicate imperfect direct repeats of 22 bp in IR2 and 16 bp in IR4, and the dotted line marks the position of a imperfect direct repeat of 15 bp in IR4. The imperfect direct repeats shown have greater than 85% base-pair matching. **B:** The IR3 repeat region (79). Numerical superscripts 1, 2, and 3 are shown above the nucleotide triplets GGG, GCA, and GGA, respectively, at position 272–979. Base-pair mismatches in two 2 4-bp repeated sequences are shown with an asterisk above the mismatched nucleotide. The repeat units 2 3 and 2 3 3 are underlined in the sequence and are interspersed with another repeat element (1 2 3)$_n$, where n varies from 1 to 4.

DNA of the P3HR-1 Isolate

P3HR-1 cells constitute a high-level virus-producing clone of cells derived from the Jijoye cell line (89). The Jijoye cell line was established from an African Burkitt tumor biopsy. As described earlier, EBV from P3HR-1 cultures differs from the virus produced by Jijoye and from all other EBV isolates in its inability to growth-transform lymphocytes *in vitro*. This inability to induce growth transformation is not abolished by end-point dilution of P3HR-1 virus, suggesting that it is not a consequence of defective interfering particles (132). Furthermore, the P3HR-1 virus can infect B lymphocytes and induce abortive or productive replication, depending in part on the presence of a latent EBV genome in the infected cell (88,211). The P3HR-1 line has been passaged for over a decade in continuous culture. Analysis of the DNA of the P3HR-1 virus indicates that it is heterogeneous (24,73,75,196). Approximately half the molecules are similar in structure to standard EBV DNAs, except for the deletion of almost the entire U2 region (Fig. 3) (10,74,77,103,106,107). In contrast, Jijoye has more of the U2 region (106). Because Jijoye virus can transform cells and P3HR-1 cannot, the data suggest that sequences within the U2 region are important in the initiation of transformation. One attempt to approach this issue has been to superinfect the latently infected, Burkitt-tumor-biopsy-derived Raji cell line with P3HR-1 and to isolate recombinants between P3HR-1 and the endogenous Raji EBV DNA (47,49,211). Small amounts of transforming virus are released following superinfection, and this DNA can be amplified by cellular growth transformation. The P3HR-1 and endogenous Raji genomes can be distinguished at several sites with two restriction endonucleases and presumably at other sites with additional enzymes (77). If transformants produced by infection with super-infection virus can be shown to harbor EBV DNA which is a recombinant between p3HR-1 and Raji U2 DNA, U2 would be clearly implicated as an important segment for the initiation of growth transformation. The role of U2 in initiation of growth transformation is complicated by the observation that the U2 region varies extensively among transformation competent virus isolates (106).

At least two minor populations of highly defective P3HR-1 molecules can be differentiated by analysis of electron micrographs of partially denatured molecules (24). The most common minor population appears to consist of a repeating unit of $35–40 \times 10^6$ d. Restriction endonuclease analysis of P3HR-1 DNA reveals the presence of defective molecules in which noncontiguous parts of UL, US, and TR have recombined in new linkage arrangements (77). The defective molecules may be important in the induction of the permissive infection observed when Raji cells are superinfected with P3HR-1 virus. The defective molecules could achieve this effect by turning on late viral functions in a manner analogous to alpha or beta genes of HSV (91) or by titrating a putative repressor of lytic infection.

Primate EBV-related Agents

Many Old World primate species, including chimpanzees, baboons, gorillas, and orangutans, are known to be latently infected with herpesviruses that are antigenically cross-reactive with EBV (42,52,54,56,57,63,114,118,169,171,190). The viruses of chimpanzees and baboons, HVPan and HVPapio, respectively, have been studied most extensively. HVPan and HVPapio are endemic in their respective primate species. Like that of EBV, the host ranges of HVPan and HVPapio are restricted to primate B lymphocytes, in which these viruses induce growth transformation and an EBNA-like intranuclear antigen (54,56,57,150,171). Although limited cross-reactions have been detected, the intranuclear antigens specified by each virus have major non-cross-reactive determinants. The VCA, MA, and early antigens specified by each of these viruses cross-react extensively with antigens of virus from the heterologous primate species.

Analyses of HVPapio and HVPan DNAs were undertaken to define the relationships of these viruses to EBV and to each other. EBV, HVPapio, and HVPan DNAs have 40% homology in each pairwise comparison (42,54,56,79–81). The sizes and organizations of HVPapio and HVPan DNAs are similar to those of EBV DNA (76,78,115). Like EBV DNA, HVPan and HVPapio DNAs have 170×10^3 bp. Tandem direct repeats of a 3,100-bp sequence, IR1, separate HVPapio and HVPan DNAs into short (14×10^3 bp) unique DNA segments, US, and long (135×10^3 bp) unique DNA segments, UL. In HVPapio and HVPan DNAs, as in EBV DNA, there is homology (DL and DR regions) between DNAs at 26–28 and 93–95 $\times 10^6$ d in UL. Restriction endonuclease fragments from both ends of HVPapio DNA vary in numbers of repeats of a 550-bp sequence, TR, which hybridize to each other. The data identifying the TR in HVPan DNA are much less complete. The terminal fragments are heterogeneous in size, suggesting that there are varying numbers of copies of the TR. Thus, both HVPan and HVPapio probably have variable numbers of copies of direct tandem TRs, similar to EBV DNA. The common features of EBV, HVPapio, and HVPan DNAs are shown in Fig. 6.

The extent of physical colinearity between EBV and HVPapio and HVPan DNAs was investigated by hybridizing labeled cloned fragments of EBV DNA (range of complexity 0.8–6.4 $\times 10^6$ d, and representing the entire EBV genome) to Southern blots of fragments of HVPapio or HVPan DNA (76). The labeled EBV DNA fragments hybridized to HVPapio and HVPan DNA fragments that correspond to the same map positions as the EBV DNA fragments (Fig. 6). EBV DNA fragments containing the duplicated region of UL of EBV DNA hybridized to both regions of UL of HVPapio and HVPan DNAs, indicating that the duplicated sequences are conserved among these DNAs. One region of nonhomology was detected in the UL of EBV and HVPapio DNAs at 54–59 $\times 10^6$ d. EBV and HVPan DNAs have homology in this region. There was no homology detected between the TR of EBV and the TR of HVPapio or HVPan. There was also no homology between the TR of HVPapio and the TR of HVPan. The lack of homology among the TRs of EBV, HVPan, and HVPapio and the difference in sizes of the TRs of EBV and HVPapio suggest that the specific nucleotide sequence of the TRs is not highly conserved among the primate EBV-related agents. Two inferences could be drawn from the lack of TR homology: First, the greater sequence divergence of TR favors the hypothesis (considered earlier) that TR may function only to facilitate circularization

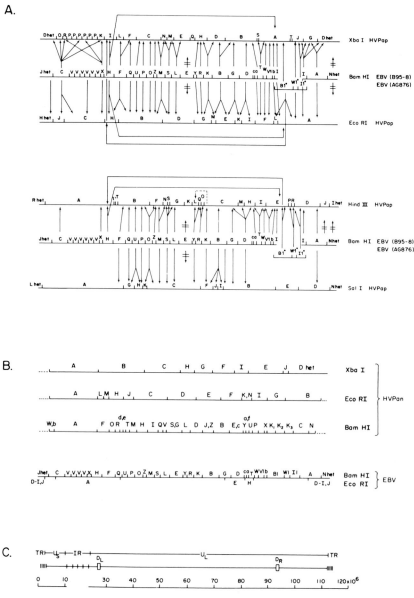

FIG. 6. Colinearity of HVPapio, HVPan, and EBV DNAs. **A:** Summary of homology between HVPapio and EBV DNAs (78). The *Bam*HI linkage map representative of a prototypical EBV genome is shown aligned with the *Xba*I, *Eco*RI, *Hind*III, and *Sal*I linkage maps of HVPapio DNA. Clones of the indicated *Bam*HI EBV DNA fragments from B95-8 and AG876 viruses were labeled *in vitro* and cross-hybridized to Southern blots of HVPapio DNA. **B:** Summary of homology of EBV and HVPan DNAs (79). The *Xba*I, *Eco*RI, and *Bam*HI maps of HVPan DNA are shown above the *Bam*HI and *Eco*RI maps of EBV DNA.

of the DNA. If TR does not encode an essential protein, its sequence may be subject to greater variation than other regions of the genome. Second, divergence might also be expected in those regions of the viral genome that may be involved in interaction with those cellular components that differ among human, chimpanzee, and baboon B lymphocytes.

The EBV-related class of herpesviruses are not endemic in New World primate species. The time of continental separation is placed at 50 million years ago. This suggests that the EBV class of agents is likely to have evolved within the last 50 million years. Apes, such as chimpanzees, and humans are believed to have developed for the past 30 million years along a different lineage from Old World monkeys, such as baboons. Chimpanzee cell DNA is more closely related to human cell DNA than is baboon cell DNA. The relatedness among primate retroviruses is similar to the cell DNA relationships (8). Retroviruses are therefore believed to have evolved with the species. The EBV-related agents do not follow this evolutionary scheme. HVPan and HVPapio are equally similar to EBV and to each other. This observation favors the hypothesis that this class of agents spread among the Old World primates within the last 30 million years and certainly after the divergence of apes and monkeys. Determination of whether the progenitor virus for the primate EBV related class of herpesviruses evolved from another herpesvirus or, less likely, from another virus group will require comparison of the nucleotide sequences of the genomes of the various classes of herpesviruses. The similarity of the IR2 and IR4 sequence to the HSV-1 terminal repeat "a" sequence suggests that there may have been a common progenitor herpesvirus (18).

TRANSFORMATION AND LATENCY WITHIN B LYMPHOCYTES

After infection with EBV, some and probably most B lymphocytes replicate perpetually in culture (55,82–84,87,157–159,194). The continued presence of the EBV intranuclear antigen (EBNA) and the EBV genome indicates that the cells remain latently infected. The frequency of spontaneous permissive infection varies with cell type and ranges from zero to 1% among cell lines derived by infection of neonatal human cells, from zero to 3% among adult human cell lines, and from zero to 10% among marmoset cell lines (54,56,128,129,142,143). Thus, on a statistical basis, marmoset lymphocytes tend to be more permissive than adult human lymphocytes, which are in turn more permissive than neonatal human lymphocytes. Within each category, some cultures are completely nonpermissive of viral replication. Maintenance of partially permissive cultures in rich media with frequent feedings usually results in rapid cell growth and selection of cells that are nonpermissive for viral replication.

In almost all latently infected cultures there are two classes of new antigenic activity. One antigen is detectable on the cell surface using immune T lymphocytes from patients recovering from primary EBV infection. This antigen, lymphocyte-derived membrane antigen (LYDMA), cannot be detected with immune sera and has not been further characterized (198). The second antigenic activity is the intranuclear antigen, EBNA (173). None of the antigens associated with abortive or productive viral infection has been identified in latently infected cells in human tissues, including latently infected normal peripheral B lymphocytes, malignant Burkitt tumor cells, and nasopharyngeal cancer cells (112,113,174,175). EBNA continues to be expressed when these cells are explanted and maintained *in vitro* or grown in nude mice. Increasing evidence suggests that EBNA is a complex of polypeptides. It is not known if EBNA and LYDMA share components.

Phosphonoacetic acid (PAA), phosphonoformic acid (PFA), and acycloguanosine (ACG) have been shown to inhibit EBV DNA replication in partially permissive cultures (16,197,203). Under the conditions used, these drugs preferentially inhibit herpesvirus DNA polymerases, suggesting that EBV DNA is replicated by a viral polymerase during productive infection (22). Although these drugs have no effect on the numbers of copies of EBV DNA in latently infected, growth-transformed cells, they can inhibit the establishment of latent infection and growth transformation. These latter data suggest that EBV polymerase-mediated DNA replication is a necessary condition to achieve latent infection and growth transformation and that once this state is achieved, the viral DNA is replicated by cellular polymerase that is less sensitive to PAA, PFA, and ACG. Alternatively, the PAA effect could be due to inhibition of a viral or cellular enzyme required for EBV DNA integration or for episome formation. The relative amount of viral DNA in synchronized cultures remains constant over the cell cycle. A slight increase during the early S phase suggests that viral DNA is replicated early during the synthesis of latently infected cell DNA (65).

The term "restringent" has been used to denote the latent state of EBV infection in growth-transformed B lymphocytes (105,107,152,160). The rationale for coining a new term was that no existing term adequately described this state. The infection is nonpermissive for viral replication, but is not entirely latent, in that the viral genome is actively transcribed, viral RNA is processed and transported, and viral protein or proteins are produced. Some viral gene product is presumed to be necessary for initiating and maintaining cellular growth transformation. Other possibilities, including a *cis*-acting effect of the viral genome, have not been rigorously excluded, but they seem unlikely, because transformation is very sensitive to ultraviolet (UV) inactivation of the virus (82). To the extent that maintenance of growth transformation requires active expression of the EBV genome, viral gene expression during primary infection and subsequent growth transformation may be different from expression in latent infections of B lymphocytes transformed prior to infection, in hybrids between EBV-infected lymphocytes and nonlymphoid cells, and in nonlymphoid cells infected by microinjection or by receptor transplantation (48,62,64,207). Whether or not the term restringent should be used for describing a latently infected African Burkitt tumor cell culture is therefore an open issue, because it is uncertain whether or not the typical infected tumor cell was initially growth-transformed by EBV. Further, even if EBV infection antedates the development of malignancy, the chromosomal change that accompanies malignant transformation (124) may be associated with a change in the state of EBV gene expression.

Viral DNA in Latently Infected Cells

Cultures of latently infected lymphocytes explanted from healthy seropositive donors, cultures of latently infected lymphocytes that were infected with EBV *in vitro*, and cultures of Burkitt tumor biopsies have been examined for the persistence of EBV DNA. In most instances the latently infected cells contain multiple copies of the EBV genome (101,102,144,146,147,163,195,214). DNA-DNA reassociation kinetics indicate that within the limits of accuracy of these analyses (5–10%), the entire EBV genome is present. In only two instances have studies indicated that an incomplete EBV genome is present in latently infected cells. The kinetics of DNA-DNA reassociation between labeled viral DNA and Namalwa cell DNA suggested that Namalwa cells have less than one complete EBV genome per cell. More recent data indicate that labeled Namalwa DNA hybridizes to all the larger *Eco*RI fragments of EBV DNA, indicating that Namalwa contains sequences spread over at least 80% of the EBV genome (M. Heller and E. Kieff, *unpublished data*). Probes from most regions of EBV DNA hybridized to EBV DNA in Namalwa cells. In a second series of studies in which labeled viral DNA was hybridized with DNA from nasopharyngeal carcinoma biopsies, the reassociation kinetics suggested that these tissues also contain less than the complete viral genome (153,154). Because nasopharyngeal carcinoma is an infiltrative malignant process, the tumor cells are mixed with normal stromal cells, and the number of EBV DNA copies per cell is lower than in Burkitt tumor tissue, which is a more uniform tumor composed primarily of infected lymphocytes. The observation of a change in reassociation kinetics in hybridizations with nasopharyngeal cancer tissue and Namalwa cell DNAs could be a consequence of degradation of the probe DNA with long intervals of hybridization. It was not demonstrated in either study that the residual labeled single-stranded viral DNA, which did not hybridize to Namalwa or nasopharyngeal carcinoma DNA, was still able to hybridize to viral DNA. Neither was it demonstrated that the unhybridized viral DNA mapped to specific "lost" region(s) of the viral genome.

The Raji cell line, a culture of nonpermissively infected Burkitt tumor cells, has been the prototype for many studies of the physical state of viral DNA in nonpermissively infected cells. By complementary RNA (cRNA) filter hybridization and by DNA-DNA reassociation kinetics, Raji cells are estimated to carry 50 copies of viral DNA. Almost all, or all, of the viral DNA in Raji cells is not covalently linked to cell DNA, although it may be loosely associated with cellular chromatin (145). Some of the episomal EBV DNA in Raji cells sediments at 65S and 100S in neutral glycerol velocity gradients, the expected values for open and supercoiled circles equal in length to EBV DNA (120). The 100S DNA sediments at 300S in alkaline glycerol gradients, indicating that it contains no nicks, gaps, or ribonucleotides (120). X-radiation converts the 100S DNA to an open 65S form that is identical in length to viral DNA (120). The Raji DNA circles are formed by covalent joining of the termini. The joining of the terminal restriction endonuclease fragments of Raji DNA into a new juncture fragment has been confirmed in Southern blots of Raji DNA (77). Viral DNA in Raji cells is partially resistant to cleavage by *Hpa*II but is sensitive to the isoschizomer *Msp*I, whereas virion DNA is sensitive to both enzymes (26,109). This strongly suggests that Raji DNA is partially methylated at CG sites and raises the possibility that methylation may play a role in control of transcription of intracellular Raji DNA. An attempt has been made to evaluate this hypothesis by examining the differential sensitivity of endogenous Raji EBV IR1 DNA to *Hpa*II and *Msp*I (S. Fennewald and E. Kieff, *unpublished data*). The sensitivity of IR1 DNA, which encodes RNA in Raji cells, was compared with that of *Bam*HI T, which does not encode messenger RNA in Raji cells. Both regions of the endogenous Raji DNA were partially resistant to *Hpa*II, indicating partial methylation. The effects of chemical induction of EBV expression in Raji cells include enhanced messenger RNA (mRNA) transcription from *Bam*HI T (105) and less methylation of *Bam*HI T DNA.

Circular episomal DNA the length of linear EBV DNA has been found in other nonpermissively infected cells and in Burkitt tumor tissue (2,99,100). The restriction endonuclease maps of intracellular DNAs from a variety of sources, including Burkitt tumor cell cultures and cultures of latently infected cells from seropositive patients, are similar to those of virion DNA except that the two terminal fragments of linear virion DNA are joined into a single fragment in intracellular DNA (20,21,77). Changes in EBV DNA during establishment of latent infection were investigated by comparing B95-8 virion DNA with intracellular EBV DNA from clones of normal neonatal lymphocytes latently infected and growth-transformed by the B95-8 virus (21,107,167). Several differences were found between the restriction endonuclease profiles of virion DNA and the intracellular DNA from the transformed cells: First, the two terminal *Eco*RI fragments of viral DNA migrate as a single larger fragment in intracellular DNA. The larger size of the terminal fragments in intracellular DNA is due in part to the covalent joining of both ends of virion DNA into a single fragment in intracellular DNA. The putative joined ends from an *in vitro* growth-transformed cell line were cloned into Charon 4A and were shown to consist of sequences from both ends of virion DNA (20). Second, there is variation in the sizes of the joined end fragments from several independently derived, latently infected, growth-transformed neonatal lymphocytes (167). This variation is in part attributable to fluctuation in the number of TRs in the joined end fragments. Some of the variation may be due to the loss of copies of TR during DNA replication. The latter phenomenon occurs commonly during propagation in *E. coli* of recombinant clones of the joined *Eco*RI termini. Digestion of the DNA of a single clone of the joined ends in Charon 4A yields molecules varying in the number of repeats of TR (20). Third, in one cell line, the fragment containing the sequences from the right terminus of EBV DNA is $12-25 \times 10^3$ bp larger than the joined terminal fragment in other cell lines. This larger size could be a consequence of 24 to 50 more copies of TR, but it could also be due to rearrangement or duplication of other viral DNA or recombination with cell DNA. Fourth, the size of the *Eco*RI A fragment varies among different cell lines from 23 to 37×10^6 d, probably because of differing numbers of repeats of IR1. Fifth, in one of the cell lines, the

*Eco*RI I and J fragments lack the *Eco*RI site between them. The size of the new *Eco*RI fragment is equal to the combined size of *Eco*RI I and J, suggesting that a single base change may have caused the loss of the *Eco*RI site.

The restriction endonuclease maps of EBV DNA were investigated in three nonpermissively infected cell lines that had been passaged for several years in culture and rapidly grown for several months prior to harvest of the intracellular viral DNA (77). Defective DNA molecules were found to accumulate as a minor population in each of the DNAs. The defective molecules consisted of sequences from various noncontiguous regions of the EBV genome linked together. Many of these defective molecules resembled the defective populations in P3HR-1 virion DNA, suggesting a common mechanism in the origins of both types of defectives. In particular, DNA in the *Eco*RI B fragment was frequently linked to DNA that maps elsewhere in standard EBV DNA. The frequent involvement of part of *Eco*RI B in defective DNA suggests that there may be an origin of DNA replication in this region. The IR3 sequence is near the center of the region that is part of the defective DNA population but is not homologous to the simian virus 40 (SV40) origin of replication. Other atypical linkages included unusual juncture fragments between the left and right ends of the DNA. None of the unusual fragments has been cloned for precise mapping and sequencing.

In nonpermissively infected cells, the EBV genome is replicated by a cellular polymerase. The generation of defective viral DNA molecules could be a consequence of replication of the viral DNA by the cellular polymerase. Rapid cell growth could enhance the generation of defective viral molecules by further stressing the cellular enzymes that are involved in viral DNA replication.

There have been a number of attempts to determine if EBV DNA is integrated into cell DNA of Raji cells (1,145). Raji cells were chosen because they have been the prototype for studies of latently infected Burkitt tumor cell lines. However, Raji cells contain numerous circular episomal copies of EBV DNA. A small fraction of EBV DNA from Raji cells bands at a lower density than virion DNA, suggesting linkage to cell DNA (1). On shearing, the less dense EBV DNA rebands at a higher density, further suggesting previous linkage to cell DNA. The data do not exclude the possibility that the small fraction of viral DNA initially banded at lower density as a consequence of tightly adherent protein or trapping by cell DNA. Studies of a malignant human B cell line infected with EBV *in vitro* have suggested that at least part of the EBV genome can integrate (4). In these experiments, the cells contained one or a few EBV DNA copies per cell, and the density of EBV DNA was near the density of cell DNA. The possibility that cytosine methylation or recombinant forms of viral DNA could lower the density of intracellular EBV DNA was not excluded in these studies.

Cytological hybridization of labeled EBV DNA fragments to metaphase chromatids of Namalwa or IB4 cells indicates that all fragments of EBV DNA are associated with a single chromosomal site in each of these two cell lines (218). EBV DNA is associated with Namalwa chromosome 1 and IB4 chromosome 4. The constant association of EBV DNA with a single chromosome site in these two cell lines suggests that EBV DNA is integrated into cell DNA. It is not known if this is a general property of latently infected cells, and viral DNA can integrate at other sites. Cloning of viral cell DNA juncture fragments would indicate which parts of the viral and cellular genomes become linked and may indicate whether or not the process requires homology between cell DNA and virus DNA. The EBV IR3 sequence has a high degree of homology to a moderately repetitive interspersed sequence in the human genome (80). The IR3-related sequences are in every human chromosome except the Y chromosome and are predominantly at centromeric and subtelomeric sites. IR3 could direct homologous recombination between viral DNA and cell DNA. To test this hypothesis, the linkage between U3 and U4 sequences was investigated in Namalwa and IB4 cells. Homologous recombination directed by IR3 would result in a loss of close linkage between U3 and U4 DNAs. The linkage remains as tight as in EBV DNA. The data therefore indicate that IR3 did not direct homologous recombination with these two cell DNAs.

Viral RNA in Latently Infected, Growth-transformed Cells and in Burkitt Tumor Cells *In Vitro*

Analyses of viral RNA from latently infected, growth-transformed B lymphocytes or from latently infected African Burkitt tumor lymphoblasts grown in culture indicate that there is extensive transcription of the viral genome (72,105,107,152,160–162). RNA from either class of latently infected B lymphocytes hybridizes to as much as 30% of randomly labeled EBV DNA. Only stable RNAs are detected in this kind of analysis. If these stable RNAs are encoded by one DNA strand or the other, but never by both complementary strands, the data would indicate that stable RNA is encoded by 60% of the single-stranded length of EBV DNA. To evaluate the possible significance of transcripts from complementary strands, RNA was permitted to anneal to itself under the same conditions used in RNA-DNA hybridizations. The RNA was then treated with pancreatic ribonuclease. The putative double-stranded RNA was then denatured and hybridized to labeled viral DNA. The RNA hybridized to less than 5% of EBV DNA, indicating that only a small part of the RNA that hybridizes to EBV DNA is encoded by complementary DNA (cDNA) strands (A. Powell, T. Dambaugh, and E. Kieff, *unpublished data*).

The polyadenylated RNA fraction from latently infected, growth-transformed cells or from cultures of Burkitt tumor lymphoblasts hybridizes to 20% of EBV DNA (105,107,152,160). The hybridization is initially rapid and reaches an early plateau, indicating that the polyadenylated RNA fraction is enriched for RNA encoded by this 20% of EBV DNA. Polyadenylated RNA does not hybridize further to viral DNA, indicating specific enrichment for those RNAs that selectively accumulate in the polyadenylated RNA fraction.

Polyribosomal RNA or cytoplasmic polyadenylated RNA from latently infected, growth-transformed cells or from cultures of Burkitt lymphocytes hybridizes to 10% of EBV DNA, indicating that a subset of the polyadenylated RNA selectively accumulates on polyribosomes (72,105,107,152,160–162). Again, additional RNAs are not detected with longer hybridizations. From the kinetics of hybridization of latently infected cellular RNAs to viral DNA, viral RNA is estimated to be 0.06% of the cellular nuclear RNA, 0.06% of the polyadenylated RNA, and 0.003% of the polyribosomal RNA. Earlier lower estimates of the abundance of viral RNA were due to degradation of the RNA during extraction and failure to correct hybridization kinetics for the effect of DNA-DNA and RNA-DNA hybridization involving the IR1 sequence in EBV DNA.

The results obtained from studies of the kinetics of hybridization of cellular RNAs to viral DNA indicate that nuclear RNAs should map more broadly in EBV DNA than should polyadenylated RNA and that polyribosomal RNA should be restricted to about 20% of the length of EBV DNA. The mapping studies that have been done are consistent with these expectations (105,107,160,219). The most precise mapping data available are for RNA from two cell lines: Raji, a Burkitt tumor cell line, and IB4, a clone of neonatal cells transformed *in vitro* by B95-8 virus (105,107,206). The results are remarkably similar and are consistent with earlier, less precise data obtained with RNA from the Namalwa Burkitt tumor cell line (104,160). Much of the increased precision of the more recent analysis is due to extensive use of cloned restriction endonuclease fragments of EBV DNA (20,21). Polyribosomal RNA is encoded by 40% of IR1 and by at least 25% of the adjacent unique region, U2 (*Bam*HI X and H fragments), and by DNA that maps at 63–66 and 110–115 × 10^6 d in EBV DNA (105,107). These results are summarized in Fig. 7. Nuclear RNA is encoded by larger fractions of those viral DNA fragments that encode polyribosomal RNA and by other fragments of EBV DNA, including the *Eco*RI F and G fragments. The finding that nuclear RNAs are encoded by larger fractions of the fragments that encode polyribosomal RNA suggests that the RNAs are derived from large nuclear precursors by cleavage or splicing. However, the possibility that the additional complexity of nuclear RNA may be due to transcripts that are not precursors for messenger RNA has not been formally excluded. The sizes of most of the nuclear RNAs encoded by the IR1-U2 region are larger than those of the cytoplasmic RNAs, as would be expected for precursor molecules (220). These RNAs are encoded by the same DNA strand of IR1-U2 that encodes messenger RNA. The large nuclear RNAs differ in size by 3-kb increments, suggesting that they vary in numbers of copies of IR1, such as would occur if they initiate from any copy of IR1, or that full copies of IR1 are spliced out. Some of the nuclear RNAs are smaller than polyadenylated polyribosomal RNA and therefore are not precursors. The smaller nuclear RNAs may be stable splicing or cleavage products of maturing RNAs. The nuclear RNA encoded by *Eco*RI F and G has been detected only by Southern blot analysis. The sizes of the *Eco*RI F and G RNAs have not been determined on Northern blots.

The sizes of the cytoplasmic polyadenylated RNAs encoded by U1, by IR1-U2, by U3-IR3-U4, and by U5 were determined by Northern blot analysis (79,206). The region of U1 from 5 to 7 × 10^6 d encodes two very low abundance RNAs of 2.3 and 2.0 kb; IR1 and U2, encode a more abundant 3-kb RNA (and a less

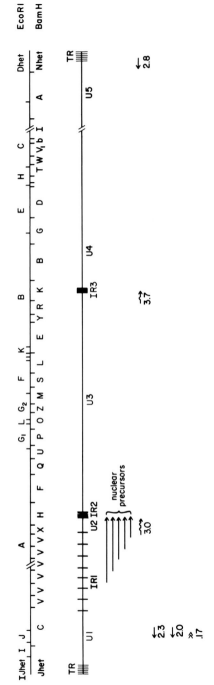

FIG. 7. EBV RNAs in latently infected cells. Arrows indicate the size and direction of transcription of RNAs from the indicated regions of B95-8 viral DNA. Nuclear precursors are shown for the IR1-U2 region; all of the other RNAs shown are cytoplasmic. The sizes in kilobases pairs of cytoplasmic RNAs are given below the arrows. All of the RNAs shown are polyadenylated, with the exception of two small 0.17-kbp RNAs (5,105,117,179). Interruptions in the 3.0- and 3.7-kbp RNAs indicate that these transcripts are spliced. The size and map position of each RNA were determined by hybridization of cloned DNA restriction endonuclease fragment probes to blots of RNA gels (206). The direction of transcription was determined by hybridization of the RNA to strand-separated DNA for the 3.0-, 3.7-, and 2.8-kbp RNAs or inferred from the hybridization pattern of oligo(dT)-primed complementary DNA for the 2.3- and 2.0-kbp RNAs (206).

abundant 1.5-kb RNA). The U3-IR3-U4 and U5 encode RNAs of 3.7 and 2.8 kb, respectively.

Two approaches have been used to determine the 5' to 3' orientation of these cytoplasmic polyadenylated RNAs (79,206,220). Short-length, oligodeoxythymi-dylic acid[oligo(dT)]-primed cDNA was synthesized as a probe for the 3' end of the RNA. The hybridization of the oligo(dT)-primed cDNA to Southern blots of recombinant EBV DNA fragments was compared with the hybridization of oligo-deoxynucleotide-primed cDNA, a probe representative of full-length RNA. The most easily interpretable data were those obtained with the 63–66 × 10^6-d region. The 3'-specific cDNA hybridized to the 63–66 × 10^6-d DNA fragment, but not to the 61–63 × 10^6 DNA fragment, whereas randomly primed cDNA hybridized to both fragments. Thus, the 3' end of the RNA encoded by this region maps to the right at 63–66 × 10^6 d, and the 5' end of the RNA maps to the left at 61–63 × 10^6 d. Both 3'-specific and randomly primed cDNA probes hybridized to the 105–110 and 110–115 × 10^6-d fragments. However, randomly primed cDNA hybridized more to the 110–115 × 10^6-d fragment, suggesting that the 3' end was in the 105–110 × 10^6-d fragment and the 5' end in the 110–115 × 10^6 fragment. Determination of orientation of the RNA encoded by the U1 or IR-U2 was not possible, because randomly primed cDNA hybridizes to all the fragments tested from this region, and the 3'-specific cDNA hybridizes to U1, to IR1 and to U2. There are more 3' ends than there are RNAs of different sizes identified by DNA from this region.

The second approach to determining the direction of transcription of these three more abundant RNAs encoded by IR1-U2, U3-IR3-U4, and U5 was to subclone the DNA fragments encoding these RNAs into pKH47, a derivative of PBR 322 that has homopolymer dAs or dTs on opposite strands. The strands of insert DNA could then be separated by chromatography on oligo(dT) and oligo(dA) cellulose. These experiments proved that the IR1-U2 3-kb RNA is transcribed from left to right, the U3-IR3-U4 3.7-kb RNA is transcribed from left to right, and the U5 2.8-kb RNA is transcribed from right to left. By S1 nuclease analysis, the 3.0- and 3.7-kb RNAs are found to be spliced; a major exon has been identified in the 2.8-kb RNA that is at least 2.3 kb. Thus, splicing of this RNA is less certain.

Two investigations led simultaneously to the discovery that EBV specifies small RNAs in latently infected cells. One group, working with sera from patients with lupus erythematosus to identify ribonucleoprotein complexes in human cells, found that ribonucleoprotein antigens from Raji cells contained a new small RNA, slightly larger than other small human cellular RNAs (117). A second group, engaged in mapping viral messenger RNAs, was attempting to resolve a discrepancy between data obtained with total cytoplasmic RNA (180) and data obtained with cytoplasmic polyadenylated RNA (105,107,160). In resolving this discrepancy, it was dem-onstrated that the most abundant viral RNA in Raji and IB4 cells is a 160-bp nonpolyadenylated RNA, encoded by the 5–7 × 10^6-d region (105,206). By both size and oligonucleotide fingerprint, the small RNA has been shown to be two distinct molecular species (5,117,179). The function of the RNA is unknown. Some of the small RNA remains associated with polyadenylated RNA through two cycles of chromatography on oligo(dT) columns and subsequently separates from the polyadenylated RNA only after heat denaturation, indicating that the small RNA hydrogen bonds to some polyadenylated RNAs (V. Van Santen and E. Kieff, *unpublished data*). The small RNA is encoded by the same DNA strand that encodes the 2.3-kbp polyadenylated RNA from this region. No homology of this region to other regions in EBV DNA is detectable by Southern blot hybridization. Therefore, the small RNA cannot bind to other EBV polyadenylated RNA by means of long regions of homology. The nature and significance of the binding of the small RNA to polyadenylated RNA remain unknown.

African Burkitt tumor biopsies from 4 patients were analyzed for EBV RNA (19). Each biopsy contained RNA that hybridized to 3 to 7% of EBV DNA. In contrast to the results obtained with the RNAs from tumor cell lines grown in culture, both polyadenylated and nonpolyadenylated RNAs from tumor tissue hybridized to only 3 to 7% of EBV DNA. These results suggest that either there is less extensive transcription of EBV DNA in tumor tissue or there is more rapid degradation of nonprocessed precursor RNAs. By Southern blot hybridization analysis and by hybridization of RNA in solution to labeled fragments of viral DNA, the polyadenylated RNA in Burkitt tumor tissue was mapped primarily to two regions: the region around and including IR1 and the region now designated U5. Some hybridization to other EBV DNA fragments was found as well.

Proteins and Antigenic Reactivities in Latently Infected, Growth-transformed Cells

The concentration of EBNA in latently infected cells is too low to be detected by direct or indirect immunofluorescence with most immune human sera. Detection of EBNA by fluorescence microscopy usually requires amplification of the antigen-antibody reactions. This has usually been done by using complement and fluorescence-labeled anticomplement antibody (173). EBNA is associated with cellular chromosomes, but it rapidly diffuses away from the chromosomes if the cells are not promptly fixed. Much of the soluble antigen that can be extracted from latently infected cells and detected with immune human sera seems to be associated with EBNA (6,116,122,123,151). Several lines of evidence indicate that EBNA is encoded by EBV: First, EBNA has been detected only in lymphocytes infected with EBV. Second, antibody to EBNA has been detected only in individuals with antibody to EBV structural antigens. Third, cells nonpermissively infected with HVPan and HVPapio also have chromosomal binding antigens (54,56,149,150,171). The HVPan antigen can be detected in the nuclei of nonpermissively infected cells by complement-enhanced immunofluorescence using chimpanzee immune sera. The HVPapio antigen cannot be detected in HVPapio-infected cells by this method, but it can be bound to acid-fixed chicken or salamander chromosomes, where it can be detected by immunofluorescence using baboon or human immune sera. Fourth, *Papio* lymphocytes infected with HVPapio can be superinfected with EBV. EBNA can then be detected in *Papio* cells using human, but not *Papio*, antisera. Fifth, human cells can be infected with HVPan, and chimpanzee lymphocytes can be infected with EBV. Both infections are nonpermissive. The nuclear antigen induced by EBV is recognized only by human sera, whereas that induced by HVPan is recognized preferentially by chimpanzee sera.

The soluble complement-fixation and the acid-fixed chromosome assays for EBNA have been used for following antigenic activity during EBNA purification (6, 116,122,123,151). The antigenic activity is stable at 80°C for 30 min and can be further purified by DNA cellulose and hydroxyapatite chromatography and by immunoprecipitation. The molecular weight of the antigenic activity in crude cellular extracts is estimated to be 180,000 by ultrafiltration and ultracentrifugation. After denaturation, the purified material consists of two polypeptides of 48×10^3 and 52×10^3 d (121). The V8 protease, cyanogen bromide products, and glycine content of the 53×10^3-d polypeptide may be similar to those of the cellular 53×10^3-d polypeptide that binds to SV40 T antigen.

Three lines of evidence indicate that there are additional polypeptides specified by EBV in the nonpermissively infected cell: First, as noted earlier, at least three relatively more abundant polyadenylated cytoplasmic RNAs have been identified in latently infected cells (206). Second, sera from latently infected rheumatoid arthritis patients and other sera from latently infected humans recognize another nuclear antigen in latently infected cells. This second nuclear antigen has been termed rheumatoid-arthritis-associated nuclear antigen (RANA) (3). The acronym perpetuates a misnomer, because neither the antibody nor the antigen is strongly associated with rheumatoid disease (13). RANA activity is maximal early in the G_1 phase and is not confined to the nucleus (187). The antigen can be detected without complement enhancement and is not altered by deoxyribonuclease treatment. Sera with high anti-RANA titers also react with latently infected cell extracts in immunodiffusion tests. There is a high correlation in terms of development and titer between anti-RANA and anti-EBNA antibodies. In an attempt to segregate EBNA and RANA, latently infected lymphocytes were fused with mouse or hamster fibroblasts (188). Nine clones of hybrid cells were EBNA-positive and RANA-negative, and 16 were RANA-positive and EBNA-negative. RANA-positive EBNA-negative clones contained DNA from at least 80% of the EBV genome. The segregation of antigens in the hybrid cells suggests that RANA and EBNA are different antigens. The third line of evidence that there are additional EBV polypeptides is from a recent study using radioimmunoelectrophoresis and fluoroimmunoelectro-phoresis procedures with sodium dodecyl sulfate extracts and immune human sera (193). Polypeptides of 73 and 81×10^3 d were detected in nonpermissively infected cells. Subcloning of a mixed population of EBNA-positive and EBNA-negative cells revealed that the 73×10^3-d polypeptide segregated with an EBNA-positive clone and was absent from an EBNA-negative clone. Furthermore, partially purified EBNA preparations from Raji cells are enriched for the 65 and 81×10^3-d poly-peptides. The $63–67 \times 10^3$-d region of denaturing polyacrylamide gels of Raji extracts removes anti-EBNA activity from human sera, suggesting that the 65×10^3-d polypeptide is an important antigenic component of EBNA.

The data are adequate to conclude that EBV specifies at least one chromatin-binding polypeptide antigen. RANA could be a separate viral gene product, a cellular protein specifically induced by EBV, or a modification of EBNA. Similarly, the 48, 53, 65, and 81×10^3-d polypeptides could be separate viral gene products, related posttranslational modifications of a common polypeptide, or cellular polypeptides induced by EBV infection. The simplest hypothesis that would account for most of the existing data is that EBNA and RANA are separate EBV-induced polypeptides. The 48×10^3-d viral polypeptide is probably a component of EBNA that complexes with a 53×10^3-d cellular polypeptide. The 65×10^3-d polypeptide may be the intact Raji EBNA polypeptide; and the 81×10^3-d polypeptide may be a component of RANA.

ABORTIVE AND PRODUCTIVE INFECTIONS

Some latently infected B lymphocytes continuously give rise to progeny cells that are permissive of viral replication. As described earlier, cell type is an important determinant of the frequency of permissive infection. The frequency of permissive infection in cultures of partially permissive infected cell lines can be increased by the addition of chemical inducers. A tumor-promoting phorbol ester, 12-O-tetra-decanoylphorbol-12-acetate (TPA), and an inducer of differentiation, sodium butyrate, are the most consistently effective inducers of permissive infection (98,215). Many other chemicals, including inhibitors of cellular DNA, RNA, and protein synthesis, hormones, cyclic nucleotides, and antibody against IgM on the cell surface, have some inducing activity (51,65–69). The variety of these chemicals makes it difficult to suggest a common mechanism for their effects. If anything, the data suggest that the regulation of viral replication in partially permissive cells is not a stringent process and is influenced by changes in cellular metabolism. A hypothesis that has been suggested is that the extent of methylation of viral DNA could be a final common path for regulating the frequency of productive viral infection. The available data dealing with CG methylation, as described earlier, indicate that the level of CG methylation of DNA is not determinative of expression. No studies have been done of methylation at specific CG sites near promoters in EBV DNA or of the level of methylation of other nucleotides.

Following exposure to butyrate or TPA, as many as 20 to 40% of the cells in a partially permissive culture become productively infected (98,217). The diffuse (D) and restricted (R) components of early antigen (EA) can be detected with some immune human sera. In addition, cellular macromolecular synthesis is inhibited, viral DNA is synthesized within the nucleus, the viral capsid antigen (VCA) complex can be detected in the cytoplasm, viral nucleocapsids assemble in the nucleus, and the membrane antigen (MA) complex can be detected on the cell surface and nuclear membrane (31). Mature virus is produced by budding through the nuclear membrane. Treatment of induced cultures with phosphonoacetic acid, acycloguanosine, or other inhibitors of viral DNA synthesis results in diminished synthesis of viral DNA, VCA, and MA. The number of cells containing EA is unchanged or is increased (58,138–140).

Some latently infected cell lines that are totally nonpermissive of viral replication can be induced to a state of abortive infection by treatment of the cultures with chemical inducers. TPA is the most effective chemical inducer. The abortive infection induced in latently infected cells by TPA is characterized by the expression of EA-D and EA-R in 10 to 40% of the cells in a culture of previously latently infected Raji cells and by the inhibition of cellular DNA, RNA, and protein synthesis. TPA does not induce synthesis of viral DNA, VCA, or MA in latently infected cultures such as the Raji cell line (138).

Superinfection of some latently infected cultures, including Raji, with the virus produced by the P3HR-1 cell line results in a more permissive state of viral infection than can be induced by TPA. In addition to EA expression, viral DNA synthesis is increased at least 100-fold (211). Low levels of viral VCA and MA can be detected in a small fraction of the cells, and some virus is produced. The released virus can be distinguished from the superinfecting P3HR-1 virus because the virus produced following superinfection can induce growth transformation of B lymphocytes (211). The Raji cell line has been the prototype for most studies on the abortive and partially permissive states of EBV infection. The extent to which viral DNA, RNA, and proteins and virus produced in superinfected Raji cells are products of the endogenous Raji EBV DNA, or of the superinfecting P3HR-1 DNA, or of putative recombinants between Raji and P3HR-1 EBV DNA, is unknown.

Viral DNA in Abortive and Productive Infections

Productive infection usually is studied by induction of viral replication in partially permissive, but largely latently infected, cell cultures. Because most viral DNA in such cells is in closed circular form before induction, replication must proceed from this as an initial substrate. The DNA could replicate as a circular molecule or go through a linear intermediate. Because viral DNAs that can circularize usually replicate through a circular intermediate, it is likely that EBV would follow this rule. Some attempt has been made to examine EBV replication in superinfected Raji cells (185). The system is favorable in that there is an enormous burst of viral DNA replication within several hours of infection of Raji cells with the P3HR-1 virus. Potential problems include inaccuracy in determining the multiplicity of superinfection and the possibility that defective P3HR-1 DNA could replicate differently than nondefective DNA. In earlier studies, restriction endonuclease digests of DNA from superinfected cells could not be differentiated from P3HR-1 viral DNA, possibly for technical reasons (183). Using pulse labels and gradient separation, first on isopycknic CsCl gradients and then on velocity glycerol gradients, 65S and possibly 80S forms of viral DNA were detected between 4 and 24 hr after superinfection of Raji cells (185). After a chase period, the 80S form was diminished, and 55–65S DNA increased, suggesting that the 80S DNA is a replication intermediate. Longer molecules were not detected with either short or long labeling periods. Evidence that longer molecules would have survived experimental manipulation was not presented. The organization of viral sequences in the 80S "intermediate" and in the 65S DNA has not been determined. The 65S DNA is presumed to be open circles. The accumulation of open-circular progeny molecules and the absence of longer molecules suggest that replication does not proceed through the generation of linear concatamers.

Viral RNA in Abortive and Productive Infections

Some of the changes in viral gene expression following chemical induction have been studied by comparing viral RNAs from cultures in which abortive infection was induced with RNAs from latently infected cultures (105,199). In these studies, which are summarized in Fig. 6, Raji cells were induced with 5-iodo-2-deoxyuridine (IUdR). EA was detected in 10% of the cells. The complexity and abundance of nuclear RNA increased slightly. Nuclear RNA from abortively infected cultures hybridized to 40% of the labeled EBV DNA, whereas nuclear RNA from latently infected cultures hybridized to 35% of labeled EBV DNA. These figures correspond to 80 and 70% of the genome, respectively, assuming that the RNAs are asymmetric transcripts. In contrast to the slight increase in the complexity of nuclear RNAs with the transition from latent to abortive infection, there was a marked increase in the complexity and abundance of stable polyadenylated and polyribosomal RNAs. The complexity of polyadenylated RNA increased from 18 to 33% and polyribosomal RNA from 10 to 30% of the DNA. Thus, whereas in latent infection there was a considerable disparity in the complexity of nuclear versus polyadenylated and polyribosomal RNAs, there was little disparity in abortive infection. Hybridization of ^{32}P-labeled cDNA synthesized from nuclear or polyribosomal RNAs to Southern blots of fragments of viral DNA confirms that nuclear RNA in abortively infected cells is encoded by most of the same fragments that encode nuclear RNA in latently infected cells. Whereas a restricted set of viral RNAs accumulates on the polyribosomes of latently infected cells, polyribosomal RNA from abortively infected cells is encoded by the same DNA fragments that encode nuclear RNAs. Thus, regions of the viral genome that encode only nuclear RNA before induction encode both nuclear and polyribosomal RNAs after induction. These data suggest that there could be a major change in the posttranscriptional processing of viral RNAs following induction. Alternatively, there could be a difference in the primary transcripts in induced or noninduced Raji cells. The comparative maps of viral polyribosomal RNAs from abortively and latently infected Raji cells are shown in Fig. 8.

Studies of the effect of actinomycin D on the induction of abortive infection indicate that the drug blocks induction (63,67,69). This suggests that new transcription is required for expression of early antigens, but it does not indicate whether or not the new transcripts differ from previously existing nuclear RNAs or encode a protein that alters RNA processing.

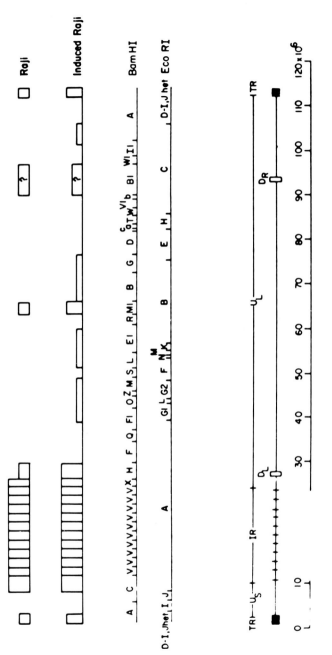

FIG. 8. Physical map of *Bam*HI and *Eco*RI restriction endonuclease fragments of the standard form of Raji EBV DNA, with the locations of DNA sequences that encode stable polyribosomal RNA in Raji and abortively infected Raji cells. The height of each bar is proportional to the extent of hybridization to blots of viral DNA of ³²P-labeled DNA complementary to Raji RNA. It is uncertain whether or not the duplications DL and DR both encode RNA (105).

Analysis of the complexity of the viral RNAs in Raji cells superinfected with P3HR-1 virus has yielded results similar to those obtained with RNA from abortively infected Raji cells induced with IUdR (152,199). These studies have not been extended to the point where new RNAs associated with the enhanced expression of the viral genome in superinfected Raji cells have been detected.

At 3 days after TPA induction of productive infection in partially permissive B95-8 cultures, MA is detected on the surfaces of 20% of the cells, and VCA is detected in the cytoplasm in 10% of the cells. Cytoplasmic polyadenylated RNAs in these cells are encoded by almost every fragment of EBV DNA, except for IR1 and U2 (92). The sizes of the RNAs encoded by each region of the EBV genome were determined by hybridization of labeled EBV DNA fragments to Northern blots of cytoplasmic polyadenylated RNAs. Comparison of RNAs from induced cultures with RNAs from induced cultures also treated with phosphonoacetic acid to inhibit viral DNA synthesis identified two RNA classes: a persistent early class of RNAs whose abundance is relatively resistant to DNA synthesis inhibition and a late class of RNAs whose abundance is sensitive to inhibition of DNA synthesis. The data are summarized in Fig. 9. Several points should be made about these data: First, persistent early and late RNAs are not clustered but are intermixed and scattered through most of the segments of U1, U3, U4, and U5. Second, cytoplasmic polyadenylated RNAs expressed during latent infection were not detected in productively infected cells. Third, some RNAs encoded by a fragment are present in high abundance (e.g., the 2.8-, 3.6-, 4.0-, and 4.5-kbp RNAs identified by labeled *Bam*HI F), whereas other RNAs encoded by the same fragment are present in lower abundance (e.g., the 9.9-, 8.0-, 6.9-, and 5.8-kbp RNAs identified by labeled *Bam*HI F). Many of the less abundant RNAs are larger in size than the more abundant RNAs and are also identified in Northern blots of nuclear RNAs. These RNAs may be nuclear precursors that leak into the cytoplasm during the extraction procedure. Fourth, nonpolyadenylated small RNAs originally identified in cells latently infected with EBV are expressed in higher abundance early in productive infection. Fifth, several DNA fragments (e.g., *Bam*HI F) encode more than one abundant RNA. In some instances, the sum of the sizes of these RNAs is more than twice the size of the fragment. Adjacent fragments do not hybridize to most of several RNAs. The data therefore indicate that the same or complementary nucleotides encode a portion of more than one RNA. Work is in progress to identify the polypeptides encoded by these RNAs.

Viral Proteins in Abortive and Productive Infections

Two strategies have been employed to identify the proteins made early in permissive EBV infection. One is to induce abortive infection in Raji cells with TPA. The second is to block late protein synthesis in superinfected Raji cells or in permissively infected cells using an inhibitor of viral DNA synthesis. As might be anticipated from data cited previously (that the viral infection induced in Raji by chemicals aborts at an earlier stage than the semipermissive infection induced by

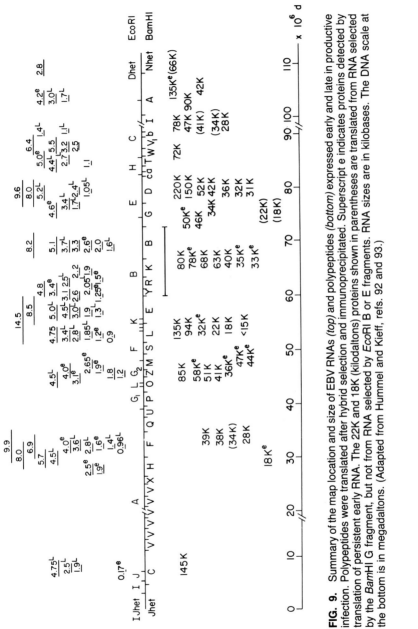

FIG. 9. Summary of the map location and size of EBV RNAs *(top)* and polypeptides *(bottom)* expressed early and late in productive infection. Polypeptides were translated after hybrid selection and immunoprecipitated. Superscript e indicates proteins detected by translation of persistent early RNA. The 22K and 18K (kilodaltons) proteins shown in parentheses are translated from RNA selected by the *Bam*HI G fragment, but not from RNA selected by *Eco*RI B or E fragments. RNA sizes are in kilobases. The DNA scale at the bottom is in megadaltons. (Adapted from Hummel and Kieff, refs. 92 and 93.)

superinfection), the two approaches have yielded different results. Two new soluble polypeptides are induced in Raji cells by TPA, and they immunoprecipitate with human anti-EA sera. These two polypeptides are 85–90 and 30–40 × 10^3 d (138).

P3HR-1-superinfected Raji cells and chemically induced P3HR-1 cultures have been prototype cultures for studies of polypeptide synthesis in permissive infection (9,43,98,140). In permissively infected cultures, the 85–90 and 30–40 × 10^3-d polypeptides are predominantly cytoplasmic in location and are synthesized in cells blocked for late polypeptide synthesis by inhibitors of viral DNA replication. Additional immunoprecipitable polypeptides are present in P3HR-1-superinfected Raji cells and in permissively infected P3HR-1 cells blocked for viral DNA replication. Human anti-EA sera immunoprecipitate 140 and 125 × 10^3-d polypeptides from induced P3HR-1 cultures. These polypeptides are all unaffected by inhibitors of viral DNA synthesis and are therefore early polypeptides that may also be components of the EA complexes.

Late viral antigen components have been identified in extracts of superinfected Raji cells and in permissively infected P3HR-1 cells (43,44,98,140). Anti-VCA and anti-MA human sera immunoprecipitate polypeptides of 150–165, 145–158, 85, 46, 34, and 18 × 10^3 d. The synthesis of these latter components and of the MAs described earlier in this chapter is prevented by treatment with inhibitors of viral DNA synthesis. All these late antigen polypeptides have been detected in extracts of both nuclei and cytoplasm. The sizes of the 150–165 and 145–158 × 10^3-d late components are compatible with those of the major viral capsid and core polypeptides.

The time course of synthesis of polypeptides in P3HR-1-superinfected Raji cells has been investigated by separating the infected cell polypeptides directly on denaturing polyacrylamide gels without prior immunoprecipitation (43,44). The effects of inhibitors of viral DNA synthesis on the synthesis of each of the polypeptides, the partitioning of the polypeptides between nucleus and cytoplasm, and the phosphorylation of the polypeptides have been evaluated. The results are summarized in Table 1. Some polypeptides similar in size to preexisting cellular polypeptides continue to be made after infection, but the synthesis of most cellular polypeptides is inhibited. These polypeptides are designated as "persistent" polypeptides and are believed to be cellular. However, the possibility that some of these polypeptides are viral and are similar in size to cellular polypeptides has not been rigorously excluded. The synthesis of these polypeptides throughout infection at the same rate as before infection favors the hypothesis that these are cellular polypeptides. During the 48-hr period following superinfection, 31 new polypeptides appear. The synthesis of only 7 of these polypeptides is inhibited by inhibitors of viral DNA synthesis. Therefore, within the context of the preceding discussion, 24 polypeptides are defined as being early polypeptides. Several polypeptides are synthesized only at specific time intervals after superinfection, suggesting that the synthesis of these polypeptides is highly regulated. Various inhibitors of cellular or viral DNA synthesis, or of both, were tested for their differential effects on viral DNA and viral protein synthesis. Several of the drugs that inhibited viral DNA synthesis resulted

TABLE 1. *Polypeptides synthesized in Raji cells after superinfection by P3HR-1 virus*

Polypeptide	Molecular weight ($\times 10^3$)	Time of maximum synthesis (hr post infection)	Effects of ACV and PAA on synthesis	Intracellular location[a]
1	155	16		N
2	145	14	Inhibition	N
2A	142	24		
3	140	10		N – C
3A	135	24		
4	125	10		C
5	123	2		4
6	122	24	Inhibition	C
7A	117	6		
8	116	2		4
10	110	24	Inhibition	N – C
10A	105	10	Stimulation[b]	
11E	100	10		C
11A	98	1		0
12	95	24	Inhibition	C
13	92	24		N
14	86	2		4
16	75	10		N + C
18	68	24		N + C
19	62	6		N
21	56	24	Inhibition	N
24	48	6		N + C
26	30	10		C
27	26	10		C
28	25	10	Inhibition	
28A	24	24		
28D	22	24		
29	21	24		

[a]Nucleus (N); cytoplasm (P).
[b]Synthesis observed only in the presence of acyclovir (ACV) and phosphonoacetic acid (PAA).
Adapted from Feighny et al. (43,44).

in overproduction of 6 early polypeptides, further suggesting that in productive infection, later polypeptides repress the synthesis of earlier polypeptides. Of the early virus-induced polypeptides, 4 are phosphorylated and accumulate to varying extents in the nucleus. Other early nuclear polypeptides are not detectably phosphorylated. The time course of the synthesis and that of the phosphorylation of specific polypeptides do not correlate well. Some proteins made early after superinfection are intensely phosphorylated very early and continue to be synthesized after their phosphorylation ceases.

Over 30 virus-specified polypeptides made early or late in virus replication have been mapped by translating RNA from B95-8 cells. The cells were induced to a permissive state of virus infection by TPA. Polypeptides were mapped to specific viral DNA fragments by hybrid selection and *in vitro* translation (93). Most of the polypeptides were reactive with immune human serum. Several components of the early antigen complex have been identified. The major core membrane, outer membrane, and viral capsid proteins have been mapped. The results are summarized in Table 2 and Fig. 9.

SUMMARY

During the first decade of EBV research, a great deal was learned about the epidemiology and biology of EBV. EBV causes infectious mononucleosis. The virus is latent in almost all adult humans. EBV is also a human cancer virus. The virus causes infected lymphocytes to grow. The growing lymphocytes can cause tumors in monkeys, in nude mice, and, as shown by recent data, in immunosuppressed humans. There is also a strong association of the virus with Burkitt lymphoma and nasopharyngeal carcinoma. It is likely that EBV is etiologically related to these two human tumors. The relationship of the virus to these human cancers may not be a simple relationship. Several steps may be involved. For Burkitt tumors, EBV may provide an initial step in growth promotion and little else. For nasopharyngeal cancer, there is even less information on the precise role of EBV.

During this second decade of EBV research there has been an explosion of information about the biochemistry of EBV, including knowledge of viral gene structure and gene function in virus replication and cellular growth transformation. EBV expression in infected cells is viewed as having three phases: latent, abortive, and permissive. Latent infection is associated with differential posttranscriptional processing of viral RNA. Thus, latently infected cells contain nuclear RNA transcribed from a significant fraction of the viral genome and mRNAs of lower complexity encoded by three separate regions of the genome. Three major mRNAs have been identified and mapped. In addition, there are two abundant small "viral-antigen-(VA)-like" RNAs in latently infected cells. A small amount of the VA-like RNA is noncovalently bound to polyadenylated RNAs. EBV specifies at least one chromatin-binding polypeptide antigen. Two distinct nulcear antigenic activities, EBNA and RANA, have been described in latently infected cells. Other lines of evidence suggest the presence of additional viral polypeptides, one of which may be a new infected cell surface antigen, LYDMA.

The abortive stage of infection can be induced in certain latently infected cell lines by treatment with chemical inducers. The appearance of viral early antigen (EA) is associated with an enhanced level of viral gene expression and inhibition of cellular macromolecular synthesis. Two major component polypeptides of the EA complex in TPA-treated cells have been identified. There is a slight increase in sequence complexity of nuclear RNA following chemical induction and a dramatic change in posttranscriptional processing that leads to an increase in the complexity and abundance of stable polyadenylated and polyribosomal RNAs. New polyribosomal RNAs are encoded by regions of the genome that do not encode the latently infected cell in RNAs. The complexity of RNA in abortively infected cells is sufficient to encode several additional viral polypeptides.

TABLE 2. *Criteria for assignment of an RNA to a polypeptide*

In vitro protein (kd/class)[a]	DNA fragment (*Bam*HI/*Eco*RI)	RNA (kbp/criteria)[b]	*In vivo* correlate
220/	/E	9.6,8.0/s,a	
150/L	/E	5.2/s,c,a	VCA
145/L	C/	4.75/s,a	Membrane
135/L	L/	4.75,3.4/s,c,a	
135/E	A/D	4.2/s,c,a,o	EA
94/L	L/	3.4,4.75/s,c,a	
90/L	A/C	3.0/s,c,o	
85/L	0,Z/	4.5/c,o	
80	/B		
78/E	/B	2.6/s,c	(EA)
72	W/		
68	/B		
63	/B		
58/E	0,Z/	3.1/c,o	
52	/E		
51	Z/	1.8/s,c,a	
50/E	G/B	4.6/c	EA
47/L	I/C	1.4/a,s	
47/E	M/	2.65,1.9/c,o	EA
44/E	M/	2.65,1.9/c,o	EA
46	G/B		
42/L	A/	1.7/s,c	
41/L	Z/	1.2/s,o,c	
40/L	/B		
39	F/		
38	F/		
36/E	Z,M/	4.0/c,a,o	EA
35/E	/B	1.5,1.25/s,c,a	EA
33/E	/B	1.5,1.25/s,c,a	EA
34/L	G/E	1.7/c,a,o	
32/E	L/	1.2/c	EA
32/L	/E		
31/L	/E		
28	F/		
28/L	I/	1.1/s,a	
22/L	L/	2.8,1.8,0.9/s,c,a	
18/L	L/	2.8,1.8,0.9/s,c,a	
15/L	L/	2.8,1.8,0.9/s,c,a	
18/E	H/	2.5/c,a	EA

[a]E, early; L, late.
[b]Criteria: s, minimum RNA size necessary to encode the polypeptide; c, correspondence between the E or L class assignment of the RNA and polypeptide; a, correspondence in relative abundance of the RNA and polypeptide; o, selection of the RNA and polypeptide by an overlapping or adjacent fragment. (Adapted from ref. 93.)

Analysis of viral gene expression during permissive infection is dependent on superinfection or TPA treatment of cells to induce viral replication. The pattern of

RNA synthesis reflects a significant change in gene expression. Nearly the entire EBV genome encodes RNA in productive infection, while the abundant mRNAs encoded by the long internal reiteration in latent and abortive infection are not detected. Some of the viral polypeptides have been identified as "late" by their sensitivity to inhibition of viral DNA synthesis. The sizes of some of these proteins are similar to the sizes of major component polypeptides of the virion.

The restricted expression of the EBV genome *in vitro* has complicated studies of EBV genetics and of the biochemical events during advanced stages of infection. The paucity of laboratory-derived mutants has hampered efforts to identify the functions of specific viral gene products. Nevertheless, recent developments in technology, including molecular cloning of EBV DNA, the development of methods for rapid DNA sequencing, *in vitro* translation systems, and monoclonal antibodies, have led to a new course in the investigation of the EBV genome. Viral polypeptides can be mapped by *in vitro* translation of viral-DNA-selected RNA, by transfection of cells with specific cloned DNA fragments, and by analysis of recombinant viruses. Cloning and sequencing of viral messenger RNAs and of the coding and control regions of viral DNA provide insight into the location of specific genes, the basis for EBV gene regulation, and the steps in RNA processing. Studies of the functions of parts of the viral genome in *in vitro* systems and in tissue culture cell lines should help to replace classic genetic analysis in understanding the physiology and chemistry of the interactions of viral and cellular genomes. Synthesis *in vitro* or in heterologous hosts of parts of the polypeptides that the viral genome encodes in latently infected, growth-transformed cells should make it possible to analyze the interaction of these proteins with the cell and virus genomes. Similarly, synthesis of important early and late virus gene products is necessary for the development of diagnostic reagents and safe polypeptide immunogens. In the appropriate population, over a long interval, a safe and effective immunogen could provide a new perspective for the evaluation of the role of EBV in lymphoma and nasopharyngeal cancer. Existing data support the expectation that tumor incidence will be reduced by preventing or limiting virus infection. The fact that latently infected cells can be induced to more advanced stages of viral gene expression is indicative of stringent control of EBV gene expression. The factors involved may be diverse, but new techniques that will permit the analysis of regulatory sites within the EBV genome and of the steps in processing of EBV RNA should lead to major advances in understanding the chemical basis for the unusual biological properties of EBV.

ACKNOWLEDGMENTS

We gratefully acknowledge research support for our laboratory from the National Cancer Institute (grants CA-19264 and CA-17281) and from the American Cancer Society (grant MV 32 G). Elliott Kieff is the recipient of an American Cancer Society Faculty Research Award (FRA-206).

REFERENCES

1. Adams, A., Lindahl, T., and Klein, G. (1973): Linear association between cellular DNA and Epstein-Barr virus DNA in a human lymphoblastoid cell line. *Proc. Natl. Acad. Sci. USA*, 70:2888–2892.
2. Adams, A., Bjursell, G., Kaschka-Dierich, C., and Lindahl, T. (1977): Circular Epstein-Barr virus genomes of reduced size in a human lymphoid cell line of infectious mononucleosis origin. *J. Virol.*, 22:373–380.
3. Alspauch, M., Jensen, F., Rabin, H., and Tan, E. (1978): Lymphocytes transformed by Epstein-Barr virus: Induction of nuclear antigen reactive with antibody in rheumatoid arthritis. *J. Exp. Med.*, 147:1018–1025.
4. Anderson-Anvret, M., and Lindahl, T. (1978): Integrated viral DNA sequences in Epstein-Barr virus-converted human lymphoma lines. *J. Virol.*, 25:710–718.
5. Arrand, J., and Rymo, L. (1982): Characterization of the major Epstein-Barr virus specific RNA in Burkitt lymphoma derived cells. *J. Virol.*, 41:376–389.
6. Baron, D., and Strominger, J. (1978): Partial purification and properties of the EBV associated nuclear antigen. *J. Biol. Chem.*, 253:2875–2881.
7. Bayliss, G., and Nonoyama, M. (1978): Mechanisms of infection with Epstein-Barr virus. III: The synthesis of proteins in superinfected Raji cells. *Virology*, 87:201–207.
8. Benveniste, R., and Todaro, G. (1976): Evolution of type C viral genes: Evidence for Asian origin of man. *Nature*, 261:101–108.
9. Bodemer, W., Summers, W., and Niederman, J. (1980): Detection of virus specific antigens in EB (P3HR-1) virus superinfection Raji cells by immunoprecipitation. *Virology*, 103:340–349.
10. Bornkamm, G. W., Delius, H., Zimber, U., Hudenwentz, J., and Epstein, M. A. (1980): Comparison of Epstein-Barr virus strains of different origin by analysis of the viral DNAs. *J. Virol.*, 35:603–618.
11. Burkitt, D. P. (1962): A tumour safari in east and central Africa. *Br. J. Cancer*, 16:379–386.
12. Burkitt, D. P. (1970): An alternative hypothesis to a vectored virus. In: *Burkitt's Lymphoma*, edited by D. Burkitt and D. Wright, pp. 210–215. Livingstone, London.
13. Catalano, M., Carson, D., Niederman, J., Feouno, P., and Vaughan, J. (1980): Antibody to the rheumatoid arthritis nuclear antigen: Its relationship to in vivo EBV infection. *J. Clin. Invest.*, 65:1238–1245.
14. Cheung, A., and Kieff, E. (1981): Epstein-Barr virus DNA. X. Direct repeat within the internal direct repeat of Epstein-Barr virus DNA. *J. Virol.*, 40:510–517.
15. Cheung, A., and Kieff, E. (1982): The long internal direct repeat in Epstein-Barr virus DNA. *J. Virol.*, 44:286–294.
16. Colby, B. M., Shaw, J. E., Elion, G. B., and Pagano, J. S. (1980): Effect of acyclovir [9-(2-hydroxyethoxymethyl)guanine] on Epstein-Barr virus DNA replication. *J. Virol.*, 34:560–568.
17. Dambaugh, T. (1980): Molecular cloning of Epstein-Barr virus DNA and analysis of RNA in human Burkitt's tumor tissue. Ph.D. thesis, University of Chicago.
18. Dambaugh, T., and Kieff, E. (1982): Identification and nucleotide sequence of two similar tandem direct repeats in Epstein-Barr virus DNA. *J. Virol.*, 44:823–833.
19. Dambaugh, T., Kieff, E., Nkrumah, F. K., and Biggar, R. J. (1979): Epstein-Barr virus RNA, in Burkitt tumor tissue. *Cell*, 16:313–322.
20. Dambaugh, T., Beisel, C., Hummel, M., King, W., Fennewald, S., Cheung, A., Heller, M., Raab-Traub, N., and Kieff, E. (1980): Epstein-Barr virus DNA. VII: Molecular cloning and detailed mapping of EBV (B95-8) DNA. *Proc. Natl. Acad. Sci. USA*, 77:2999–3003.
21. Dambaugh, T., Raab-Traub, N., Heller, M., Beisel, C., Hummel, M., Cheung, A., Fennewald, S., King, W., and Kieff, E. (1980): Variations among isolates of Epstein-Barr virus. *Ann. N.Y. Acad. Sci.*, 602:711–719.
22. Datta, A. K., Feighny, R. J., and Pagano, J. S. (1980): Induction of Epstein-Barr virus-associated DNA polymerase by 12-*O*-tetradecanoylphorbol-13-acetate. Purification and characterization. *J. Biol. Chem.*, 255:5120–5125.
23. Deinhart, F., Falk, L., Wolfe, L., Paciza, J., and Johnson, D. (1975): Response of marmosets to experimental infection with Epstein-Barr virus. In: *Oncogenesis and Herpesviruses II*, edited by G. de Thé, M. Epstein, and H. zur Hausen, pp. 161–168. IARC, Lyon.
24. Delius, H., and Bornkamm, G. W. (1978): Heterogeneity of Epstein-Barr virus. III. Comparison

of a transforming and a non-transforming virus by partial denaturation mapping of their DNAs. *J. Virol.*, 27:81–89.

25. Desgranges, C., Wolf, H., de Thé, G., Shanmugaratnam, K., Cammoun, N., Ellouz, R., Klein, G., Lennert, K., Munoz, N., and zur Hausen, H. (1975): Nasopharyngeal carcinoma. X. Presence of Epstein-Barr genomes in separated epithelial cells of tumours in patients from Singapore, Tunisia and Kenya. *Int. J. Cancer*, 16:7–15.

26. Desrosiers, R., Mulder, C., and Fleckenstein, B. (1979): Methylation of herpesvirus saimiri-DNA in lymphoid tumor cells lines. *Proc. Natl. Acad. Sci. USA*, 76:3839–3843.

27. de Thé, G. (1979): Demographic studies implicating the virus in the causation of Burkitt's lymphoma: Prospects for nasopharyngeal carcinoma. In: *The Epstein-Barr Virus*, edited by M. Epstein and B. Achong, pp. 418–435. Springer-Verlag, Berlin.

28. de Thé, G., Geser, A., Day, N., Tukei, P., Williams, E., Beri, D., Smith, P., Dean, A., Bornkamm, G., Feorino, P., and Henle, W. (1978): Epidemiologic evidence for causal relationship between Epstein-Barr virus and Burkitt's lymphoma from Ugandan prospective study. *Nature*, 274:756–761.

29. Dolyniuk, M., Pritchett, R., and Kieff, E. (1976): Proteins of Epstein-Barr virus. I. Analysis of the polypeptides of purified enveloped Epstein-Barr virus. *J. Virol.*, 17:935–949.

30. Dolyniuk, M., Wolff, E., and Kieff, E. (1976): Proteins of Epstein-Barr virus. II: Electrophoretic analysis of the polypeptides of the nucleocapsid and the glucosamine and polysaccharide containing components of the enveloped virus. *J. Virol.*, 18:289–297.

31. Edson, C., and Thorley-Lawson, D. (1981): Epstein-Barr virus membrane antigens: Characterization, distribution and strain differences. *J. Virol.*, 39:172–184.

32. Einhorn, L., and Ernberg, I. (1978): Induction of EBNA precedes the first cellular S phase after EBV infection of human lymphocytes. *Int. J. Cancer*, 21:157–160.

33. Epstein, M. A., and Achong, B. G. (1968): Specific immunofluorescence test for the herpes type EB virus of Burkitt lymphoblasts, authenticated by electron microscopy. *J. Natl. Cancer Inst.*, 40:593–607.

34. Epstein, M. A., and Achong, B. G. (1970): The EB virus. In: *Burkitt's Lymphoma*, edited by D. Burkitt and D. Wright, pp. 231–248. Livingstone, London.

35. Epstein, M. A., and Achong, B. G. (1979): Morphology of the virus and of virus induced cytopathologic changes. In: *The Epstein-Barr Virus*, edited by M. Epstein and B. Achong, pp. 24–33. Springer-Verlag, Berlin.

36. Epstein, M. A., and Achong, B. G. (1979): Discovery and general biology of the virus. In: *The Epstein-Barr Virus*, edited by M. Epstein and B. Achong, pp. 1–22. Springer-Verlag, Berlin.

37. Epstein, M. A., and Barr, Y. M. (1964): Cultivation in vitro of human lymphoblasts from Burkitt's malignant lymphoma. *Lancet*, 1:252–253.

38. Epstein, M. A., Achong, B. G., and Barr, Y. M. (1964): Virus particles in cultured lymphoblasts from Burkitt's lymphoma. *Lancet*, 1:702–703.

39. Epstein, M. A., Achong, B. G., and Pope, J. (1967): Virus in cultured lymphoblasts from a New Guinea Burkitt lymphoma. *Br. Med. J.*, 21:290–291.

40. Epstein, M. A., Hunt, R. D., and Rabin, H. (1973): Pilot experiments with EB virus in owl monkeys *(Aotus trivirgatus).* I. Reticuloproliferative disease in an inoculated animal. *Int. J. Cancer*, 12:309–318.

41. Epstein, M. A., Henle, G., Achong, B. G., and Barr, Y. M. (1965): Morphological and biological studies on a virus in cultured lymphoblasts from Burkitt's lymphoma. *J. Exp. Med.*, 121:761–770.

42. Falk, L., Deinhardt, F., Nonoyama, M., Wolfe, L. G., Bergholz, C., Lapin, B., Yakovleva, L., Agrba, V., Henle, G., and Henle, W. (1976): Properties of a baboon lymphotropic herpesvirus related to Epstein-Barr virus. *Int. J. Cancer*, 18:798–807.

43. Feighny, R., Farrell, M., and Pagano, J. (1980): Polypeptide synthesis and phosphorylation in EBV infected cells. *J. Virol.*, 34:455–463.

44. Feighny, R., Henry, B., and Pagano, J. (1981): EBV polypeptides: Effect of inhibition of viral DNA replication on their synthesis. *J. Virol.*, 37:68–71.

45. Fialkow, P., Klein, E., Klein, G., Clifford, P., and Singh, S. (1973): Immunoglobulin and glucose 6 phosphate dehydrogenase as markers of cellular origin in Burkitt's lymphoma. *J. Exp. Med.*, 138:89–102.

46. Fischer, D., Miller, G., Gradoville, L., Heston, L., Westrate, M., Maris, W., Wright, J., Brandsma, J., and Summers, W. (1981): Genome of a mononucleosis EBV contains fragments previously regarded to be unique to Burkitt's lymphoma isolates. *Cell*, 24:543–554.

47. Fresen, K. O., and zur Hausen, H. (1976): Establishment of EBNA-expressing cell lines by

infection of Epstein-Barr virus (EBV)-genome-negative human lymphoma cells with different EBV strains. *Int. J. Cancer*, 17:161–166.

48. Fresen, K. O., and zur Hausen, H. (1977): Transient induction of a nuclear antigen unrelated to Epstein-Barr nuclear antigen in cells of two human B-lymphoma lines converted by Epstein-Barr virus. *Proc. Natl. Acad. Sci. USA*, 74:363–366.

49. Fresen, K. O., Cho, M.-S., Gissmann, L., and zur Hausen, H. (1979): NC 37-R1 EB-virus: A possible recombinant between intracellular NC 37 viral DNA and superinfecting P3HR-1 EBV. *Intervirology*, 12:303–310.

50. Furlong, D., Swift, H., and Roizman, B. (1972): Arrangement of herpes virus deoxyribonucleic acid in the core. *J. Virol.*, 10:1071–1074.

51. Gerber, P. (1972): Activation of Epstein-Barr virus by 5'-bromo-deoxyuridine in virus free human cells. *Proc. Natl. Acad. Sci. USA*, 69:83–85.

52. Gerber, P., and Birch, S. M. (1967): Complement-fixing antibodies in sera of human and non-human primates to viral antigens derived from Burkitt's lymphoma cells. *Proc. Natl. Acad. Sci. USA*, 58:478–484.

53. Gerber, P., and Hoyer, B. (1971): Induction of cellular DNA synthesis in human leukocytes by Epstein-Barr virus. *Nature*, 231:46–47.

54. Gerber, P., Pritchett, R., and Kieff, E. (1976): Antigens and DNA of a chimpanzee agent related to Epstein-Barr virus. *J. Virol.*, 19:1090–1100.

55. Gerber, P., Whang-Peng, J., and Monroe, J. H. (1969): Transformation and chromosome changes induced by Epstein-Barr virus in normal human leukocyte cultures. *Proc. Natl. Acad. Sci. USA*, 63:740–747.

56. Gerber, P., Nkrumah, F., Pritchett, R., and Kieff, E. (1976): Comparative studies of Epstein-Barr virus strains from Ghana and the United States. *Int. J. Cancer*, 17:71–81.

57. Gerber, P., Kalter, S. S., Schidlovsky, G., Peterson, W. D., Jr., and Daniel, M. D. (1977): Biologic and antigenic characteristics of Epstein-Barr virus-related herpesvirus of chimpanzees and baboons. *Int. J. Cancer*, 20:448–459.

58. Gergely, L., Klein, G., and Ernberg, I. (1971): The action of DNA antagonists on Epstein-Barr virus (EBV)-associated early antigen (EA) in Burkitt's lymphoma lines. *Int. J. Cancer*, 7:293–302.

59. Given, D., and Kieff, E. (1978): DNA of Epstein-Barr virus. IV. Linkage map for restriction enzyme fragments of the B95-8 and W91 strains of EBV. *J. Virol.*, 28:524–542.

60. Given, D., and Kieff, E. (1979): DNA of Epstein-Barr virus. VI. Mapping of the internal tandem reiteration. *J. Virol.*, 31:315–324.

61. Given, D., Yee, D., Griem, K., and Kieff, E. (1979): DNA of Epstein-Barr virus. V. Direct repeats at the ends of EBV DNA. *J. Virol.*, 30:852–862.

62. Glaser, R., and O'Neill, F. J. (1972): Hybridization of Burkitt lymphoblastoid cells. *Science*, 176:1245–1247.

63. Goldman, N., Landon, H. C., and Reisher, J. I. (1968): Fluorescent antibody and gel diffusion reactions of human and chimpanzee sera with cells cultured from Burkitt tumors and normal chimpanzee blood. *Cancer Res.*, 28:2489–2495.

64. Graessman, A., Wolf, H., and Bornkamm, G. (1980): Expression of EBV genes in different cell types after microinjection of viral DNA. *Proc. Natl. Acad. Sci. USA*, 77:433–436.

65. Hampar, B., Derge, J. G., and Showalter, S. D. (1974): Enhanced activation of the repressed Epstein-Barr viral genome by inhibitors of DNA synthesis. *Virology*, 58:298–301.

66. Hampar, B., Derge, J. G., Martos, L. M., and Walker, J. L. (1972): Synthesis of Epstein-Barr virus after activation of the viral genome in a "virus-negative" human lymphoblastoid cell (Raji) made resistant to 5-bromodeoxyuridine. *Proc. Natl. Acad. Sci. USA*, 69:78–82.

67. Hampar, B., Tanaka, A., Nonoyama, M., and Derge, J. G. (1974): Replication of the resident repressed EBV genome during early S phase (S-1 period) of non-producer Raji cells. *Proc. Natl. Acad. Sci. USA*, 71:631–633.

68. Hampar, B., Lenoir, G., Nonoyama, M., Derge, J. G., and Chang, S.-Y. (1976): Cell cycle dependence for activation of Epstein-Barr virus by inhibitors of protein synthesis or medium deficient in arginine. *Virology*, 69:660–668.

69. Hampar, B., Derge, J. G., Nonoyama, M., Chang, S.-Y., Tagamets, M., and Showalter, S. D. (1974): Programming of events in Epstein-Barr virus-activated cells induced by 5-iododeoxyuridine. *Virology*, 62:71–89.

70. Hanto, D., Frizera, G., Purtilo, D., Sakamoto, K., Sullivan, J., Saemundsen, A., Klein, G., Simmons, R., and Najarian, J. (1981): Clinical spectrum of lymphproliferative disorders in renal transplant recipients and evidence for the role of EBV. *Cancer Res.*, 41:4253–4271.

71. Haynes, B., Schooley, R., Grouse, J., Payling, W. C., Dolin, R., and Fauci, A. (1979): Characterization of thymus derived lymphocyte subsets in acute Epstein-Barr virus induced infectious mononucleosis. *J. Immunol.*, 122:699–702.

72. Hayward, S. D., and Kieff, E. (1976): Epstein-Barr virus-specific RNA. I. Analysis of viral RNA in cellular extracts and in the polyribosomal fraction of permissive and nonpermissive lymphoblastoid cell lines. *J. Virol.*, 18:518–525.

73. Hayward, S. D., and Kieff, E. (1977): The DNA of Epstein-Barr virus. II. Comparison of molecular weights of restriction endonuclease fragments of the DNA of strains of EBV and identification of end fragments of the B95-8 strain. *J. Virol.*, 23:421–429.

74. Hayward, S. D., Nogge, L., and Hayward, G. (1980): Organization of repeated regions within the Epstein-Barr virus DNA molecule. *J. Virol.*, 33:507–521.

75. Hayward, S. D., Pritchett, R., Orellana, T., King, W., and Kieff, E. (1976): The DNA of Epstein-Barr virus fragments produced by restriction enzymes: Homologous DNA and RNA in lymphoblastoid cells. In: *Animal Virology 4*, edited by D. Baltimore, A. Huang, and C. F. Fox, pp. 619–639. Academic Press, New York.

76. Heller, M., and Kieff, E. (1981): Colinearity between the DNAs of Epstein-Barr virus and herpesvirus papio. *J. Virol.*, 37:821–826.

77. Heller, M., Dambaugh, T., and Kieff, E. (1981): Epstein-Barr virus DNA. IX: Variation among viral DNAs from producer and non-producer infected cells. *J. Virol.*, 38:632–648.

78. Heller, M., Gerber, P., and Kieff, E. (1981): Herpesvirus papio DNA is similar in organization to Epstein-Barr virus DNA. *J. Virol.*, 37:698–709.

79. Heller, M., Henderson, A., and Kieff, E. (1982): A repeat sequence in Epstein-Barr virus DNA is related to interspersed repeated cell DNAs which are at specific sites on human chromosome. *Proc. Natl. Acad. Sci. USA*, 79:5916–5920.

80. Heller, M., Gerber, P., and Kieff, E. (1982): DNA of herpesvirus pan, a third member of the Epstein-Barr virus-herpesvirus papio group. *J. Virol.*, 41:931–939.

81. Heller, M., Van Santen, V., and Kieff, E. (1982): A simple repeat sequence in Epstein-Barr virus DNA is transcribed in latent and productive infection. *J. Virol.*, 44:311–320.

82. Henderson, E., Heston, L., Grogon, E., and Miller, G. (1978): Radiobiologic inactivation of Epstein-Barr virus. *J. Virol.*, 25:51–59.

83. Henderson, E., Miller, G., Robinson, J., and Heston, L. (1977): Efficiency of transformation of lymphocytes by Epstein-Barr virus. *Virology*, 76:152–163.

84. Henderson, E., Robinson, J., Frank, A., and Miller, G. (1977): Epstein-Barr virus: Transformation of lymphocytes separated by size or exposed to bromodeoxyuridine and light. *Virology*, 82:196–205.

85. Henle, G., and Henle, W. (1966): Immunofluorescence in cells derived from Burkitt's lymphoma. *J. Bacteriol.*, 91:1248–1256.

86. Henle, W., and Henle, G. (1979): Seroepidemiology of the virus. In: *The Epstein-Barr Virus*, edited by M. Epstein and B. Achong, pp. 61–78. Springer-Verlag, Berlin.

87. Henle, W., Diehl, V., Kohn, G., zur Hausen, H., and Henle, G. (1967): Herpes-type virus and chromosome marker in normal lymphocytes after growth with irradiated Burkitt cells. *Science*, 157:1064–1065.

88. Henle, W., Henle, G., Zajac, B., Pearson, G., Waubke, R., and Scriba, M. (1970): Differential reactivity of human serums with early antigens induced by Epstein-Barr virus. *Science*, 169:188–190.

89. Hinuma, Y., Konn, M., Yamaguchi, J., Wudarski, D., Blaskeslee, J., and Grace, J. (1967): Immunofluorescence and herpes type virus particles in the P3 HR-1 Burkitt's lymphoma clone. *J. Virol.*, 1:1045–1051.

90. Hoffman, G., Lazarowitz, S., and Hayward, D. (1980): Monoclonal antibody against a 250,000 dalton glycoprotein of EBV identifies a membrane antigen and a neutralized antigen. *Proc. Natl. Acad. Sci. USA*, 77:2979–2983.

91. Honess, R., and Roizman, B. (1974): Regulation of herpes virus macromolecular synthesis. I. Cascade regulation of the synthesis of three groups of viral proteins. *J. Virol.*, 14:8–18.

92. Hummel, M., and Kieff, E. (1982): Epstein-Barr virus RNA. VIII: Viral RNA in permissively infected B95-8 cells. *J. Virol.*, 43:262–272.

93. Hummel, M., and Kieff, E. (1982): Mapping of polypeptides encoded by the Epstein-Barr virus genome in productive infection. *Proc. Natl. Acad. Sci. USA*, 79:5698–5702.

94. Hummeler, K., Henle, G., and Henle, W. (1966): Fine structure of a virus in cultured lymphoblasts from Burkitt's lymphoma. *J. Bacteriol.*, 91:1366–1368.

95. Jat, P., and Arrand, J. (1982): In vitro transcription of two Epstein-Barr virus specified small RNA molecules. *Nucleic Acids Res.*, 10:3407–3425.

96. Jehn, U., Lindahl, T., and Klein, G. (1972): Fate of virus DNA in the abortive infection of human lymphoid cell lines by Epstein-Barr virus. *J. Gen. Virol.*, 16:409–412.

97. Jondal, M., and Klein, G. (1973): Surface markers on human B and T lymphocytes. II. Presence of Epstein-Barr virus receptors on B lymphocytes. *J. Exp. Med.*, 138:1365–1378.

98. Kallin, B., Luka, J., and Klein, G. (1979): Immunochemical characterization of Epstein-Barr virus-associated early and late antigens in butyrate treated P3HR-1 cells. *J. Virol.*, 32:710–716.

99. Kaschka-Dierich, C., Falk, L., Bjursell, G., Adams, A., and Lindahl, T. (1977): Human lymphoblastoid cell lines derived from individuals without lymphoproliferative disease contain the same latent forms of Epstein-Barr virus DNA as those found in tumor cells. *Int. J. Cancer*, 20:173–180.

100. Kaschka-Dierich, C., Adams, A., Lindahl, T., Bornkamm, G., Bjursell, G., and Klein, G. (1976): Intracellular forms of Epstein-Barr virus DNA in human tumor cells in vivo. *Nature*, 260:302–306.

101. Kawai, Y., Nonoyama, M., and Pagano, J. (1973): Reassociation kinetics for EBV DNA: Nonhomology to mammalian DNA and homology of viral DNA in various diseases. *J. Virol.*, 12:1006–1012.

102. Kieff, E., and Levine, J. (1974): Homology between Burkitt herpes viral DNA and DNA in continuous lymphoblastoid cells from patients with infectious mononucleosis. *Proc. Natl. Acad. Aci. USA*, 71:355–358.

103. Kieff, E., Given, D., Powell, A. L. T., King, W., Dambaugh, T., and Raab-Traub, N. (1979): Epstein-Barr virus: Structure of the viral DNA and analysis of viral RNA in infected cells. *Biochim. Biophys. Acta*, 560:355–373.

104. Kieff, E., Raab-Traub, N., Given, D., King, W., Powell, A. L. T., Pritchett, R., and Dambaugh, T. (1978): Mapping of putative transforming sequences of EBV DNA. In: *Oncogenesis and Herpesviruses*, edited by P. M. Biggs, G. de Thé, and L. N. Payne, pp. 527–552. IARC, Lyon.

105. King, W., Van Santen, V., and Kieff, E. (1981): Epstein-Barr virus RNA. IV. Viral RNA in restringently and abortively infected Raji cells. *J. Virol.*, 38:649–660.

106. King, W., Dambaugh, T., Heller, M., Dowling, J., and Kieff, E. (1982): A variable region of the EBV genome is included in the P3HR-1 deletion. *J. Virol.*, 43:979–986.

107. King, W., Powell, A. L. T., Raab-Traub, N., Hawke, M., and Kieff, E. (1980): Epstein-Barr virus RNA. V. Viral RNA in a restringently infected, growth-transformed cell line. *J. Virol.*, 36:506–518.

108. Kintner, C., and Sugden, B. (1979): The structure of the termini of the DNA of Epstein-Barr virus. *Cell*, 17:661–671.

109. Kintner, C., and Sugden, B. (1981): Conservation and progressive methylation of EBV DNA sequences in transformed cells. *J. Virol.*, 38:305–316.

110. Kirsch, I., Morton, C., Nakahara, K., and Leder, P. (1982): Human immunoglobulin heavy chain genes map to a region of translocations in malignant B lymphocytes. *Science*, 216:301–303.

111. Klein, G. (1979): The relationship of the virus to nasopharyngeal carcinoma. In: *The Epstein-Barr Virus*, edited by M. Epstein and B. Achong, pp. 340–350. Springer-Verlag, Berlin.

112. Klein, G., Svedmyr, E., Jondal, M., and Persson, P. (1976): EBV determined nuclear antigen (EBNA) positive cells in the peripheral blood of infectious mononucleosis patients. *Int. J. Cancer*, 23:746–751.

113. Klein, G., Giovanella, B. C., Lindahl, T., Fialkow, P. J., Singh, S., and Stehlin, J. (1974): Direct evidence for the presence of Epstein-Barr virus DNA and nuclear antigen in malignant epithelial cells from patients with anaplastic carcinoma of the nasopharynx. *Proc. Natl. Acad. Sci. USA*, 71:4737–4741.

114. Landon, J. C., Ellis, L. B., Zene, H. C., and Frabrizio, D. P. A. (1968): Herpes-type virus in cultured leukocytes from chimpanzees. *J. Natl. Cancer Inst.*, 40:181–192.

115. Lee, Y. S., Tanaka, A., Law, R., Nonoyama, M., and Rabin, H. (1981): Linkage map of the fragments of herpes virus papio DNA. *J. Virol.*, 37:710–720.

116. Lenoir, G., Berthelon, M.-C., Favre, M.-C., and de Thé, G. (1976): Characterization of Epstein-Barr virus antigens. I. Biochemical analysis of the complement-fixing soluble antigen and relationship with Epstein-Barr virus-associated nuclear antigens. *J. Virol.*, 17:672–674.

117. Lerner, M., Andrews, N., Miller, G., and Steitz, J. (1981): Two small RNAs encoded by EBV and complexed with protein are precipitated by antibodies from patients with systemic lupus erythematosus. *Proc. Natl. Acad. Sci. USA*, 78:805–809.

118. Levy, J. A. S., Levy, D. B., Hirshaut, Y., Kafuko, G., and Prince, A. (1971): Presence of EBV antibodies in sera from wild chimpanzees. *Nature*, 233:559–560.

119. Lindahl, T., Klein, G., Reedman, B. M., Johansson, B., and Singh, S. (1974): Relationship between Epstein-Barr virus (EBV) DNA and the EBV determined nuclear antigen (EBNA) in Burkitt's lymphoma biopsies and other lymphoproliferative malignancies. *Int. J. Cancer*, 13:764–772.

120. Lindahl, T., Adams, A., Bjursell, G., Bornkamm, G. W., Kaschka-Dierich, C., and Jehn, U. (1976): Covalently closed circular duplex DNA of Epstein-Barr virus in human lymphoid cell line. *J. Mol. Biol.*, 102:511–530.

121. Luka, J., Jornvall, H., and Klein, G. (1980): Purification and biochemical characterization of the EBV determined nuclear antigen and associated protein with a 53,000 d subunit. *J. Virol.*, 35:592–602.

122. Luka, J., Lindahl, T., and Klein, G. (1978): Purification of the Epstein-Barr virus determined nuclear antigen from EBV transformed human lymphoid cells. *J. Virol.*, 27:604–611.

123. Luka, J., Siegert, W., and Klein, G. (1977): Solubilization of the Epstein-Barr virus-determined nuclear antigen and its characterization as a DNA-binding protein. *J. Virol.*, 22:1–8.

124. Manolov, G., and Manolova, Y. (1972): Marker band in one chromosome 14 from Burkitt lymphomas. *Nature*, 237:33–34.

125. Mayyasi, S., Schidlovsky, G., Bulferre, L., and Buschek, F. (1967): Coating reaction of herpes type virus isolated from malignant tissues with an antibody present in sera. *Cancer Res.*, 27:2020–2023.

126. Menezes, J., Leibold, W., and Klein, G. (1975): Biological differences between different Epstein-Barr virus (EBV) strains with regard to lymphocyte transforming ability. *Exp. Cell Res.*, 92:478–484.

127. Miller, G. (1979): Experimental carcinogenicity by the virus in vivo. In: *The Epstein-Barr Virus*, edited by M. Epstein and B. Achong, pp. 352–372. Springer-Verlag, Berlin.

128. Miller, G., and Lipman, M. (1973): Comparison of the yield of infectious virus from clones of human and simian lymphoblastoid lines transformed by EBV. *J. Exp. Med.*, 138:1398–1412.

129. Miller, G., and Lipman, M. (1973): Release of infectious Epstein-Barr virus by transformed marmoset leukocytes. *Proc. Natl. Acad. Sci. USA*, 70:190–194.

130. Miller, G., Niederman, J. C., and Andrews, L. (1973): Prolonged oropharyngeal excretion of EB virus following infectious mononucleosis. *N. Engl. J. Med.*, 288:229–232.

131. Miller, G., Coope, D., Niederman, J., and Pagano, J. (1976): Biological properties and viral surface antigens of Burkitt lymphoma and mononucleosis derived strains of EBV released from transformed marmoset cells. *J. Virol.*, 18:1071–1080.

132. Miller, G., Robinson, J., Heston, L., and Lipman, M. (1974): Differences between laboratory strains of Epstein-Barr virus based on immortalization, abortive infection and interference. *Proc. Natl. Acad. Sci. USA*, 71:4006–4010.

133. Miller, G., Grogan, E., Heston, L., Robinson, J., and Smith, D. (1981): Epstein-Barr viral DNA: Infectivity for human placental cells. *Science*, 212:452–455.

134. Miller, G., Shope, T., Lisco, H., Still, D., and Lipman, M. (1972): Epstein-Barr virus: Transformation, cytopathic changes, and viral antigens in squirrel monkey and marmoset leukocytes. *Proc. Natl. Acad. Sci. USA*, 69:383–387.

135. Mocarski, E. S., and Roizman, B. (1981): Site-specific inversion sequence of the herpes simplex virus genome: Domain and structural features. *Proc. Natl. Acad. Sci. USA*, 78:7047–7051.

136. Moss, D., and Pope, J. (1972): Assay of the infectivity of Epstein-Barr virus by transformation of human leukocytes in vitro *J. Gen. Virol.*, 17:233–236.

137. Moss, D., and Pope, J. (1975): EB virus associated nuclear antigen production and cell proliferation in adult peripheral blood leukocytes inoculated with QiMR-W1L strain of EB virus. *Int. J. Cancer*, 15:503–511.

138. Mueller-Lantzsch, N., Yamamoto, N., and zur Hausen, H. (1979): Analysis of early and late Epstein-Barr virus associated polypeptides by immunoprecipitation. *Virology*, 97:378–387.

139. Mueller-Lantzsch, N., Georg, B., Yamamoto, N., and zur Hausen, H. (1980): Epstein-Barr virus-induced proteins. II. Analysis of surface polypeptides from EBV-producing and superinfected cells by immunoprecipitation. *Virology*, 102:401–411.

140. Mueller-Lantzsch, N., Georg, B., Yamamoto, N., and zur Hausen, H. (1980): Epstein-Barr virus-induced proteins. III. Analysis of polypeptides from P3HR-1-EBV superinfected NC37 cells by immunoprecipitation. *Virology*, 102:231–233.

141. Nilsson, K. (1979): The nature of lymphoid cell lines and their relationship to the virus. In: *The Epstein-Barr Virus*, edited by M. Epstein and B. Achong, pp. 225–282. Springer-Verlag, Berlin.

142. Nilsson, K., Klein, G., Henle, W., and Henle, G. (1971): The establishment of lymphoblastoid lines from adult and fetal human lymphoid tissue and its dependence on EBV. *Int. J. Cancer*, 8:443–450.

143. Nilsson, K., Klein, G., Henle, G., and Henle, W. (1972): The role of EBV in the establishment of lymphoblastoid cell lines from adult and foetal lymphoid tissue. In: *Oncogenesis and Herpesviruses*, edited by P. M. Biggs, G. de Thé, and L. N. Payne, pp. 285–290. IARC, Lyon.

144. Nonoyama, M., and Pagano, J. S. (1971): Detection of Epstein-Barr viral genome in nonproductive cells. *Nature [New Biol.]*, 233:103–106.

145. Nonoyama, M., and Pagano, J. S. (1972): Separation of Epstein-Barr virus DNA from large chromosomal DNA in non-virus producing cells. *Nature [New Biol.]*, 238:169–171.

146. Nonoyama, M., and Pagano, J. S. (1973): Homology between Epstein-Barr virus DNA and viral DNA from Burkitt's lymphoma and nasopharyngeal carcinoma determined by DNA-DNA reassociation kinetics. *Nature*, 242:44–47.

147. Nonoyama, M., Huang, C. H., Pagano, J. S., Klein, G., and Singh, S. (1973): DNA of Epstein-Barr virus detected in tissue of Burkitt's lymphoma and nasopharyngeal carcinoma. *Proc. Natl. Acad. Sci. USA*, 70:3265–3268.

148. O'Conor, G. T., and Rabson, A. S. (1965): Herpes-like particles in an American lymphoma: Preliminary note. *J. Natl. Cancer Inst.*, 35:899–903.

149. Ohno, S., Luka, J., Falk, L., and Klein, G. (1978): Serologic reactivities of human and baboon sera against EBNA and herpes virus papio determined nuclear antigen. *Eur. J. Cancer*, 14:955–960.

150. Ohno, S., Luka, J., Falk, L., and Klein, G. (1979): Detection of a nuclear, EBNA-type antigen in apparently EBNA negative herpesvirus papio (HVP)-transformed lymphoid lines by the acid fixed nuclear binding technique. *Int. J. Cancer*, 20:941–946.

151. Ohno, S., Luka, J., Lindahl, T., and Klein, G. (1977): Identification of a purified complement-fixing antigen as the EBV determined nuclear antigen (EBNA) by its binding to metaphase chromosomes. *Proc. Natl. Acad. Sci. USA*, 74:1605–1609.

152. Orellana, T., and Kieff, E. (1977): Epstein-Barr virus specific RNA. II. Analysis of polyadenylated viral RNA in restringent, abortive and productive infection. *J. Virol.*, 22:321–330.

153. Pagano, J. S., and Juang, C.-H. (1976): Epstein-Barr virus genome in infectious mononucleosis. *Nature*, 263:787–789.

154. Pagano, J. S., Huang, C.-H., Klein, G., de Thé, G., Shanmugaratnam, K., and Yang, C.-S. (1975): Homology of Epstein-Barr virus DNA in nasopharyngeal carcinoma from Kenya, Taiwan, Singapore and Tunisia. In: *Oncogenesis and Herpesviruses II*, edited by G. de Thé, M. Epstein, and H. zur Hausen, pp. 179–190. IARC, Lyon.

155. Pearson, G., and Qualtiere, L. (1978): Papain solubilization of the Epstein-Barr virus induced membrane antigen. *J. Virol.*, 28:344–351.

156. Pizzo, P. A., Magrath, I. T., Chattopadhyay, S. K., Biggar, R. J., and Gerber, P. (1978): A new tumor-derived transforming strain of Epstein-Barr virus. *Nature*, 272:629–631.

157. Pope, J. H., Achong, B., and Epstein, M. (1968): Cultivation and fine structure of virus bearing lymphoblasts from a second New Guinea Burkitt lymphoma. *Int. J. Cancer*, 3:171–182.

158. Pope, J. H., Horne, M. K., and Scott, W. (1968): Transformation of fetal human leukocytes in vitro in filtrates of a human leukemic cell line containing herpes-like virus. *Int. J. Cancer*, 3:857–866.

159. Pope, J. H., Scott, W., Reedman, B. M., and Water, M. K. (1971): EB virus as a biologically active agent. In: *Recent Advances in Human Tumor Virology and Immunology*, edited by W. Nakahara, K. Nishioka, T. Hirayama, and Y. Ito, pp. 177–188. University of Tokyo Press.

160. Powell, A. L. T., King, W., and Kieff, E. (1979): Epstein-Barr virus specific RNA. III. Mapping of the DNA encoding viral specific RNA in restringently infected cells. *J. Virol.*, 29:261–274.

161. Pritchett, R. F., Hayward, S. D., and Kieff, E. (1975): DNA of Epstein-Barr virus. I. Comparison of DNA of virus purified from P3HR-1 and B95-8 cells. *J. Virol.*, 15:556–569.

162. Pritchett, R. F., Hayward, S. D., and Kieff, E. (1975): Analysis of the DNA of Epstein-Barr

viruses and transcriptional products in transformed cells. In: *Oncogenesis and Herpesviruses*, edited by G. de Thé, M. Epstein, and H. zur Hausen, pp. 177–191. IARC, Lyon.

163. Pritchett, R. F., Pedersen, M., and Kieff, E. (1976): Complexity of EBV homologous DNA in continuous lymphoblastoid cell lines. *Virology*, 74:227–231.

164. Purtilo, D., Deflorio, D., Yang, J., Otto, R., and Edwards, W. (1977): Variable phenotypic expression of an X-linked recessive lympho-proliferative syndrome. *N. Engl. J. Med.*, 297:1087–1091.

165. Qualtiere, L., and Pearson, G. (1979): Epstein-Barr virus induced membrane antigens: Immunochemical characterization of Triton X-100 solubilized viral membrane antigens from EBV-superinfected Raji cells. *Int. J. Cancer*, 23:808–817.

166. Qualtiere, L., and Pearson, G. (1980): Radioimmune precipitation study comparing the Epstein-Barr virus membrane antigens expressed on P3HR-1 virus-superinfected Raji cells to those expressed on cells in a B95-8 virus transformed producer culture activated with tumor promoting agent (TPA). *Virology*, 102:360–369.

167. Raab-Traub, N., Dambaugh, T., and Kieff, E. (1980): DNA of Epstein-Barr virus. VIII. B95-8, the previous prototype, is an unusual deletion derivative. *Cell*, 22:257–267.

168. Raab-Traub, N., Pritchett, R., and Kieff, E. (1978): DNA of Epstein-Barr virus. III. Identification of restriction enzyme fragments which contain DNA sequences which differ among strains of EBV. *J. Virol.*, 27:388–398.

169. Rabin, H., Neubauer, R., Hopkins, F., and Nonoyama, M. (1978): Further characterization of a herpes virus-positive orangutan cell line and comparative aspects of in vitro transformation with lymphotropic Old World primate herpesviruses. *Int. J. Cancer*, 21:762–767.

170. Rabin, H., Neubauer, R. H., Hopkins, R. F., III, Dzhikidze, E. K., Shevtsova, Z. V., and Lapin, B. A. (1977): Transforming activity and antigenicity of an Epstein-Barr like virus from lymphoblastoid cell lines of baboons with lymphoid disease. *Intervirology*, 8:240–249.

171. Rabin, H., Strnad, B. C., Neubauer, R. H., Brown, A. M., Hopkins, R. F., and Mazur, R. A. (1980): Comparison of nuclear antigens of Epstein-Barr virus (EBV) and EBV-like simian viruses. *J. Gen. Virol.*, 48:265–272.

172. Ragona, G., Ernberg, I., and Klein, G. (1980): Induction and biological characterization of the Epstein-Barr virus (EBV) carried by the Jijoye lymphoma line. *Virology*, 101:553–557.

173. Reedman, B. M., and Klein, G. (1973): Cellular localization of an Epstein-Barr virus (EBV)-associated complement-fixing antigen in producer and non-producer lymphoblastoid cell lines. *Int. J. Cancer*, 11:499–520.

174. Reedman, B. M., Klein, G., Pope, J. H., Walters, M. K., Hilgers, J., Singh, S., and Johansson, B. (1974): Epstein-Barr virus-associated complement-fixing and nuclear antigens in Burkitt lymphoma biopsies. *Int. J. Cancer*, 13:755–763.

175. Robinson, J., and Smith, D. (1981): Virus associated cell transformation and host alteration. Infection of human B lymphocytes with high multiplicities of Epstein-Barr virus: Kinetics of EBNA expression, cellular DNA synthesis and mitosis. *Virology*, 109:336–343.

176. Robinson, J., Smith, D., and Niederman, J. (1981): Plasmacytic differentiation of circulating EBV infected B lymphocytes during acute infectious mononucleosis. *J. Exp. Med.*, 153:235–244.

177. Robinson, J., Brown, N., Anderman, W., Halliday, K., Francke, U., Robert, M., Anderson-Anvret, M., Horstmann, D., and Miller, G. (1980): Diffuse polyclonal B cell lymphoma during primary infection by Epstein-Barr virus. *N. Engl. J. Med.*, 307:1293–1295.

178. Roizman, B., and Kieff, E. (1975): Herpes simplex and Epstein-Barr viruses in human cells and tissues: A study in contrasts. In: *Cancer: A Comprehensive Treatise 2*, edited by F. F. Becker, pp. 241–322. Plenum Press, New York.

179. Rosa, M., Gottlieb, E., Lerner, M., and Steitz, J. (1981): Striking similarities are exhibited by two small EBV encoded RNAs and adenovirus associated RNAs VAI and VAII. *Mol. Cell. Biol.*, 1:785–796.

180. Rymo, L. (1979): Identification of transcribed regions of Epstein-Barr virus DNA in Burkitt lymphoma-derived cells. *J. Virol.*, 32:8–18.

181. Rymo, L., and Forsblum, S. (1978): Cleavage of Epstein-Barr virus DNA by restriction endonuclease EcoRI, HindIII and BamI. *Nucleic Acids Res.*, 5:1387–1402.

182. Sawyer, R., Evans, A., Niederman, J., and McCollum, R. (1971): Prospective studies of a group of Yale University freshman and the occurrence of infectious mononucleosis. *J. Infect. Dis.*, 123:263–270.

183. Shaw, J., Seebeck, T., Li, J.-L., and Pagano, J. S. (1977): Epstein-Barr virus DNA synthesized in superinfected Raji cells. *Virology*, 77:762–771.
184. Shope, T., Dechairo, D., and Miller, G. (1973): Malignant lymphoma in cotton-top marmosets following inoculation of Epstein-Barr virus. *Proc. Natl. Acad. Sci. USA*, 70:2487–2491.
185. Siegel, P., Clough, W., and Strominger, J. (1981): Sedimentation characterisitics of newly synthesized Epstein-Barr virus viral DNA in superinfected cells. *J. Virol.*, 38:880–885.
186. Skare, J., and Strominger, J. (1980): Cloning and mapping of *Bam*HI endonuclease fragments from the transforming B95-8 strain of Epstein-Barr virus. *Proc. Natl. Acad. Sci. USA*, 77:3860–3864.
187. Slovin, S., Vaughan, J., and Carson, D. (1980): Expression of EBNA and RANA during different phases of cell growth cycle. *Int. J. Cancer*, 26:9–15.
188. Slovin, S., Glassy, M., Dambaugh, T., Catalano, M., Ewing, R., Ferrone, S., Kieff, E., Vaughan, T., and Carson, D. (1981): Discordant expression of two Epstein-Barr virus associated antigens EBNA and RANA in man-rodent somatic cell hybrids. *J. Immunol.*, 127:585–590.
189. Spear, P. G. (1980): Composition and organization of herpes viruses virions and properties of some of the structural proteins. In: *Oncogenesis and Herpesviruses Vol. 1*, edited by F. Rapp, pp. 53–84. CRC Press, Boca Raton, Fla.
190. Stevens, D. A., Pry, T. W., Blackman, E., and Manaker, R. (1970): Comparison of antigens from human and chimpanzee herpes-type virus-infected hemic cell lines. *Proc. Soc. Exp. Biol. Med.*, 133:678–683.
191. Stewart, S., Lovelace, E., Whang, J., and Ngu, V. (1965): Burkitt tumor, tissue culture, cytogenetic and viral studies. *J. Natl. Cancer Inst.*, 34:319–328.
192. Strnad, B., Neubauer, R., Rabin, H., and Mazur, R. (1979): Correlation between EBV membrane antigen and three large cell surface glycoproteins. *J. Virol.*, 32:885–894.
193. Strnad, B., Schuster, T., Hopkins, R., Neubauer, R., and Rabin, H. (1981): Identification of an EBV nuclear antigen by fluoroimmunoelectrophoresis and radioimmunoelectrophoresis. *J. Virol.*, 38:996–1004.
194. Sugden, B., and Mark, W. (1977): Clonal transformation of adult human leukocytes by Epstein-Barr virus. *J. Virol.*, 23:503–508.
195. Sugden, B., Phelps, M., and Domoradzki, J. (1979): EBV DNA is amplified in transformed lymphocytes. *J. Virol.*, 31:590–595.
196. Sugden, B., Summers, W. C., and Klein, G. (1976): Nucleic acid renaturation and restriction endonuclease cleavage analyses show that the DNAs of a transforming and nontransforming strain of Epstein-Barr virus share approximately 90% of their nucleotide sequences. *J. Virol.*, 18:765–775.
197. Summers, W., and Klein, G. (1976): Inhibition of Epstein-Barr virus DNA synthesis late gene expression by phosphonacetic acid. *J. Virol.*, 18:151–155.
198. Svedmyr, E., and Jondal, M. (1975): Cytotoxic effector cells specific for B cell lines transformed by Epstein-Barr virus are present in patients with infectious mononucleosis. *Proc. Natl. Acad. Sci. USA*, 72:1622–1626.
199. Tanaka, A., Nonoyama, M., and Glaser, R. (1977): Transcription of latent Epstein-Barr virus genomes in human epithelial/Burkitt hybrid cells. *Virology*, 82:63–68.
200. Thorley-Lawson, D. (1979): Characterization of cross reacting antigens on the Epstein-Barr virus envelope and plasma membrane of producer cells. *Cell*, 16:33–42.
201. Thorley-Lawson, D., and Edson, C. (1979): Polypeptides of the Epstein-Barr virus membrane antigen complex. *J. Virol.*, 32:458–467.
202. Thorley-Lawson, D., and Geilinger, K. (1980): Monoclonal antibodies against the major glycoprotein (gp350/220) of Epstein-Barr virus neutralize infectivity. *Proc. Natl. Acad. Sci. USA*, 77:5307–5311.
203. Thorley-Lawson, D., and Strominger, J. L. (1976): Transformation of human lymphocytes by Epstein-Barr virus is inhibited by phosphonoacetic acid. *Nature*, 263:332–334.
204. Toplin, I., and Schidlovsky, G. (1966): Partial purification and electron microscopy of the virus in the EB-3 cell line derived from a Burkitt lymphoma. *Science*, 152:1084–1085.
205. Tosato, G., Magrath, I., Koski, I., Dooley, N., and Blasese, M. (1979): Activation of suppression T cells during Epstein-Barr virus induced infectious mononucleosis. *N. Engl. J. Med.*, 301:1133–1137.
206. Van Santen, V., Cheung, A., and Kieff, E. (1981): Epstein-Barr virus RNA. VII. Size and

direction of transcription of virus specified cytoplasmic RNA in a cell line transformed by EBV. *Proc. Natl. Acad. Sci. USA*, 78:1930–1934.

207. Volsky, D. J., Shapiro, I. M., and Klein, G. (1980): Transfer of Epstein-Barr virus receptors to receptor-negative cells permits virus penetration and antigen expression. *Proc. Natl. Acad. Sci. USA*, 77:5453–5457.

208. Volsky, D. J., Klein, G., Volsky, B., and Shapiro, I. M. (1981): Production of infectious EBV in mouse lymphocytes. *Nature*, 293:399–401.

209. Wagner, E. K., Roizman, B., Savage, T., Spear, P. G., Mizell, M., Darr, F., and Sypowicz, D. (1970): Characterization of the DNA of the herpesvirus associated with Lucke adenocarcinoma of the frog and Burkitt lymphoma of man. *Virology*, 42:257–261.

210. Wolf, H., zur Hausen, H., Klein, G., Becker, Y., Henle, G., and Henle, W. (1975): Attempts to detect virus-specific DNA sequences in human tumors. III. EBV DNA in nonlymphoid nasopharyngeal carcinoma cells. *Med. Microbiol. Immunol.*, 161:15–21.

211. Yajima, Y., and Nonoyama, M. (1976): Mechanisms of infection with Epstein-Barr virus. I. Viral DNA replication and formation of non-infectious virus particles in superinfected Raji cells. *J. Virol.*, 19:187–194.

212. Yamamoto, N., and Hinuma, Y. (1976): Clonal transformation of human leukocytes by Epstein-Barr virus in soft agar. *Int. J. Cancer*, 17:191–196.

213. Yi, Z., Yuxi, L., Chumen, L., Sanwen, C., Jihneng, W., Jisong, Z., and Hauyong, Z. (1980): Application of an immunoenzymatic method and an immunoautoradiographic method for a mass survey of nasopharyngeal carcinoma. *Intervirology*, 13:162–168.

214. zur Hausen, H., and Schulte-Holthausen, H. (1970): Presence of EB virus nucleic acid homology in a "virus free" line of Burkitt's tumor cells. *Nature*, 227:245–248.

215. zur Hausen, H., Hecker, E., O'Neill, F. J., and Freese, U. K. (1978): Persisting oncogenic herpesvirus induced by tumor promoter TPA. *Nature*, 272:373–375.

216. zur Hausen, H. H., Schulte-Holthausen, J., Klein, G., Henle, W., Henle, G., Clifford, P., and Santesson, L. (1970): EB virus DNA in biopsies of Burkitt tumors and anaplastic carcinomas of the nasopharynx. *Nature*, 228:1056–1057.

217. zur Hausen, H., Bornkamm, G., Schmidt, R., and Hecker, E. (1979): Tumor initiators and promoters in the induction of EBV. *Proc. Natl. Acad. Sci. USA*, 76:782–785.

218. Henderson, A., Ripley, S., Heller, M., and Kieff, E. (1983): *Proc. Natl. Acad. Sci. USA, (in press)*.

219. Van Santen, V., Cheung, A., Hummel, M., and Kieff, E. (1983): *J. Virol., (in press)*.

220. Van Santen, V., Cheung, A., Hummel, M., and Kieff, E. (1983): *J. Virol., (in press)*.

Advances in Viral Oncology, Volume 3, edited by
George Klein. Raven Press, New York © 1983.

Epstein-Barr Virus Transformation: Biological and Functional Aspects

Jesper Zeuthen

Institute of Human Genetics, University of Aarhus, DK-8000 Aarhus, and Department of Immunology and Cell Biology, Pharmaceuticals R&D, Novo Industri A/S DK-2880 Bagsvaerd, Denmark

The Epstein-Barr virus (EBV) is a lymphotropic virus in humans. EBV causes infectious mononucleosis (IM) and is associated with two very different types of human malignant neoplastic disease: African Burkitt lymphoma (BL), caused by malignant proliferation of B lymphocytes, and nasopharyngeal carcinoma (NPC), caused by malignant proliferation of epithelioid cells. The association of EBV with African BL as well as NPC has been documented by serology (55,56) and by detection of EBV DNA in tumor material (103,137,229). The most extensive evidence concerns African BL. About 97% of BL cases from the highly endemic regions of Africa involved EBV-carrying clones of B lymphocyte origin (79). Both BL tumor cells *in vivo* and BL-derived cell lines carry multiple copies of EBV genomes, often of the order of 30 to 40 copies per cell. Some of these multiple copies of EBV genomes appear to be integrated in the cellular DNA, but the majority are present as free nonintegrated DNA copies (74). BL cells show no detectable viral antigen expression *in vivo*, with the exception of the EBV-determined nuclear antigen, EBNA (156), which is present in all cells that carry the EBV genome. EBNA is a DNA-binding protein (6,106), and its binding to chromosomes (140) was noted in the original report by Reedman and Klein (156). In its properties, EBNA resembles the nuclear antigens (T antigens) induced by oncogenic papovaviruses like SV40 or polyoma virus (88), although this resemblance may be superficial.

In most cases the BL-derived cell lines are derived from *in vitro* growth of the tumorigenic cell clone found *in vivo* (30,31). These cell lines express EBNA similarly to the original tumor cells. In addition to EBNA, some cell lines of BL origin also contain a low fraction of cells that express antigens characteristic of the viral productive cycle (so-called producer cell lines), whereas other cell lines do not express such antigens at all (so-called nonproducer lines) (134). These antigens are the viral capsid antigens (VCA) (54), the early antigen (EA) complex (59), and the membrane antigen (MA) (84,85). These antigens have been defined mainly by means of direct and indirect immunofluorescence. The nuclear EBNA antigen usually can be detected only by the highly sensitive anticomplement immunofluorescence method (60).

MA was first identified on BL biopsy cells and later on BL-derived cell lines (84). Expression of MA was dependent on the expression of VCA in such cells; however, MA was also detected on the membrane of VCA-negative cells. There was a correlation between the EBV-neutralizing titer and anti-MA titers (145), which suggested that MA probably could be present on the viral envelope. This was confirmed by electron microscopy (176). Several laboratories have attempted to identify MA. Qualtière and Pearson (154) identified four polypeptides from superinfected Raji cells. Källin et al. (70) identified six glycosylated polypeptides in induced P3HR-1 cells, four of these (275K, 236K, 168K, and 90K) possibly corresponding to MA polypeptides. Similar polypeptides were described by Thorley-Lawson and Edson (198), with molecular weights of 350K, 220K, 140K, and 85K. At least the 350K and 220K polypeptides were antigenically related, and the 220K protein probably was a degradation product. Recently, monoclonal antibodies have been produced against the 350K and 220K glycoproteins (62,199) that also have neutralizing activity against the virus.

VCA was the first EBV antigen to be detected by immunofluorescence (54). It has been shown that anti-VCA antibodies react with naked virus but not enveloped virus and that VCA therefore probably corresponds to structural components of the virus capsid (176). Antibodies against VCA are present in all EBV-seropositive individuals, but they have also been raised in rabbits (206). Dolyniuk et al. (22) showed nucleocapsids of EBV to be composed of seven polypeptides ranging in molecular weight from 200K to 28K. Kallin et al. (70) showed that two polypeptides of 165K and 158K are late components in induced cells and are precipitated by anti-VCA positive sera.

EA was first identified by differences in immunofluorescence staining using either sera from healthy donors or sera from acute IM patients (59). The sera from healthy donors often failed to react with superinfected cells, and superinfection appeared to induce an EA different from VCA. EA consists of two components: One antigen, designated restricted (R), is found in the cytoplasm; the other, designated diffuse (D), is dispersed and is found in both nucleus and cytoplasm (57). In viral infection, the R component appears shortly before the D component (177). The R component is destroyed by methanol or ethanol fixation, in contrast to the D component. EA has been shown to consist of at least 15 polypeptides with molecular weights in the range of 152K to 31K (70,77,133).

In contrast to BL, IM is a self-limiting disease, and the finding by Svedmyr and Jondal (194) of cytotoxic T lymphocytes specific for EBV-transformed cell lines in blood from IM patients during the acute phase of the disease suggests that this self-limitation results in part from the cell-mediated immune response of the host. These workers named the structure expressed on EBV-transformed cells that was recognized by specific cytotoxic T cells LYDMA (lymphocyte-determined membrane antigen). It has also been shown that T cells with proper education in culture specifically kill autochtonous EBV-transformed LCL lines (157). This response is HLA-restricted (131) and can be blocked by monoclonal antibodies directed against HLA-A, -B, and -C common determinants (209). Cloned T cells recognize the

LYDMA antigen in association with one particular HLA-A or -B determinant (210). Monoclonal antibodies that appear to identify the target structure appear now to have been identified (78). Immunodeficiencies can lead to uncontrolled proliferation of EBV-infected cells in IM, leading to lymphoproliferative disease (153,171).

RECOGNITION, ADSORPTION, AND TRANSFORMATION

Recognition and adsorption of EBV involves an interaction between the viral envelope and the membrane of the cell that is infected. Thus, both viral envelope proteins and some proteins on the surface of the cell participate in this process.

It has been known for several years that the receptor for EBV is present on peripheral B lymphocytes, but not on T lymphocytes (46,66,125). It is noteworthy that the P3HR-1 strain of EBV, a nontransforming strain, apparently can bind to the EBV receptor of peripheral B cells, because its adsorption prevents any subsequent effect of the addition of the transforming B95-8 strain of EBV (182). Various experiments have suggested that this receptor for EBV on B cells either is virtually identical with or is closely associated with the receptor for the C3 component of complement (24,67,91,202,216–218). The occurrence of the EBV receptor is closely correlated with the occurrence of the complement receptor in both normal B cells and a variety of B lymphoid lines. The cell line Jijoye is an EBV-receptor- and complement-receptor-positive line from which the virus-producing subclone P3HR-1 was isolated. P3HR-1 cells are EBV-receptor- as well as complement-receptor-negative. In spontaneous nonproducing revertants of P3HR-1, the reappearances of EBV receptors and complement receptors are closely linked (91). Moreover, there is a complete overlap of the two receptors by immunofluorescence and cocapping of these receptors, and the binding of C3 prevents the binding of EBV (67,217).

Earlier work on the EBV receptors was performed mainly with the virus adsorption bioassay test developed by Sairenji and Hinuma (172). Most studies used only one of the two main viral prototypes, usually P3HR-1 virus, in spite of the fact that antigenic and envelope protein variations had been observed between substrains of the virus (132,154,196). The question arises whether or not the variations between the viral substrains are reflected by corresponding variations in the nature and binding properties of the EBV receptor. A defective EBV receptor (the U698 cell) is capable of binding P3HR-1 but not B95-8 virus. The existence of this receptor, detected by indirect envelope immunofluorescence, was not detected by the virus-adsorption bioassay (67,218). By means of a radiolabeled EBV-binding assay (96) a receptor of a similar specificity was demonstrated on this cell line as well as on a nonproducer variant of P3HR-1 (211). Biochemical studies of the envelope components of EBV have suggested that two high-molecular-weight polypeptides (350K and 229K) of the four major EBV envelope components are necessary for cell binding (212).

It has been known for several years that all EBV-transformed lines are B cell lines and that essentially all peripheral B cells bind EBV. More recent experiments have suggested that only a small fraction of B cells that bind EBV can be transformed. Several experiments have indicated that a maximum of 5% of peripheral B cells are transformable even at high multiplicity of infection and that the fraction transformed may have surface IgM and may contain an unusually high density of HLA antigens (115,161,182). The increase in the number of IgM-bearing cells in IM patients may be related to these facts (1). The only apparent exception to the B cell specificity of EBV receptors is the Molt-4 T cell, which does express complement receptors on 65% of the cells and adsorbs EBV, but the adsorbed virus does not induce EBNA or stimulate DNA synthesis (118). The reason for this is not understood.

EBV infects human B lymphocytes (24,66,117). Katsuki et al. (76) and Steele et al. (180) have shown that the target cells most likely are the IgM-bearing B lymphocytes in cord blood, whereas the target cells may be IgG-, IgM-, or IgA-bearing B cells in adult peripheral blood (76). The infection leads to polyclonal, continuously growing B lymphoblastoid cell lines (14,35,58,121,148,173). Several assays have been used to follow the EBV-directed transformation (immortalization): stimulation of DNA synthesis, outgrowth of cells, growth on feeder layers, and growth in agarose after infection (13,52,75,126,159,192,214). In these studies, between 0.1 and 10% of the target lymphocytes were estimated to be transformed. Henderson et al. (52) and Sugden and Mark (192) found that the transformation of the target cells followed a linear response with dilution of EBV. The dose–response relationship closely followed theoretical "one-hit" kinetics. Earlier studies did not use purified target B cells, but mixed lymphocyte populations, which must have resulted in low efficiencies of transformation, because transformation in mixed lymphocyte populations has been shown to be suppressed by T cells (197). Zerbini and Ernberg (220) studied the responses of purified B cells after infection with B95-8 virus; 19 to 97% of the B cells showed EBNA after infection. This could suggest different susceptibilities of subpopulations of target cells. A nonlinear response was seen in EBNA induction that could not be compared with one-hit or multi-hit kinetics; 50 to 95% of the infected cells continued growing when incubated on a human fibroblast feeder layer in microwells. In soft agarose, a small proportion of these cells (less than 4%) established growing colonies that could be picked and recloned.

Studies of the early events occurring after transformation of lymphocytes of EBV have indicated that EBNA is synthesized very early after addition of the virus, after 12 to 18 hr (5,23). The appearance of EBNA is followed at 24 hr by morphological transformation characteristics of blast cells without DNA synthesis or increase in cell number. At 36 hr, the initiation of DNA synthesis can be detected by auto-radiography in the presence of ^{3}H-thymidine, followed by cell proliferation. The drug phosphonoacetic acid (PAA) blocks viral DNA replication and virus production (139,193) and also prevents transformation of B lymphocytes by EBV if added before 3 days (201). The EBV-specific DNA polymerase suggested by these experiments has been purified and characterized (43). The simplest interpretation of the sensitivity of transformation to PAA is that EBV DNA replication must precede integration and that this replication requires a specific DNA polymerase. Several other viral DNA polymerases have also been found to be sensitive to PAA, including the polymerases of HSV, cytomegalovirus, and Marek's disease virus.

The early events after EBV infection have been characterized in some detail. Viral adsorption and penetration are followed by the induction of EBNA, RNA synthesis, expression of LYDMA, activation of polyclonal immunoglobulin production, DNA synthesis, and cell division (5,23,130,159,161) (Fig. 1). The activation of immunoglobulin production is T-cell-independent, in contrast to the usual polyclonal B cell activators (11).

Following recognition and adsorption to the cell membrane, the virus enters the cell and is uncoated. The entry of the virus may occur either by pinocytosis or by fusion of the viral envelope with the membrane of the host cell, which is suggested from electron microscopy (174). The time of penetration of the virus is less than 1 hr, as measured by the loss of ability of anti-EBV serum to inhibit transformation or by the ability to abort transformation by separation of cells and virus by centrifugation (201).

LYMPHOID CELL LINES

Infection of B lymphocytes by EBV regularly leads to transformation (immortalization) (147) of B cells into lymphoblastoid cell lines (LCL) (135). These lines show many differences from cell lines established from BL tumors. Normally, B lymphocytes are transitory cells located within a sequence of differentiation that proceeds from primitive stem cells toward mature immunoglobulin-secreting end cells, i.e., plasma cells. EBV cannot infect either stem cells or plasma cells, because infection of B cells by EBV is sharply restricted to surface-immunoglobulin- and complement(C3)-receptor-positive B cells.

The phenotypic changes induced by EBV itself have been studied by comparing EBV-negative B lymphoma lines that can be infected and converted to EBV-positive derivatives with such EBV-positive sublines. EBV conversion of the two EBV-

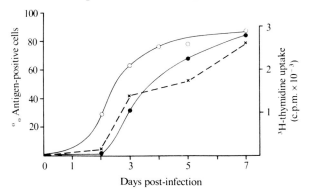

FIG. 1. Induction of EBNA-positive cells (●), LYDMA-positive cells (○), and DNA synthesis (×) in cultures of T-cell-depleted lymphocytes infected with EBV. EBNA was detected by immunofluorescence, LYDMA by cytotoxicity, and DNA synthesis by ^{3}H-thymidine pulse labeling (18 hr) prior to harvest. (From Moss et al., ref. 130, with permission.)

negative lymphoma lines, Ramos and BJAB, was found to cause no cytogenetic changes (92), but it did cause several phenotypic alterations, i.e., increased resistance to saturation, decreased serum dependence, decreased capping of surface markers, increased lectin agglutinability, and increased ability to activate the alternative complement pathway (114,129,184–186,215). Most of these effects are surprisingly similar to the phenotypic changes induced by the classic transforming viruses in monolayer cultures. Recent studies have shown that EBV conversion in EBV-negative cells induces several new antigens, including some antigens regarded as specific for human T cells (163).

In contrast to LCL cells, cell lines of BL origin appear to represent clones of proliferating neoplastic cells (7,30,205). BL-derived cell lines correspond to an intermediate step in B cell differentiation, and they synthesize immunoglobulins (usually IgM) that appear almost exclusively to be destined for plasma membrane integration (28,87) and are not secreted at the high rates characteristic of myeloma cell lines that are equivalent to fully differentiated plasma cells (112).

An interesting monoclonal antibody that appears to differentiate between LCL and BL cells has been described recently (213). The antibody, which was obtained by immunization with BL (Daudi) cells, appears to react with high fractions of different BL cell lines, and although it has been found to react with some normal cell types, it has not been observed to react with LCL cell lines.

LCL cells appear to represent a step in differentiation that is intermediate between BL and myeloma cells, and some immunoglobulin secretion can be observed (135). The rosetting of human B cells with antigen-coated erythrocytes prior to *in vitro* EBV transformation has permitted establishment of LCL clones that produce human monoclonal antibodies with different specificities (187), such as hapten (99), RH blood group antigen (97), and streptococcal carbohydrate (188), as well as rheumatoid factor (IgM anti-IgG) (183). Like other LCL lines, these grow to a density of about 10^6 cells/ml. Their supernatants contain 5 to 20 g of antibody per milliliter. It has also been possible to adapt the fusion of lymphocytes with myeloma cells to obtain monoclonal-antibody-producing hybridoma cells (100) in the human system (18,141), and such hybridomas produce larger amounts of secreted human immunoglobulins. Recently, Kozbor et al. (98) succeeded in fusing antibody-producing LCL cell lines with a human myeloma, and these hybridomas produced high amounts of the anti-tetanus-toxoid monoclonal antibody produced by the anti-tetanus-toxoid-specific LCL line employed for the fusion.

CYTOGENETICS OF LCL AND BL CELLS

Parallel cytogenetic and nude mouse inoculation studies (136,219) have dispelled earlier notions that all EBV-transformed lines could be tumorigenic, irrespective of their origin. Virally immortalized LCL lines remain purely diploid during several months of cultivation *in vitro*; they fail to grow subcutaneously in nude mice, and they have a low (<2%) cloning efficiency in agarose. After prolonged passage *in vitro*, they usually become aneuploid and might become capable of tumor formation after nude mouse inoculation. In contrast to this, BL biopsied cells and their derived cell lines are aneuploid and tumorigenic from the beginning and have a high cloning efficiency in agarose.

The chromosomal changes of long-passaged LCL lines show no apparent specific features, although secondary changes toward aneuploidy are frequently observed. Gains of chromosomes appear to be more frequent than losses. The chromosome gains are not completely random, because trisomy is often found for chromosomes 3, 7, 8, 9, and 12; the trisomy 7 is of particular interest because it is also found in both BL and non-BL lymphoma lines (181,219).

In contrast, most BL cells contain the same highly specific marker. This marker was first identified as 14q +, with an extra band at the distal end of the long arm of one chromosome 14 (107). 14q + markers have subsequently been described in a variety of other lymphoreticular neoplasias (32,33,109,113,123,124,219). More detailed studies revealed important differences between the 14q + markers of BL and non-BL lymphomas. In BL, the extra band is derived from chromosome 8 (219) [t(8;14)(q24;q32)] and represents exactly identical breaking points in different cases (108). In non-BL with a 14q + marker the donor chromosomes are often variable; pieces can be derived from chromosomes 1, 4, 10, 11, 14, 15, and 18, in addition to chromosome 8; for reviews, see Fukuhara and Rowley (33) and Mitelman (124).

The BL-associated reciprocal t(8;14) translocation is not limited to EBV-carrying BL (Fig. 2). It was also found in EBV-negative American BL (219) and in the rare B cell form of acute lymphocytic leukemia (ALL) (123), believed to represent neoplastic growth of similar cell type as BL. Together with the fact that EBV-transformed LCL of non-BL origin do not carry the t(8;14) chromosome, this suggests that EBV is not involved in causing the translocation, but other factors must be involved. It is a question which chromosome is more important in the association of this translocation with BL.

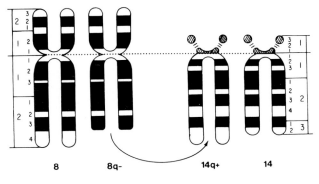

TRANSLOCATION

FIG. 2. Schematic diagram of the BL-associated t(8;14) reciprocal translocation. The dash line designates the position of the centromeres. (From Epstein et al., ref. 26, with permission.)

Recently, variant forms of the BL translocation have been described. In these cases, the same distal part of the chromosome 8 becomes translocated, but to chromosome 2 or 22 rather than to chromosome 14 (10,124,127,204). This situation is reminiscent of the Philadelphia chromosome, where a t(22;9) translocation is found in most cases, whereas a minority (~10%) show a chromosome 22 deletion with the same breakpoint, but with either no identifiable translocation site or a translocation to other recipient chromsomes (167). The variant BL translocations suggest that the distal part of chromosome 8, rather than chromosome 14, carries the gene(s) responsible for development of BL. Because chromosome 14 is known to contain the immunoglobulin heavy-chain loci in humans (19,61), it is possible that the translocation is affected by the immunoglobulin gene region, an area obviously highly active in B lymphocytes. Manolova et al. (108) and Hecht and Kaiser-McCaw (51) have demonstrated that the translocated band of chromosome 8 changes its stainability in a typical BL-associated 8;14 translocation, suggesting that such a position effect would be compatible with such a direct effect of the position on chromosome 14 of the translocated segment of chromosome 8. This same concept is further supported by the recent demonstration that the human κ light-chain gene is on chromosome 2 and the human λ light-chain gene is on chromosome 22 (27,107)—the same two chromosomes that were involved as recipients of the distal chromosome 8 fragment in the variant BL translocations. A very similar observation has been made with murine plasmacytomas that carry t(12;15) or t(6;15) translocations. Mouse chromosome 12 carries the immunoglobulin heavy-chain locus, and chromosome 6 carries the κ light-chain locus (53), and the segment of chromosome 15 involved in these translocations could be associated with regulation of lymphocyte differentiation and growth, because murine B and T cell leukemias frequently are trisomic for the involved segment of chromosome 15 (81).

The mechanism by which the t(8;14) translocation develops in BL is not understood, although it is rather clear that EBV cannot be directly involved. Klein (80) has suggested that BL develops in at least three different steps. In African BL associated with EBV, a first step could be EBV-induced immortalization of some B lymphocytes on primary infection with EBV. A second step could be associated with environment-dependent factors that would allow latent EBV-carrying cells chronic proliferation and could further facilitate this by relative immunosuppression. The third and final step would take place if and when the "right" reciprocal t(8;14) translocation was generated; this would lead to the outgrowth of an autonomous monoclonal tumor.

It is interesting to note that chromosome 14 anomalies frequently are involved in ataxia-telangiectasia (AT), a condition noted for a markedly increased incidence of lymphoreticular neoplasia (113) as well as agammaglobulinemia (116). Most AT patients have clones of lymphocytes marked by translocations involving chromosome 14 (113). The breaks observed in chromosome 14 have always been in the long arm in the q11-q12 region, and the other chromosomes involved as partners in translocations have been chromsomes 7, 8, and 14 and the X chromosome.

Chromosome 14 rearrangements are found in varying proportions (2–5%) in lymphocytes, and they were found to be reduced in frequency in LCL lines, as compared with normal lymphocyte cultures. In recent unpublished work (I. Ernberg, B. G. Giovanella, and J. Zeuthen) we observed LCL lines derived from AT patients clone at slightly increased frequencies as compared with LCL lines from AT carriers or normal individuals. By successive cloning of an AT-derived LCL line, subclones that cloned at very high frequencies (up to 42% cloning efficiency in agarose) were isolated, and their cloning efficiencies in agarose correlated with their tumorigenicity in nude mice. Chromosome studies on these subclones showed increased frequencies of chromosome breakage, but no evidence for the generation of any translocations involving chromosome 14 *in vitro* was found. Therefore, no associations with chromosome 14 translocations and increased transformed phenotype are indicated by these *in vitro* studies, but it is, of course, still highly possible that such mechanisms might operate *in vivo*.

EBV TRANSFORMATION AND EBNA

In recent years, considerable progress has been made toward understanding the transforming proteins of the small papovaviruses such as SV40 and polyoma virus. In the SV40 system, large T antigen is the main candidate for a transforming protein, either alone or with small T antigen (110). In addition to its function in transformation, it is also involved in initiation of the late viral replication cycle. Large T antigen binds to the origin of viral DNA replication and also inhibits early mRNA synthesis. In experiments where different amounts of large T antigen were measured in infected cells, a critical amount of T antigen was found to be necessary before viral DNA replication and synthesis of late viral antigens could occur (45). SV40 T antigen is complexed to a cellular protein of molecular weight 53,000 (53K) in the nucleus of the transformed cell (101). Very similar and possibly identical 53K proteins have now been identified in a wide variety of transformed cells and tumor cells. These proteins have recently been shown to share extensive sequence homologies (68). Small amounts of 53K protein have also been detected in normal mouse tissues. Nondividing lymphocytes (in G_0) do not produce 53K unless stimulated by mitogen to enter the division cycle (G_m). The induction of 53K protein is at the level of gene transcription and occurs within 4 hr of mitogenic stimulation. This correlates with the time required for lymphocytes to become committed to enter the division cycle and is consistent with 53K protein functioning early during the transition from G_0 to G_m (122). A comparison of turnover rates suggests that the role of the SV40 large T antigen in transformation may relate to its ability to stabilize 53K protein. The ability of large T antigen to promote the viral cycle would not interfere with transformation of nonpermissive cells.

In the case of EBV-transformed cells, it now seems that a similar situation could account for transformation. EBNA is, as already mentioned, the only antigen regularly found in cells carrying the EBV genome. In similarity to the T antigens of SV40 and polyoma virus, it is a DNA-binding protein (106), and it is now known to consist of a probably virus-specific 48K subunit that is complexed with a 53K protein of cellular origin (88,104). More recent studies have shown the 48K component of EBNA to be a degradation product of a larger 65K to 70K polypeptide (191; J. Luka, *personal communication*). A similar and probably identical 53K protein, not complexed with 48K, is also present in some EBV-negative B-cell-derived lymphoma lines, but in smaller quantities than in the EBV-carrying lines. EBV conversion of these lines into stable EBNA-positive sublines has been shown to increase their content of 53K protein (88), and, as already mentioned, to result in parallel increased transformed phenotypes in these EBV-converted sublines. Work in other laboratories has demonstrated purified EBNA to have two activities that correlate with transformation of malignant cells, i.e., to stimulate the template activity of chromatin (72) and to have an associated protein kinase activity similar to that associated with transforming proteins in other systems (73). Other early DNA-binding proteins have been described in the EBV system (165) that could have other roles in the establishment of transformation. Recent measurements of replicon sizes in EBV-negative B-cell-derived lymphoma lines and their EBV-converted sublines indicate that the presence of the EBV genome, and possibly of EBNA, activates new initiation points for cellular DNA replication (142), in similarity to what has previously been observed for SV40-transformed cells (111).

By microinjection of cells with microcapillaries, Tjian et al. (203) showed that SV40 large T antigen stimulated DNA synthesis in quiescent (G_0) fibroblasts. Similar results have been obtained by microinjection of G_0 fibroblast monolayers with purified EBNA using a special method (71) based on the fusion of cells with protein-filled erythrocyte ghosts (88,224). This experiment was repeated with the two purified 48K and 53K subunits of EBNA, and stimulation of cellular DNA synthesis in 3T3 cells was observed only with the purified 53K protein, indicating that the activation of DNA synthesis, presumably by activation of new DNA initiation points, is associated with the 53K subunit rather than the 48K subunit (J. Zeuthen and J. Luka, *unpublished data*). In similarity to the case of SV40 T antigen, it is likely that the function of the 48K protein could be stabilization of the cellular 53K component, rather than a direct function. Similar results have been obtained by EBNA fusion-microinjection of human lymphocytes, which are also activated to DNA synthesis. Also in this case it appears that it is the 53K component that is active in stimulating growth, because similar results have been obtained with complete EBNA and with 53K proteins purified from several different cell lines (EBV-negative and -positive BL cells as well as transformed mouse cell lines) (Fig. 3) (J. Zeuthen and J. Luka, *unpublished data*).

Whereas SV40 and EBV show surprising homologies, the transformation of cells by polyoma virus appears to occur by a different mechanism. For polyoma virus there is now extensive evidence that large T antigen in itself is neither necessary nor sufficient for transformation (64). In all probability, middle T antigen, a 56K protein coded for by the early region of the viral genome, is involved in the transformation function. The polyoma virus middle T antigen has protein kinase activity (64) and could function similarly to the transforming proteins of retroviruses that also have protein kinase activity (63).

STRUCTURE AND FUNCTION OF EBV DNA

Because of lack of a permissive tissue culture system for propagation of EBV, only a limited number of isolates have been studied and characterized. More detailed biochemical studies have been restricted to those strains that can be propagated in sufficient amounts to allow purification of the virus and viral DNA. This approach is clearly necessary in order to obtain genetic information on the coding capacity of individual EBV DNA fragments, although some information has already been obtained using UV inactivation kinetic data (25).

EBV of the transforming B95-8 strain was inactivated by UV-irradiation to establish the dose–response relationship for early virus-induced functions in human B lymphocytes. Based on the dose–response curves, the target-size cross sections for viral DNA for the induction of EBNA expression, DNA synthesis, and IgM synthesis were established (Fig. 4). The relative target sizes were found to be small in relation to the size of the whole genome (100 megadaltons): around 8 Md for the induction of EBNA as well as IgM synthesis, and about 3 Md for the induction of DNA synthesis. The relative target sizes are reasonable in view of the amount of viral information transcribed by immortalized non-virus-producing cells (21,49,143,150,168). In these studies, transcription from three or four regions of the genome corresponded to between 17 and 30% of viral DNA found in

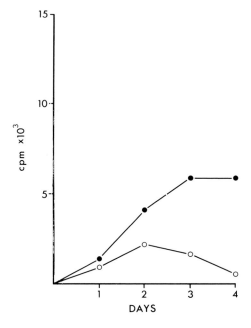

FIG. 3. Stimulation of DNA synthesis in human cord blood lymphocytes injected with 53K protein from EBV-negative Ramos cells by fusion with protein-loaded autologous erythrocyte ghosts: (●) injected with 53K protein (○) fusion with mock-loaded ghosts. DNA synthesis was measured by ^{3}H-thymidine pulse labeling (4 hr) prior to harvest. (J. Zeuthen and J. Luka, *unpublished data*.)

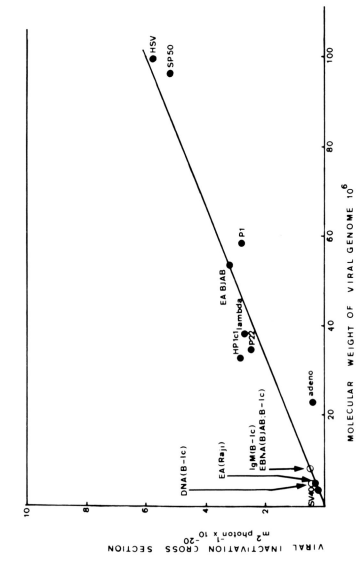

FIG. 4. Relationship between viral DNA cross section and molecular weight of viral DNA for different double-stranded DNA viruses in repair-competent hosts, compared with various EBV-induced functions/antigens. Indicated are induction of DNA synthesis [DNA(B-Ic)], induction of EBNA [EBNA(BJAB;B-Ic)], induction of EA in Raji cells by P3HR-1 superinfection [EA(Raji)], and induction of IgM synthesis [IgM(B-Ic)]. Also shown is induction of EA in BJAB cells by P3HR-1 superinfection (EA BJAB), which shows a much larger target size than for Raji cells. (From Engblom and Ernberg, ref. 25, data based in part on ref. 19a, with permission.)

poly(A) + nuclear RNA transcripts, while only 3 to 6% was represented in cytoplasmic, virus-specific poly(A) + transcripts.

The characterization of the EBV genome in molecular terms has benefited considerably from modern molecular cloning techniques. The genome, as mentioned, is close to 100 Md (151,152) and has been analyzed mainly using EBV DNA from the B95-8 producer line (120). Although B95-8 virus is similar to other isolates of EBV in its ability to induce EBNA and enhance the growth of lymphocytes (117), it is known to be missing DNA contained in other BL tumor isolates of EBV (155). The size and sequence arrangements of B95-8 and other isolates have been determined, and detailed restriction enzyme cleavage maps and cloned EBV DNA are available (4,12,20,37,50,169,170). For further discussion of the structure of EBV DNA, see the chapter by Kieff and associates in this volume (77).

Studies by Rymo (168) have shown that most of the EBV-encoded RNA is transcribed from the 2×10^6-d *Eco*RI J fragment in both Raji cells and BL biopsy material. To a lesser extent, two other regions (the *Hin*dIII C fragment and the *Eco*RI G_1 or G_2 fragments have also been observed to be transcribed. Because the *Eco*RI J fragment encodes RNA sequences abundant in EBV-transformed cell lines, one might ask if it contains the information for EBNA. This is not the case, because the *Eco*RI J fragment encodes for two small RNA species (166 and 172 nucleotides) (3,160) that are not polyadenylated and probably are present in ribonucleoprotein particles. We have analyzed the function of the *Eco*RI J fragment in human lymphocytes in a more direct way. By fusion of DNA-loaded erythrocyte ghosts using a newly developed method [a modification of the method of Kaltoft and Celis (71)] it was possible to transfer cloned *Eco*RI J DNA into human cord blood lymphocytes and determine if it has any stimulating activity when injected into lymphocytes in this way (J. Zeuthen, G. Bjursell, and J. Arrand, *unpublished data*). Injection of cells with *Eco*RI J fragments has a clearly stimulating effect on DNA synthesis in lymphocytes, in contrast to other EBV DNA fragments tested. The *Eco*RI-J-fragment-injected lymphocytes continued to divide for up to 8 weeks after injection, but no stable transformed cells were obtained. Also, the growing cells were found to be negative for EBNA. The failure to obtain stable transformed cells could be due either to lack of integration of the transferred EBV *Eco*RI J fragment or to lack of some other factor necessary for stable transformation of cells (Fig. 5).

Recently, the *Eco*RI J fragment has been subdivided by additional cloning into two subfragments (J1 and J2) that carry the information for the two small RNA molecules mentioned (65). These two cloned DNAs have also been tested by fusion-microinjection into cord blood lymphocytes, and both have been found to be effective in stimulating growth of lymphocytes (J. Zeuthen, G. Bjursell, and J. Arrand, *unpublished data*). The mechanism for the stimulation of lymphocytes by microinjection of *Eco*RI J DNA remains obscure. One likely explanation would be that the small RNAs could serve as initiator RNAs for DNA synthesis. The results from these experiments, when compared with our results from the microinjection of EBNA and the host-cell-specified 53K protein, point to the possibility that EBV uses several different mechanisms to achieve growth promotion and transformation of lymphocytes.

By Ca^{2+}-dependent transfection techniques, Grogan et al. (47) succeeded in mapping EA expression to the 17.2-Md *Eco*RI B fragment, and it is beyond doubt that similar approaches will help to clarify the genetic mapping of EBV DNA.

Other recent transfection experiments where the DNAs from two different strains of EBV (one transforming, non-EA-inducing strain; one nontransforming, EA-inducing strain) were used to transform epithelial cells showed that transfection of epithelial cells with DNA from both of these sources resulted in EA expression (190). This result can be explained either by epithelial cells presenting a more permissive system for lytic infection or by an artifact of the Ca^{2+} transfection procedure. It must be stressed that it cannot *a priori* be assumed that DNA transferred by Ca^{2+} transfection is expressed in a normal physiological fashion.

It is still debated whether or not EBV codes for a viral thymidine kinase (tk) enzyme similar to that of the other herpesviruses like herpes simplex (146). There is some circumstantial evidence that this might be the case, because EBV-super-infected tk cells do not express a tk enzyme activity (15,164). After microinjection of tk-deficient mouse 3T3 fibroblasts with EBV, we have been able to select tk$^+$ cells that appear to contain a small fragment of EBV DNA defined only by hybridization with the *Eco*RI H and *Bam*HI X and V^d cloned fragments (E. T. Sørensen, J. Arrand, and J. Zeuthen, *unpublished data*). The presence of this relatively small fragment and evidence from other closely related herpesviruses (144) could suggest that this region indeed carries an EBV-specified tk gene.

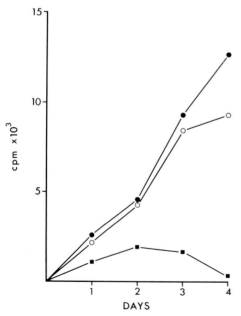

FIG. 5. Stimulation of DNA synthesis in human cord blood lymphocytes injected with two plasmid DNA preparations of cloned EBV DNA using fusion with DNA-loaded autologous erythrocyte ghosts: (○) injected with a subfragment of the *Eco*RI J fragment (J1), (●) injected with a different subfragment of *Eco*RI J (J2), and (■) injected with a cloned *Eco*RI B fragment. The two different subfragments of *Eco*RI J each code for one of two small RNA species (166 and 172 nucleotides) (65). DNA synthesis was measured by ³H-thymidine pulse labeling (4 hr) prior to harvest. (J. Zeuthen, G. Bjursell, and J. Arrand, *unpublished data*.)

CHARACTERIZATION AND DIFFERENTIATION OF HYBRID CELLS

The regulatory mechanisms that control the differentiation of BL cell lines, as well as EBV genome expression, are not understood at the molecular level. As a first approach to characterizing some of these properties of BL cells, somatic cell genetics can at least provide some insight. Somatic cell hybrids [for an extensive review, see Ringertz and Savage (158)] can be isolated between different parental lines carrying appropriate selective markers and can be identified in several ways, i.e., by their isoenzyme patterns, HLA markers, and chromosomal markers, as well as other phenotypic markers. Analysis of chromosomal markers has proved especially useful for hybrids with BL cell lines, because many of these lines carry several characteristic markers that can be identified by means of chromosome banding techniques.

In hybrids between the two BL-derived lines Raji and Namalwa (which express small amounts of IgM kappa and large amounts of IgM lambda, respectively, on their surfaces) it was possible to quantitate the amounts of kappa and lambda chains expressed on the surfaces of Raji/Namalwa hybrids and clones (162). In spite of some variability, the hybrids showed almost the same levels of surface kappa and lambda chains as the parental lines from which they were formed. The BL-derived Daudi line expresses very high levels of surface IgM kappa (28), and high levels of surface IgM kappa are also expressed in hybrids of Daudi with both P3HR-1 (9) and Raji (225). This last result differs from the results of a previous study on another Daudi/Raji hybrid that was selected for an adherent phenotype (16) and showed reduced IgM kappa expression (89). It has been shown that cell shape is an important factor for expression of the differentiated phenotype (2), and it is therefore possible that selection of adherent cells has worked against expression of the differentiated marker. In hybrids of lymphoid cells with cells of other lineages, immunoglobulin synthesis may be totally extinguished (221), and this is also observed immediately after fusion of immunoglobulin-producing cells with other cell types (223). Hybrids of BL cells with other hematopoietic cells have been isolated to analyze further this type of restriction. A hybrid between the human erythroleukemic cell line K562 [inducible for hemoglobin synthesis by hemin (166)] and P3HR-1 showed complete suppression of EBV receptors (93), and another hybrid of K562 with Daudi showed complete suppression of surface IgM as well as other lymphoid markers (225). Both of the hybrids with K562 contained high levels of heme and were inducible for hemoglobin synthesis. The presence of Ia-like antigens on the two hybrids was analyzed by a very sensitive technique using staining of the cells with *Staphylococcus aureus* coupled to different monoclonal antibodies against Ia, and less than 1% of the hybrid cells expressed Ia (227). An additional hybrid between the human promyelocytic leukemic cell line HL-60 (17) and P3HR-1 has been analyzed and has been shown to strongly express Ia-like antigens, but it has lost the myeloid markers that were characteristic of the HL-60 parent (95). These results show that the erythroid phenotype dominates at the expense of the B cell phenotype in the two hybrids with K562 and that the B cell phenotype dominates in the hybrid with HL-60. The differentiation patterns appear to be mutually exclusive and also to be dependent on the state of differentiation of the nonlymphoid parent, because the primitive K562 line dominates, whereas the HL-60 line does not express its myeloid markers in hybrids with BL cells.

Isoenzymes are usually coexpressed in hybrid cells and can be used to identify them. In the case of BL cells, one curious deficiency noted is the total absence of one enzyme, soluble malic enzyme (ME_S), although this enzyme is expressed in lymphocytes as well as other cell types (149), arguing that the absence of this enzyme in BL cells is related to the specific phenotype of BL cells. HLA-A,B,C antigens of the parental cells are also coexpressed in hybrids. The hybrids with the Daudi line constitute a special case, because this line is negative for β_2-microglobulin and HLA (29,89,222). In hybrids with Raji cells that express HLA and β_2-microglobulin, expression of new HLA specificities (A10, B38, B17) has been observed (29,89). This argues in agreement with biochemical evidence that β_2-microglobulin is a component of surface-expressed HLA on cells and that the consequence of loss of β_2-microglobulin in Daudi cells is loss of HLA expression, which can be reexpressed if β_2-microglobulin is supplied by another cell. K562 cells express β_2-microglobulin and HLA very weakly on the surface (222), although HLA-A,B,C heavy chains can be detected using sensitive assays (226,227). The membrane defect of K562 is partially dominant in both hybrids between BL cells and K562 (93,225,227).

VIRUS EXPRESSION IN HYBRID CELLS

As already mentioned, EBV-carrying BL-derived cell lines can be divided into nonproducer, abortive producer, and producer cell lines on the basis of their expression of EBV lytic cycle antigens. The number of cells entering the lytic cycle can be amplified by the inducers BUdR (34), IUdR (48), n-butyrate (105), the phorbol ester tetradecanoylphorbol acetate (TPA) (203), and azacytidine (8), whose only common denominator is a known effect on differentiation in a variety of cell types. Somatic cell hybrids have been employed for studying the control of EBV expression. These hybrids have furnished information not readily obtained with EBV-carrying cells alone. Hybrids between BL cells and human nonlymphoid cells have been produced by fusion of producer P3HR-1 cells and epithelial-like D98 (D98/ P3HR-1), and nonproducer Raji cells and D98 cells (D98/Raji) (39–41). Both D98/ P3HR-1 and D98/Raji hybrids contain multiple copies of the EBV genome, express EBNA, and show no evidence of spontaneous virus activation. Because producer P3HR-1 cells do show spontaneous virus activation, often at relatively high levels, the lack of spontaneous activation in the D98/P3HR-1 hybrid suggests the presence of a factor(s) that maintains the virus genome in a repressed state. Treatment of D98/P3HR-1 hybrids with IUdR results in virus activation similar to that seen when P3HR-1 cells are treated with the drug. The IUdR-activated hybrid cells synthesize EA in the presence of the analogue, and "free" viral DNA, VCA, and virus particles are formed following removal of the drug (40). The levels of virus activation in IUdR-treated hybrid cells may be higher than those observed in drug-treated P3HR-

1 cells. Further, dibutyryl cyclic AMP (cAMP), known to affect cellular regulation, can induce low levels of virus activation in D98/P3HR-1 hybrid cells and may enhance the levels of virus activation induced by IUdR (228). A similar effect of cAMP on BL cells themselves has not been observed. Abortive producers such as Raji cells switch on EA production in only a small proportion of cells, but these do not proceed further to viral DNA synthesis and synthesis of VCA (34,36). The block in viral antigen production in Raji cells is not complemented after hybridization to EBV-negative lymphoma cells (BJAB), in spite of the fact that EA production is amplified (82), showing that the defect in Raji cells is primarily viral rather than cellular. This is in agreement with recent results showing that Raji EBV DNA carries two deletions (170) that could be responsible for this defectiveness.

As mentioned, the inducibility for EA is amplified in the Raji/BJAB hybrid (82), in spite of the absence of VCA production. It has been suggested that similar control mechanisms are involved in the response of BL cells to superinfection with EBV and inducibility with IUdR with respect to EA synthesis (82,86). Results consistent with this suggestion have been obtained by comparing the inducibility of EA by superinfection and IUdR using Raji cells and tetraploid Raji cells obtained by Colcemid® treatment (175). The levels of EA synthesis following superinfection of IUdR treatment are significantly lower in the tetraploid cells than in the diploid Raji cells. Further tetraploidization of Raji cells does not result in the expected doubling of EBV DNA copies. These observations are consistent with the reported correlation between IUdR inducibility and number of viral DNA copies (152,195). Other types of hybrid cells have given information with respect to the controls that could be involved in EBV antigen expression. With certain minor variations, the picture is consistent. When producer BL lines are hybridized with nonproducers, producer status tends to dominate over nonproducer status, and inducibility over noninducibility (9,82,83,128,138). This suggests that many controls are of a positive nature, and the observation that the inducers used interfere with differentiation, whereas standard mutagenic or carcinogenic agents are noninducers (8,230), strongly suggests that at least some controls may be cellular rather than viral. It is of interest that EBV production and inducibility in many cases parallel the behavior of other B cell markers in the cell hybrids studied. In cases where BL cells were hybridized to fibroblasts, virus production and inducibility were switched off in spite of the continued presence of EBV DNA in multiple copies and uninfluenced expression of EBNA (38,90). In the course of serial propagation of hybrids between mouse fibroblasts and EBV-carrying cells, detectable EBV genomes and EBNA are lost concomitantly with the loss of human chromosomes (90,179,189). The consensus reached from these studies is that the presence of EBV genomes and EBNA cannot be associated with one particular human chromosome in hybrids of mouse fibroblasts with human cells that carry multiple copies of EBV genomes. Exceptions do occur, however, as evidenced by the isolation of hybrid clones that contain viral DNA and EBNA in the absence of recognizable human chromosomes, but because these do retain some human isoenzymes, it suggests the possibility that some human DNA has been translocated to mouse chromosomes (189). The viral DNA could be carried along with the human DNA in an integrated state or could persist in an episomal state independent of the retained human DNA. In the P3HR-1/K562 hybrid, a similar complete block against EA and VCA inducibility was observed using the three inducers IUdR, sodium butyrate, and TPA (93) that parallels the loss of other B cell functions, but in the other Daudi/K562 hybrid this was not observed; this difference could be due to a very high number (84 genome equivalents/cell) of EBV genomes in the last hybrid that could override the negative controls imposed by the nonlymphoid parent (94). In spite of the fact that IUdR failed to induce viral antigen synthesis in P3HR-1/K562 hybrid cells, viral transcription was shown to increase from 10 to 25% after IUdR induction (102). In the Daudi/K562 hybrid cells, IUdR induced viral transcription from more than 40% of the viral genome. RNAs extracted from polyribosomes of the two induced hybrids both contained about 20% of the viral RNA sequences found in whole cell extracts, whereas for P3HR-1 cells most viral RNA transcripts can be found in polysomes (102). These findings could indicate the presence of some additional translational control mechanisms that could contribute to the suppression of EBV genome expression in these hybrids.

Exceptions to the rule of extinction of EBV inducibility in hybrids of BL cells with other lineages are the hybrids with human epithelial-like carcinoma cells (42,39,195), where the hybrids have been observed to be completely permissive. This observation might be of some relevance to NPC, because epithelial carcinoma cells might be more compatible with EBV production than other human cells of non-B-cell origin. Whereas the virus shows exquisite specificity for B lymphocytes *in vitro*, this is clearly not the case for NPC, in which squamous epithelial cells of the nasopharynx undergo malignant transformation *in vivo* and subsequently carry the EBV genome. Purified EBV DNA has been introduced into cells using both microinjection (44) and Ca^{2+}-dependent transfection producers (47,119), and the complete virus has been brought to infect cells lacking EBV receptors by transplantation of virus receptors into cells that do not normally express such structures (207,208). A transient low level of EBNA expression was noted by Volsky et al. (208), but otherwise all the data available suggest that different types of cells produce late viral antigens in the absence of EBNA, in stark contrast to what is usually the case with lymphocytes and epithelial cells from NPC. However, in microinjection experiments using amnion epithelial cells injected with EBV, we have found evidence suggesting that such cells can express EBNA, which might be a prerequisite for transformation of epithelial cells in NPC.

ACKNOWLEDGMENTS

I thank Miss Doris Jepsen for excellent secretarial assistance. Work in the author's laboratory was generously supported by grants from the Danish Natural Science Council, the Danish Medical Research Council, and the Danish Cancer Society, and by an award from the Boel Foundation.

REFERENCES

1. Aiuti, F., Ciarla, M. V., D'Asero, R., and Garafalo, J. A. (1973): Surface markers on lymphocytes of patients with infectious diseases. *Infect. Immun.*, 8:110–117.
2. Allan, M., and Harrison, P. (1980): Co-expression of differentiation markers in hybrids between Friend cells and lymphoid cells and the influence of cell shape. *Cell*, 19:437–447.
3. Arrand, J., and Rymo, L. (1982): Characterization of the major Epstein-Barr virus-specific RNA in Burkitt lymphoma-derived cells. *J. Virol.*, 41:376–389.
4. Arrand, J. R., Rymo, L., Walsh, J. E., Björck, E., Lindahl, T., and Griffin, B. E. (1981): Molecular cloning of the complete Epstein-Barr virus genome as a set of overlapping restriction endonuclease fragments. *Nucleic Acids Res.*, 9:2999–3014.
5. Aya, T., and Osato, T. (1974): Early events in transformation of human cord lymphocytes by Epstein-Barr virus: Induction of DNA synthesis mitosis and the virus-associated nuclear antigen synthesis. *Int. J. Cancer*, 14:341–347.
6. Baron, D., and Strominger, L. (1978): Partial purification and properties of the Epstein-Barr virus-associated nuclear antigen. *J. Biol. Chem.*, 253:2875–2881.
7. Béchet, J. M., Fialkow, P., Nilsson, K., and Klein, G. (1974): Immunoglobulin synthesis and glucose-6-phosphate dehydrogenase as cell markers in human lymphoblastoid cell lines. *Exp. Cell Res.*, 89:275–282.
8. Ben-Sasson, S. A., and Klein, G. (1981): Activation of the Epstein-Barr virus genoma by 5-aza-cytidine in latently infected human lymphoid lines. *Int. J. Cancer*, 28:131–135.
9. Ber, R., Klein, G., Moar, M., Povey, S., Rosén, A., Westman, A., Yefenof, E., and Zeuthen, J. (1978): Somatic cell hybrids between human lymphoma lines. IV. Establishment and characterization of a P3HR-1/Daudi hybrid. *Int. J. Cancer*, 21:707–719.
10. Berger, R., Bernheim, A., Weh, H.-J., Flandria, G., Daniel, M.-T., Brouet, J.-C., and Colbert, N. (1979): A new translocation in Burkitt's tumor cells. *Hum. Genet.*, 53:111–112.
11. Bird, A. G., Britton, S., Ernberg, I., and Nilsson, K. (1981): Characteristics of Epstein-Barr virus activation of human B lymphocytes. *J. Exp. Med.*, 154:832–839.
12. Bornkamm, G. W., Delius, H., Zimber, U., Hudewentz, J., and Epstein, M. A. (1980): Comparison of Epstein-Barr virus strains of different origin by analysis of the viral DNAs. *J. Virol.*, 35:603–618.
13. Chang, R. S., Fillingame, R. A., Paglieroni, T., and Glassy, F. J. (1976): A procedure for quantifying susceptibility of human lymphocytes to transformation by Epstein-Barr virus. *Proc. Soc. Exp. Biol. Med.*, 153:193–196.
14. Chang, R. S., and Golden, H. D. (1971): Transformation of human leukocytes by throat wash from infectious mononucleosis patients. *Nature*, 234:359–360.
15. Chen, S.-T., Estes, J. E., Huang, E.-S., and Pagano, J. S. (1978): Epstein-Barr virus associated thymidine kinase. *J. Virol.*, 26:203–208.
16. Clements, G. B., Klein, G., Zeuthen, J., and Povey, S. (1976): The selection of somatic cell hybrids between human lymphoma cell lines. *Somatic Cell Genet.*, 2:309–324.
17. Collins, S. J., Gallo, R. C., and Galagher, R. E. (1977): Continuous growth and differentiation of human myeloid leukemia cells in suspension culture. *Nature*, 270:347–350.
18. Croce, C., Linnenbach, A., Hall, W., Steplewski, Z., and Koprowski, H. (1980): Production of human hybridomas secreting antibodies to measles virus. *Nature*, 288:488–489.
19. Croce, C. M., Shander, M., Martinis, J., Cicurel, L., D'Ancona, G. G., and Koprowski, H. (1980): Preferential retention of human chromosome 14 in mouse × human B cell hybrids. *Eur. J. Immunol.*, 10:486–488.
19a. Dalens, M., and Adams, A. (1977): Induction of Epstein-Barr associated early antigen in different lymphoid cell lines with ultra-violet-irradiated P3HR-1 virus. *Virol.*, 83:305–312.
20. Dambaugh, T., Beisel, C., Hummel, M., King, W., Fennewald, S., Cheung, A., Heller, M., Raab-Traub, N., and Kieff, E. (1980): EBV (B95-8) DNA: Molecular cloning and detailed mapping. *Proc. Natl. Acad. Sci. USA*, 77:2999–3003.
21. Dambaugh, T., Nkrumah, F. K., Biggar, R. J., and Kieff, E. (1979): Epstein-Barr virus RNA in Burkitt tumor tissue. *Cell*, 16:313–322.
22. Dolyniuk, M., Wolff, E., and Kieff, E. (1976): Proteins of Epstein-Barr virus. II. Electrophoretic analysis of the polypeptides of the nucleocapsid and the glucosamine and polysaccharide-containing components of the enveloped virus. *J. Virol.*, 17:935–949.

23. Einhorn, L., and Ernberg, I. (1978): Induction of EBNA precedes the first cellular S-phase after EBV-infection of human lymphocytes. *Int. J. Cancer*, 21:157–160.

24. Einhorn, L., Steinitz, M., Yefenof, E., Ernberg, I., Bakacs, T., and Klein, G. (1978): Epstein-Barr virus receptors, complement receptors, and EBV infectability of different lymphocyte fractions of peripheral blood. II. Epstein-Barr virus studies. *Cell. Immunol.*, 35:43–58.

25. Engblom, I., and Ernberg, I. (1981): Ultraviolet inactivation of Epstein-Barr virus induces nuclear antigen (EBNA), DNA and IgM synthesis in human B lymphocytes. *Virology*, 112:228–239.

26. Epstein, A. L., Kaiser-McCaw, B., Hecht, F., and Kaplan, H. S. (1978): Functional and cyto-genetic characterization of established human malignant lymphoma cell lines. In: *Human Lymphocyte Differentiation: Its Application to Cancer*, INSERM Symposium No. 8, edited by B. Serrou, and C. Rosenfeld, pp. 327–336. Elsevier/North Holland, Amsterdam.

27. Erikson, I., Martinis, I., and Croce, C. M. (1981): Assignment of the genes for human λ im-munoglobulin chains to chromosome 22. *Nature*, 294:173–175.

28. Eskeland, T., and Klein, E. (1971): Isolation of 7S IgM and kappa chains from the surface membrane of tissue culture cells derived from Burkitt lymphoma. *J. Immunol.*, 107:1368–1375.

29. Fellous, M., Kamoun, M., Wiels, J., Dausset, J., Clements, G., Zeuthen, J., and Klein, G. (1977): Induction of HLA expression in Daudi cells after cell fusion. *Immunogenetics*, 5:423–436.

30. Fialkow, P. J., Klein, G., Gartler, S. M., and Clifford, P. (1970): Clonal origin for individual Burkitt tumors. *Lancet*, 1:384–386.

31. Fialkow, P. J., Klein, E., Klein, G., Clifford, P., and Singh, S. (1973): Immunoglobulin and glucose-6-phosphate dehydrogenase as markers of cellular origin in Burkitt lymphome. *J. Exp. Med.*, 138:89–102.

32. Fleischman, E. W., and Prigogina, E. L. (1977): Karyotype abnormalities of malignant lympho-mas. *Hum. Genet.*, 35:269–279.

33. Fukuhara, S., and Rowley, J. D. (1978): Chromosome 14 translocations in non-Burkitt lymphomas. *Int. J. Cancer*, 22:14–21.

34. Gerber, P., and Lucas, S. (1972): Epstein-Barr virus associated antigens activated in human cells by 5-bromo-deoxyuridine. *Proc. Soc. Exp. Biol. Med.*, 141:431–435.

35. Gerber, P., Whang-Peng, J., and Monroe, J. H. (1969): Transformation and chromosome changes induced by Epstein-Barr virus in normal leukocyte cultures. *Proc. Natl. Acad. Sci. USA*, 63:740–747.

36. Gergely, L., Klein, G., and Ernberg, I. (1971): Appearance of Epstein-Barr virus associated antigens in infected Raji cells. *Virology*, 45:10–21.

37. Given, D., and Kieff, E. (1978): DNA of Epstein-Barr virus. VI. Mapping of the internal tandem reiteration. *J. Virol.*, 31:315–324.

38. Glaser, R., Ablashi, D. V., Nonoyama, M., Henle, W., and Easton, J. (1977): Enhanced on-cogenic behavior of human and mouse cells after cellular hybridization with Burkitt tumor cells. *Proc. Natl. Acad. Sci. USA*, 74:2574–2578.

39. Glaser, R., and Nonoyama, M. (1973): Epstein-Barr virus: Detection of genome in somatic cell hybrids of Burkitt lymphoblastoid cells. *Science*, 179:492–493.

40. Glaser, R., Nonoyama, M., Becker, B., and Rapp, F. (1973): Synthesis of Epstein-Barr virus antigens and DNA in activated somatic cell hybrids. *Virology*, 55:62–69.

41. Glaser, R., and O'Neil, F. J. (1972): Hybridization of Burkitt lymphoblastoid cells. *Science*, 176:1245–1247.

42. Glaser, R., and Rapp, F. (1972): Rescue of Epstein-Barr virus from somatic cell hybrids of Burkitt lymphoblastoid cells. *J. Virol.*, 10:288–296.

43. Goodman, S. R., Prezyna, C., and Benz, W. C. (1978): Two Epstein-Barr virus associated DNA polymerase activities. *J. Biol. Chem.*, 253:8617–8628.

44. Graessmann, A., Wolf, H., and Bornkamm, G. W. (1980): Expression of Epstein-Barr virus genes in different cell types after microinjection of viral DNA. *Proc. Natl. Acad. Sci. USA*, 77:433–436.

45. Graessmann, A., Graessmann, M., and Mueller, C. (1981): Regulation of SV40 gene expression. *Adv. Cancer Res.*, 35:111–149.

46. Greaves, M. F., and Brown, G. (1975): Epstein-Barr virus binding sites on lymphocyte subpop-ulations and the origin of lymphoblasts in cultured lymphoid cell lines and in the blood of patients with infectious mononucleosis. *Clin. Immunol. Immunopathol.*, 3:514–524.

47. Grogan, E., Miller, G., Henle, W., Rabson, M., Shedd, D., and Niedermann, J. C. (1981):

Expression of Epstein-Barr viral early antigen in monolayer tissue cultures after transfection with viral DNA and DNA fragments. *J. Virol.*, 40:861–869.

48. Hampar, B., Deree, J. G., Nonoyama, M., Chang, S. Y., Tagamets, M. A., and Showalter, S. D. (1974): Programming of events in Epstein-Barr virus-activated cells induced by 5-iododeoxyuridine. *Virology*, 62:71–89.

49. Hayward, S., and Kieff, E. (1976): Epstein-Barr virus specific RNA. I. Analysis of viral RNA in cellular extracts and in polyribosomal fraction of permissive and non-permissive lymphoblastoid cell lines. *J. Virol.*, 18:518–525.

50. Hayward, S. D., and Kieff, E. (1977): DNA of Epstein-Barr virus. II. Comparison of the molecular weights of restriction endonuclease fragments of the DNA of Epstein-Barr virus strains and identification of end fragments of the B95-8 strain. *J. Virol.*, 23:421–429.

51. Hecht, F., and Kaiser-McCaw, B. (1981): Position effect of 8;14 translocation in Burkitt's lymphoma. *N. Engl. J. Med.*, 304:174–175.

52. Henderson, E., Miller, G., Robinson, J., and Heston, L. (1977): Efficiency of transformation of lymphocytes by Epstein-Barr virus. *Virology*, 76:152–163.

53. Hengartner, H., Meo, T., and Müller, E. (1978): Assignment of genes for immunoglobulin K and heavy chains to chromosomes 6 and 12 in mouse. *Proc. Natl. Acad. Sci. USA*, 75:4494–4498.

54. Henle, G., and Henle, W. (1966): Immunofluorescence in cells derived from Burkitt's lymphoma. *J. Bacteriol.*, 91:1248–1256.

55. Henle, G., Henle, W., Clifford, P., Diehl, V., Kafuko, G. W., Kirya, B. G., Klein, G., Morrow, R. H., Munube, G. M. R., Pilo, P., Takle, P. M., and Ziegler, J. L. (1969): Antibodies to Epstein-Barr virus in Burkitt's lymphoma and control groups. *J. Natl. Cancer Inst.*, 43:1147–1157.

56. Henle, G., Henle, W., Klein, G., Gunvén, P., Clifford, P., Morrow, R. H., and Ziegler, J. L. (1971): Antibodies to early EBV-induced antigens in Burkitt's lymphoma. *J. Natl. Cancer Inst.*, 46:861–871.

57. Henle, G., Henle, W., and Klein, G. (1971): Demonstration of two distinct components in the early antigen complex of Epstein-Barr virus infected cells. *Int. J. Cancer*, 8:272–282.

58. Henle, W., Diehl, V., Kohn, G., zur Hausen, H., and Henle, G. (1967): Herpes-type virus and chromosome markers in normal leukocytes after growth with irradiated Burkitt cells. *Science*, 157:1064–1065.

59. Henle, W., Henle, G., Zajac, B., Pearson, G., Waubke, R., and Scriba, M. (1970): Differential reactivity of human sera with early antigens induced by Epstein-Barr virus. *Science*, 168:188–190.

60. Hinuma, Y., Ohta, R., Miyamoto, T., and Ishida, N. (1962): Evaluation of the complement method of fluorescent antibody technique with myxoviruses. *J. Immunol.*, 89:19–26.

61. Hobart, M. J., Rabbitts, T. H., Goodfellow, P. N., Solomon, E., Chambers, A., Spurr, N., and Povey, S. (1981): Immunoglobulin heavy chain genes in humans are located on chromosome 14. *Ann. Hum. Genet.*, 45:331–335.

62. Hoffman, G. J., Lazarowits, S. G., and Hayward, S. D. (1980): Monoclonal antibody against a 250,000-dalton glycoprotein of Epstein-Barr virus identifies a membrane antigen and a neutralizing antigen. *Proc. Natl. Acad. Sci. USA*, 77:2979–2983.

63. Hunter, T. (1980): Proteins phosphorylated by the RSV transforming function. *Cell*, 22:647–648.

64. Ito, Y. (1980): Organization and expression of the genomes of polyoma virus. In: *Viral Oncology*, edited by G. Klein, pp. 447–480. Raven Press, New York.

65. Jat, P., and Arrand, J. R. (1982): In vitro transcription of two Epstein-Barr virus specified small RNA molecules. *Nucleic Acids Res.*, 10:3407–3425.

66. Jondal, M., and Klein, G. (1973): Surface markers of human B and T lymphocytes. II. Presence of Epstein-Barr virus receptors on B lymphocytes. *J. Exp. Med.*, 138:1365–1378.

67. Jondal, M., Klein, G., Oldstone, M., Bokish, V., and Yefenof, E. (1976): Surface markers on human B and T lymphocytes. VIII. Association between complement and Epstein-Barr virus (EBV) receptors on human lymphoid cells. *Scand. J. Immunol.*, 5:401–410.

68. Jörnvall, H., Luka, J., Klein, G., and Apella, E. (1982): A 53K protein common to chemically and virally transformed cells shows extensive sequence similarities between species. *Proc. Natl. Acad. Sci. USA*, 79:287–291.

69. Kaiser-McCaw, B., Epstein, A. L., Kaplan, A. L., and Hecht, F. (1977): Chromosome 14 translocation in African and North American Burkitt's lymphomas. *Int. J. Cancer*, 19:482–486.

70. Källin, B., Luka, J., and Klein, G. (1979): Immunochemical characterization of Epstein-Barr virus-associated early and late antigens in *n*-butyrate-treated P3HR-1 cells. *J. Virol.*, 32:710–716.
71. Kaltoft, K., and Celis, J. E. (1978): Ghost-mediated transfer of human hypoxanthine guanine phosphoribosyl transferase into deficient Chinese hamster ovary cells by means of polyethylene glycol-induced fusion. *Exp. Cell Res.*, 115:423–427.
72. Kamata, T., Tanaka, S., Aikawa, S., Hinuma, Y., and Watanabe, Y. (1979): A possible function of Epstein-Barr virus-determined nuclear antigen (EBNA): Stimulation of chromatin template activity *in vitro*. *Virology*, 95:222–226.
73. Kamata, T., Takaki, K., Hinuma, Y., and Watanabe, Y. (1981): Protein kinase activity associated with the Epstein-Barr virus-determined nuclear antigen. *Virology*, 113:512–520.
74. Kaschka-Dierich, C., Adams, A., Lindahl, T., Bornkamm, G. W., Bjursell, G., Klein, G., Giovanella, B. C., and Singh, S. (1976): Intracellular forms of Epstein-Barr virus DNA in human tumor cells *in vitro*. *Nature*, 260:302–306.
75. Katsuki, T., and Hinuma, Y. (1976): A quantitative analysis of the susceptibility of human leukocytes to transformation by Epstein-Barr virus. *Int. J. Cancer*, 18:7–13.
76. Katsuki, T., Hinuma, Y., Yamamoto, N., Abo, T., and Kumagai, K. (1977): Identification of the target cells in human B lymphocytes for transformation by Epstein-Barr virus. *Virology*, 83:287–294.
77. Kieff, E., Dambaugh, T., Hummel, M., and Heller, M. (1983): Epstein-Barr virus transformation and replication. In: *Advances in Viral Oncology, Vol. 3*, edited by G. Klein, Raven Press, New York.
78. Kintner, C., and Sugden, B. (1981): Identification of antigenic determinants unique to the surface of cells transformed by Epstein-Barr virus. *Nature*, 294:458–460.
79. Klein, G. (1978): Cancer, viruses, and environmental factors. In: *Viruses and Environment*, edited by E. Kurstak and K. Maramorosch, pp. 1–12. Academic Press, New York.
80. Klein, G. (1979): Lymphoma development in mice and humans: Diversity of initiation is followed by convergent cytogenetic evolution. *Proc. Natl. Acad. Sci. USA*, 76:2442–2446.
81. Klein, G. (1981): The role of gene dosage and genetic transpositions in carcinogenesis. *Nature*, 294:313–318.
82. Klein, G., Clements, G., Zeuthen, J., and Westman, A. (1976): Somatic cell hybrids between human lymphoblastoid cell lines. II. Spontaneous and induced patterns of Epstein-Barr virus (EBV) cycle. *Int. J. Cancer*, 17:715–724.
83. Klein, G., Clements, G., Zeuthen, J., and Westman, A. (1977): Spontaneous and induced patterns of the Epstein-Barr virus (EBV) cycle in a new set of somatic cell hybrids. *Cancer Letters*, 3:91–98.
84. Klein, G., Clifford, P., Klein, E., and Stjernswärd, J. (1966): Search for tumor specific immune reactions in Burkitt lymphoma patients by the membrane immunofluorescence reaction. *Proc. Natl. Acad. Sci. USA*, 55:1628–1635.
85. Klein, G., Clifford, P., Klein, E., and Stjernswärd, J. (1967): Membrane immunofluorescence reactions of Burkitt's lymphoma cells from biopsy specimens and tissue culture. *J. Natl. Cancer Inst.*, 39:1027–1044.
86. Klein, G., and Dombos, L. (1973): Relationship between the sensitivity of EBV-carrying lymphoblastoid lines to superinfection and the inducibility of the resident viral genome. *Int. J. Cancer*, 11:327–337.
87. Klein, G., Eskeland, T., Inoue, M., Strom, R., and Johansson, B. (1970): Surface immunoglobulin moieties on lymphoid cells. *Exp. Cell Res.*, 62:133–148.
88. Klein, G., Luka, J., and Zeuthen, J. (1980): Transformation induced by Epstein-Barr virus and the role of the nuclear antigen. *Cold Spring Harbor Symp. Quant. Biol.*, 44:253–261.
89. Klein, G., Terasaki, P., Billing, R., Honig, R., Jondal, M., Rosén, A., Zeuthen, J., and Clements, G. (1977): Somatic cell hybrids between human lymphoma lines. III. Surface markers. *Int. J. Cancer*, 19:66–76.
90. Klein, G., Wiener, F., Zech, L., zur Hausen, H., and Reedman, B. (1974): Segregation of the EBV-determined nuclear antigen (EBNA) in somatic cell hybrids derived from the fusion of a mouse fibroblast and a human Burkitt lymphoma line. *Int. J. Cancer*, 14:54–64.
91. Klein, G., Yefenof, E., Falk, K., and Westman, A. (1978): Relationship between Epstein-Barr virus (EBV)-production and the loss of the EBV receptor/complement receptor complex in a series of sublines derived from the same original Burkitt's lymphoma. *Int. J. Cancer*, 21:552–560.
92. Klein, G., Zeuthen, J., Terasaki, P., Billing, R., Honig, R., Jondal, M., Westman, A., and

Clements, G. (1976): Inducibility of the Epstein-Barr virus (EBV) cycle and surface marker properties of EBV-negative lymphoma lines and their *in vitro* EBV-converted sublines. *Int. J. Cancer*, 18:639–652.

93. Klein, G., Zeuthen, J., Eriksson, I., Terasaki, P., Bernoco, M., Rosén, A., Masucci, G., Povey, S., and Ber, R. (1980): Hybridization of a myeloid leukemia derived cell line (K562) with a Burkitt lymphoma line (P3HR-1). *J. Natl. Cancer Inst.*, 64:725–738.

94. Klein, G., Zeuthen, J., Ber, R., and Ernberg, I. (1982): Human lymphoma-lymphoma hybrids and lymphoma-leukemia hybrids. II. Epstein-Barr virus induction patterns. *J. Natl. Cancer Inst.*, 68:197–202.

95. Koeffler, H. P., Sparkes, R. S., Billings, R., and Klein, G. (1981): Somatic cell hybrid analysis of hematopoietic differentiation. *Blood*, 58:1159–1163.

96. Koide, N., Wells, A., Volsky, D. J., Shapiro, I. M., and Klein, G. (1981): The detection of Epstein-Barr virus receptors utilizing radiolabelled virus. *J. Gen. Virol.*, 54:191–195.

97. Koskimies, S. (1980): A human lymphoblastoid cell line producing specific antibody against Rh-D antigen. *Scand. J. Immunol.*, 11:73–77.

98. Kozbor, D., Lagarde, A. E., and Roder, J. C. (1982): Human antitetanus toxoid monoclonal antibodies produced by a human myeloma hybridized with an EB-virus transformed cell line. *Proc. Natl. Acad. Sci USA*, 79:6651–6655.

99. Kozbor, D., Steinitz, M., Klein, G., Koskimies, S., and Mäkelä, O. (1979): Establishment of anti-TNP antibody producing human lymphoid lines by preselection for hapten binding followed by EBV transformation. *Scand. J. Immunol.*, 10:187–194.

100. Köhler, G., and Milstein, C. (1976): Derivation of specific antibody-producing tissue culture and tumor lines by cell fusion. *Eur. J. Immunol.*, 6:511–519.

101. Lane, D. P., and Crawford, L. V. (1979): T antigen is bound to a host protein in SV40-transformed cells. *Nature*, 278:261–263.

102. Lau, R., Nonoyama, M., and Klein, G. (1981): Somatic cell hybrids between human lymphoma and human myeloid leukemia cells. I. Induction of resident viral genome transcription and antigen formation by IUdR and TPA. *Virology*, 110:259–269.

103. Lindahl, T., Klein, G., Reedman, B. M., Johansson, B., and Singh, S. (1974): Relationship between Epstein-Barr virus (EBV) DNA and the EBV-determined nuclear antigen (EBNA) in Burkitt lymphoma biopsies and other lymphoproliferative malignancies. *Int. J. Cancer*, 13:764–772.

104. Luka, J., Jörnvall, H., and Klein, G. (1980): Purification and biochemical characterization of the EBV-determined nuclear antigen (EBNA) and an associated protein with a 53K subunit. *J. Virol.*, 35:592–602.

105. Luka, J., Källin, B., and Klein, G. (1979): Induction of the Epstein-Barr (EBV) cycle in latently infected cells by *n*-butyrate. *Virology*, 94:228–251.

106. Luka, J., Siegert, W., and Klein, G. (1977): Solubilization of the Epstein-Barr virus-determined nuclear antigen and its characterization as a DNA-binding protein. *J. Virol.*, 22:1–8.

107. Manolov, G., and Manolava, Y. (1972): Marker band in one chromosome 14 from Burkitt lymphomas. *Nature*, 237:33–34.

108. Manolova, Y., Manolov, G., Kieler, J., Levan, A., and Klein, G. (1979): Genesis of the 14q+ marker in Burkitt lymphoma. *Hereditas*, 90:5–10.

109. Mark, J., Ekedahl, C., and Hagman, A. (1977): Origin of the translocated segment of the 14q+ marker in non-Burkitt lymphomas. *Humangenetik*, 36:277–282.

110. Martin, R. G. (1981): The transformation of cell growth and transmogrification of DNA synthesis of simian virus 40. *Adv. Cancer Res.*, 34:1–68.

111. Martin, R. G., and Oppenheim, A. (1977): Initiation points for DNA replication in non-transformed and simian virus SV40-transformed Chinese hamster lung cells. *Cell*, 11:859–869.

112. Matsuoka, Y., Takahashi, Y., Yagi, Y., Moore, G. E., and Pressman, D. (1968): Synthesis and secretion of immunoglobulins by established cell lines of human hematopoietic origin. *J. Immunol.*, 101:1111–1120.

113. McCaw, K. B., Hecth, F., Harnden, D. G., and Teplitz, R. J. (1975): Somatic rearrangement of chromosome 14 in human lymphocytes. *Proc. Natl. Acad. Sci. USA*, 72:2071–2075.

114. McConnell, I., Klein, G., Lint, T. F., and Lachman, P. J. (1978): Activation of the alternative complement pathway by human B cell lymphoma lines is associated with Epstein-Barr virus transformation of the cells. *Eur. J. Immunol.*, 8:453–460.

115. McCune, J. M., Humphreys, R. E., Yocum, R. R., and Strominger, J. L. (1975): Enhanced

representation of HL-A antigens on human lymphocytes after mitogenesis induced by phytohe-magglutinin or Epstein-Barr virus. *Proc. Natl. Acad. Sci. USA*, 72:3206–3209.

116. McKusick, V. A., and Cross, H. E. (1966): Ataxia-telangiectasia and Swiss-type agammaglob-ulinemia. *J.A.M.A.*, 195:739–745.

117. Menezes, J., Jondal, M., Leibold, W., and Dorval, G. (1976): Epstein-Barr virus interaction with human lymphocyte subpopulations: Virus adsorption, kinetics of expression of EBV-associated nuclear antigen (EBNA) and lymphocyte transformation. *Infect. Immun.*, 13:303–310.

118. Menezes, J., Seigneurin, J. M., Patel, P., Bourkas, A., and Lenoir, G. (1977): Presence of Epstein-Barr virus receptors, but absence of virus penetration, in cells of an Epstein-Barr virus genome-negative human lymphoblastoid T line (Molt 4). *J. Virol.*, 22:816–821.

119. Miller, G., Grogan, E., Heston, L., Robinson, J., and Smith, D. (1981): Epstein-Barr viral DNA: Infectivity for human placental cells. *Science*, 212:452–455.

120. Miller, G., and Lipman, M. (1973): Release of infectious Epstein-Barr virus by transformed marmoset leukocytes. *Proc. Natl. Acad. Sci. USA*, 70:190–194.

121. Miller, G., Lisco, H., Kohn, H. T., and Stitt, D. (1971): Establishment of cell lines from normal adult human blood leukocytes by exposure to Epstein-Barr virus and neutralization by human sera with Epstein-Barr virus antibody. *Proc. Soc. Exp. Biol. Med.*, 137:1459–1465.

122. Milner, J., and Milner, S. (1981): SV40-53K antigen: A possible role for 53K in normal cells. *Virology*, 112:785–788.

123. Mitelman, F., Anvret-Andersson, M., Brandt, L., Catovsky, D., Klein, G., Manolov, G., Man-olova, Y., Mark-Vendel, E., and Nilsson, P. G. (1979): Reciprocal 8;14 translocation of EBV-negative B-cell acute lymphocytic leukemia and in a leukemic nonendemic Burkitt lymphoma. *Int. J. Cancer*, 24:27–33.

124. Mitelman, R. (1981): Marker chromosome 14q+ in human cancer and leukemia. *Adv. Cancer Res.*, 34:141–167.

125. Mizuno, F., Aya, T., and Osato, T. (1974): B-lymphocytes as targets for EB virus transformation. *Br. Med. J.*, 3:689.

126. Mizuno, F., Aya, T., and Osato, T. (1976): Growth in semisolid agar medium of human cord leukocytes freshly transformed by Epstein-Barr virus. *J. Natl. Cancer Inst.*, 56:171–173.

127. Miyoshi, I., Kiraki, S., Kimura, I., Miyamoto, K., and Sato, J. (1979): 2/8 Translocation in a Japanese Burkitt's lymphoma. *Experientia*, 35:742–743.

128. Moar, M. H., Ber, R., Klein, G., Westman, A., and Eriksson, I. (1978): Somatic cell hybrids between human lymphoma lines. V. IUdR inducibility and P3HR-1 superinfectability of Daudi/HeLa (DAD) and Daudi/P3HR-1 (DIP-1) cell lines. *Int. J. Cancer*, 22:669–680.

129. Montagnier, L., and Gruest, J. (1979): Cell density-dependence for growth in agarose of two human lymphoma lines and its decrease after Epstein-Barr virus conversion. *Int. J. Cancer*, 23:71–76.

130. Moss, D. J., Rickinson, A. B., Wallace, L. E., and Epstein, M. A. (1981): Sequential appearance of Epstein-Barr virus nuclear and lymphocyte-detected membrane antigens in B cell transformation. *Nature*, 29:664–666.

131. Moss, D. J., Wallace, L. E., Rickinson, A. B., and Epstein, M. A. (1981): Cytotoxic T cell recognition of Epstein-Barr virus-infected B cells. I. Specificity and HLA restriction of effector cells reactivated *in vitro*. *Eur. J. Immunol.*, 11:686–693.

132. Mueller-Lantzsch, N., Georg-Fries, B., Herbst, H., zur Hausen, H., and Braun, D. G. (1981): Epstein-Barr virus strain- and group-specific antigenic determinants detected by monoclonal an-tibodies. *Int. J. Cancer*, 28:321–327.

133. Mueller-Lantzsch, N., Yamamoto, N., and zur Hausen, H. (1979): Analysis of early and late Epstein-Barr virus-associated polypeptides by immunoprecipitation. *Virology*, 97:378–387.

134. Nadkarni, J. S., Nadkarni, J. J., Clifford, P., Manolov, G., Fenyö, E. M., and Klein, E. (1969): Characteristics of new cell lines derived from Burkitt lymphomas. *Cancer*, 23:64–79.

135. Nilsson, K., and Pontén, J. (1975): Classification and biological nature of established human hematopoietic cell lines. *Int. J. Cancer*, 15:321–341.

136. Nilsson, K., Giovanella, B. C., Stehlin, J. S., and Klein, G. (1977): Tumorigenicity of human hematopoietic cell lines in athymic nude mice. *Int. J. Cancer*, 20:337–344.

137. Nonoyama, M., and Pagano, J. S. (1973): Homology between Epstein-Barr virus DNA and viral DNA from Burkitt's lymphoma and nasopharyngeal carcinoma determined by DNA-DNA reas-sociation kinetics. *Nature*, 242:44–47.

138. Nyormoi, O., Klein, G., Adams, A., and Dombos, L. (1973): Sensitivity to EBV superinfection

and IUdR inducibility of hybrid cells formed between a sensitive and a relatively resistant Burkitt lymphoma cell line. *Int. J. Cancer*, 12:396–408.

139. Nyormoi, O., Thorley-Lawson, D. A., Elkington, J., and Strominger, J. L. (1976): Differential effect of phosphonoacetic acid on the expression of Epstein-Barr viral antigens and virus production. *Proc. Natl. Acad. Sci. USA*, 73:1745–1748.

140. Ohno, S., Luka, J., Lindahl, T., and Klein, G. (1977): Identification of a purified complement-fixing antigen as the Epstein-Barr virus nuclear antigen (EBNA) by its binding to metaphase chromosomes. *Proc. Natl. Acad. Sci. USA*, 74:1605–1609.

141. Olsson, L., and Kaplan, H. S. (1980): Human hybridomas producing monoclonal antibodies of predefined antigenic specificity. *Proc. Natl. Acad. Sci. USA*, 77:5429–5431.

142. Oppenheim, A., Shlomai, Z., and Ben-Bassat, H. (1981): Initiation points for cellular deoxyribonucleic acid replication in human lymphoid cells converted by Epstein-Barr virus. *Mol. Cell Biol.*, 1:753–762.

143. Orellana, T., and Kieff, E. (1977): Epstein-Barr virus specific RNA. II. Analysis of polyadenylated viral RNA in restringent, abortive and productive infections. *J. Virol.*, 22:321–330.

144. Otsuka, H., Hazell, M., Kit, M., Quavi, H., and Kit, S. (1981): Cloning of the marmoset herpesvirus thymidine kinase gene and analysis of the boundaries of the coding region. *Virology*, 113:196–213.

145. Pearson, G., Dewey, F., Klein, G., Henle, G., and Henle, W. (1970): Relation between neutralization of Epstein-Barr virus and antibodies to cell membrane antigens induced by the virus 1,2. *J. Natl. Cancer Inst.*, 45:989–997.

146. Pellicer, A., Wigler, M., Axel, R., and Silverstein, S. (1978): The transfer and stable integration of the HSV thymidine kinase gene into mouse cells. *Cell*, 14:133–141.

147. Pope, J. H. (1979): Transformation by the virus *in vitro*. In: *The Epstein-Barr Virus*, edited by M. Epstein, and B. Achong, pp. 205–223. Springer-Verlag, Berlin.

148. Pope, J. H., Horne, M. K., and Scott, W. (1968): Transformation of foetal human leukocytes in vitro by filtrates of a human leukemic cell line containing herpes-like virus. *Int. J. Cancer*, 3:857–866.

149. Povey, S., Jeremiah, S., Arthur, E., Ber, R., Fialkow, P. J., Gardiner, E., Goodfellow, P. N., Karande, A., Klein, G., Quintero, M., Steel, C. M., and Zeuthen, J. (1981): Deficiency of malic enzyme: A possible marker for malignancy in lymphoid cells. *Ann. Hum. Genet.*, 45:237–252.

150. Powell, A. L. T., King, W., and Kieff, E. (1979): Epstein-Barr virus specific RNA. III. Mapping of DNA encoding viral specific RNA in restringently infected cells. *J. Virol.*, 29:261–274.

151. Pritchett, R. F., Hayward, S. D., and Kieff, E. D. (1975): DNA of Epstein-Barr virus. I. Comparative studies of the DNA of Epstein-Barr virus from HR-1 and B95-8 cells. Size, structure, and relatedness. *J. Virol.*, 15:556–569.

152. Pritchett, R., Pedersen, M., and Kieff, E. (1976): Complexity of EBV homologous DNA in continuous lymphoblastoid cell lines. *Virology*, 74:227–231.

153. Purtilo, D. T., Sakamoto, K., Saemundsen, A. K., Sullivan, J. L., Synnerholm, A. C., Anvret, M., Pritchard, M., Sloper, C., Sieff, C., Pincott, J., Pachman, L., Rich, K., Cruzi, F., Cornet, J. A., Collins, R., Barnes, N., Knight, J., Sandstedt, B., and Klein, G. (1981): Documentation of Epstein-Barr virus infection in immunodeficient patients with life-threatening lymphoproliferative diseases by clinical virological, and immunopathological studies. *Cancer Res.*, 41:4226–4236.

154. Qualtière, L. F., and Pearson, G. R. (1980): Radioimmune precipitation study comparing the Epstein-Barr virus membrane antigens expressed on P3HR-1 virus superinfected Raji cells to those expressed on cells in a B95-8 virus transformed producer culture activated with tumor-promoting agent (TPA). *Virology*, 102.360–369.

155. Raab-Traub, N., Pritchett, R., and Kieff, E. (1978): DNA of Epstein-Barr virus. III. Identification of restriction enzymes that contain DNA sequences which differ among strains of Epstein-Barr virus. *J. Virol.*, 27:388–398.

156. Reedman, B. M., and Klein, G. (1973): Cellular localization of an Epstein-Barr virus (EBV)-associated complement-fixing antigen in producer and non-producer lymphoblastoid cell lines. *Int. J. Cancer*, 11:499–520.

157. Rickinson, A. B., Moss, D. J., Wallace, L. E., Rowe, M., Misko, I. S., Epstein, M. A., and Pope, J. H. (1981): Long-term T-cell mediated immunity to Epstein-Barr virus. *Cancer Res.*, 41:4216–4221.

158. Ringertz, N. R., and Savage, R. E. (1976): *Cell Hybrids*. Academic Press, New York.

159. Robinson, J., and Miller, G. (1975): Assay for Epstein-Barr virus based on the stimulation of DNA synthesis in mixed leukocytes from human umbilical blood. *J. Virol.*, 15:1065–1072.

160. Rosa, M. D., Gottlieb, E., Lerner, M. R., and Steitz, J. A. (1981): Striking similarities are exhibited by two small Epstein-Barr virus-encoded ribonucleic acids and the adenovirus-associated ribonucleic acids VAI and VAII. *Mol. Cell Biol.*, 1:785–796.

161. Rosén, A., Britton, S., Gergely, P., Jondal, M., and Klein, G. (1977): Epstein-Barr virus infection of human lymphocytes *in vivo*. *Nature*, 267:52–54.

162. Rosén, A., Clements, G., Klein, G., and Zeuthen, J. (1977): Double immunoglobulin production in cloned somatic cell hybrids between two human lymphoid lines. *Cell*, 11:139–147.

163. Rosental, K. S., Shuman, H., and Strominger, J. L. (1981): Induction of several new antigens including a T cell-associated antigen, following conversion of the EBV-negative B cell line Ramos to EHR-B Ramos by Epstein-Barr virus. *J. Immunol.*, 127:746–754.

164. Roubal, J., and Klein, G. (1981): Synthesis of thymidine kinase (TK) in Epstein-Barr virus-superinfected Raji TK-negative cells. *Intervirology*, 15:43–48.

165. Roubal, J., Källin, B., Luka, J., and Klein, G. (1981): Early DNA-binding polypeptides of Epstein-Barr virus. *Virology*, 113:285–292.

166. Rutherford, T. R., Clegg, J. B., and Weatherall, D. J. (1979): K562 human leukaemic cells synthesize embryonic haemoglobin in response to haemin. *Nature*, 280:164–165.

167. Rowley, J. D. (1980): Chromosome abnormalities in cancer. *Cancer Genet. Cytogenet.*, 2:175–198.

168. Rymo, L. (1979): Identification of transcribed regions of Epstein-Barr virus DNA in Burkitt lymphoma derived cells. *J. Virol.*, 32:8–18.

169. Rymo, L., Lindahl, T., and Adams, A. (1979): Sites of sequence variability in Epstein-Barr virus DNA from different sources. *Proc. Natl. Acad. Sci. USA*, 76:2794–2798.

170. Rymo, L., Lindahl, T., Povey, S., and Klein, G. (1981): Analysis of restriction endonuclease fragments of intracellular Epstein-Barr virus DNA and isoenzymes indicate a common origin of the Raji, NC-37 and F-265 human lymphoid cell lines. *Virology*, 115:115–124.

171. Saemundsen, A. K., Purtilo, D. T., Sakamoto, K., Sullivan, J. L., Synnerholm, A. C., Hanto, D. C., Simmons, R., Anvret, M., Collins, R., and Klein, G. (1981): Documentation of Epstein-Barr virus infection in immunodeficient patients with life-threatening lymphoproliferative diseases by Epstein-Barr virus complementary RNA/DNA and viral DNA/DNA hybridization. *Cancer Res.*, 41:4237–4242.

172. Sairenji, T., and Hinuma, Y. (1973): Modes of Epstein-Barr virus infection in human floating cell lines. *Gann*, 64:583–590.

173. Schneider, U., and zur Hausen, H. (1975): Epstein-Barr virus induced transformation of human leukocytes after cell fractionation. *Int. J. Cancer*, 15:59–65.

174. Seigneurin, J.-M., Vuillaume, M., Lenoir, G., and de Thé, G. (1977): Replication of Epstein-Barr virus: Ultrastructural and immunofluorescent studies of P3HR-1 superinfected Raji cells. *J. Virol.*, 234:836–845.

175. Shapiro, I., Andersson-Anvret, M., and Klein, G. (1978): Polyploidization of EBV-carrying lymphoma lines decreases the inducibility of EBV-determined early antigen following P3HR-1 virus superinfection of iododeoxyuridine treatment. *Intervirology*, 10:94–101.

176. Silvestre, D., Kourilsky, F. M., Klein, G., Yata, J., Neauport-Sautes, C., and Levy, J. P. (1971): Relationship between EBV-associated membrane antigen on BL cells and viral envelope demonstrated by immunoferritin labelling. *Int. J. Cancer*, 8:222–233.

177. Simonova, I., Zavadova, H., and Vonka, V. (1977): Differential expression of D and R components of Epstein-Barr virus early antigen after superinfection and after induction with 5-iododeoxyuridine. *Acta Virol.*, 21:184–188.

178. Skare, J., and Strominger, J. L. (1980): Cloning and mapping of *Bam* HI endonuclease fragments of DNA from the transforming B95-8 strain of EBV. *Proc. Natl. Acad. Sci. USA*, 77:3860–3864.

179. Spira, J., Povey, S., Wiener, F., Klein, G., Andersson-Anvret, M. (1977): Chromosome banding, isoenzyme studies and determination of Epstein-Barr virus DNA content on human Burkitt lymphoma/mouse hybrids. *Int. J. Cancer*, 20:849–853.

180. Steele, C. M., Philipsson, J., Arthur, E., Gardiner, S. E., Newton, M. M., and McIntosh, R. V. (1977): Possibility of EB virus preferentially transforming a subpopulation of human B lymphocytes. *Nature*, 270:729–730.

181. Steele, C. M., Woodward, M. A., Davidson, C., Philipson, J., and Arthur, E. (1977): Nonrandom chromosome gains in human lymphoblastoid cell lines. *Nature*, 270:349–351.

182. Steinitz, M., Bakacs, T., and Klein, G. (1978): Interaction of B95-8 and P3HR-1 substrains of Epstein-Barr virus (EBV) with peripheral human lymphocytes. *Int. J. Cancer*, 22:251–258.

183. Steinitz, M., Izak, G., Cohen, S., Ehrenfeld, M., and Flechner, J. (1980): Continuous production of rheumatoid factor by *in vitro* EBV-transformed lymphocytes. *Nature*, 287:443–445.

184. Steinitz, M., and Klein, G. (1975): Comparison between growth characteristics of an Epstein-Barr virus (EBV)-genome-negative lymphoma line and its EBV-converted subline *in vitro*. *Proc. Natl. Acad. Sci. USA*, 72:3518–3520.

185. Steinitz, M., and Klein, G. (1976): Epstein-Barr virus (EBV)-induced change in the saturation sensitivity and serum dependence of established, EBV-negative lymphoma lines *in vitro*. *Virology*, 70:570–573.

186. Steinitz, M., and Klein, G. (1977): Further studies on the difference in serum dependence in EBV negative lymphoma lines and their *in vitro* converted, virus-genome carrying sublines. *Eur. J. Cancer*, 13:1269–1275.

187. Steinitz, M., Klein, G., Koskimies, S., and Mäkelá, O. (1977): Epstein-Barr virus-induced B-lymphocyte cell lines producing specific antibody. *Nature*, 269:420–422.

188. Steinitz, M., Seppälä, I., Eichmann, K., and Klein, G. (1979): Establishment of a human lymphoblastoid cell line with specific antibody production against group A streptococcal carbohydrate. *Immunobiology*, 156:41–47.

189. Steplewski, Z., Koprowski, H., Andersson-Anvret, M., and Klein, G. (1978): Epstein-Barr virus in somatic cell hybrids between mouse cells and human nasopharyngeal carcinoma cells. *J. Cell. Physiol.*, 97:1–8.

190. Stoerker, J., Parris, D., Yajima, Y., and Glaser, R. (1981): Pleiotropic expression of Epstein-Barr virus DNA in human epithelial cells. *Proc. Natl. Acad. Sci. USA*, 78:5852–5855.

191. Strnad, B. C., Schuster, T. C., Hopkins, R. F., III, Neubauer, R. H., and Rabin, H. (1981): Identification of an Epstein-Barr virus nuclear antigen by fluorimmunoelectrophoresis and radioimmunoelectrophoresis. *J. Virol.*, 38:996–1004.

192. Sugden, B., and Mark, W. (1977): Clonal transformation of adult human leukocytes by Epstein-Barr virus. *J. Virol.*, 23:270–273.

193. Summers, W. C., and Klein, G. (1976): Inhibition of Epstein-Barr virus DNA synthesis and late antigen expression by phosphonoacetic acid. *J. Virol.*, 18:151–155.

194. Svedmyr, E., and Jondal, M. (1975): Cytotoxic cells specific for B cell lines transformed by Epstein-Barr virus are present in patients with infectious mononucleosis. *Proc. Natl. Acad. Sci. USA*, 72:1622–1626.

195. Tanaka, A., Nonoyama, M., and Hampar, B. (1976): Partial elimination of latent Epstein-Barr virus genomes from virus producing cells by cycloheximide. *Virology*, 70:164–170.

196. Thorley-Lawson, D. (1979): Characterization of cross-reacting antigens on the Epstein-Barr virus envelope and plasma membrane of producer cells. *Cell*, 16:33–42.

197. Thorley-Lawson, D., Chess, L., and Strominger, J. L. (1978): Suppression of in vitro Epstein-Barr virus infection: A new role for adult human T lymphocytes. In: *Advances in Comparative Leukemia Research*, edited by P. Bentvelzen et al., pp. 219–222. Elsevier/North Holland, Amsterdam.

198. Thorley-Lawson, D. A., and Edson, C. (1979): Polypeptides of the Epstein-Barr virus membrane antigen complexes. *J. Virol.*, 32:458–467.

199. Thorley-Lawson, D. A., and Geilinger, K. (1980): Monoclonal antibodies against the major glycoprotein (gp 350/220) of Epstein-Barr virus neutralize infectivity. *Proc. Natl. Acad. Sci. USA*, 77:5307–5311.

200. Thorley-Lawson, D. A., and Strominger, J. L. (1976): Transformation of human lymphocytes by Epstein-Barr virus is inhibited by phosphonoacetic acid. *Nature*, 263:332–334.

201. Thorley-Lawson, D. A., and Strominger, J. L. (1978): Reversible inhibition by phosphonoacetic acid of human B lymphocyte transformation by Epstein-Barr virus. *Virology*, 86:432–441.

202. Trowbridge, I. S., Hyman, R., and Klein, G. (1977): Human B cell line deficient in the expression of B-cell specific proteins (gp 27,35). *Eur. J. Immunol.*, 7:640–645.

203. Tjian, R., Fey, G., and Graessmann, G. (1978): Biological activity of purified simian virus 40 T antigen proteins. *Proc. Natl. Acad. Sci. USA*, 75:1279–1284.

204. Van den Berghe, H., Parloir, C., Gosseye, S., Englebienne, V., Cornu, G., and Sokal, G. (1979): Variant translocation in Burkitt lymphoma. *Cancer Genet. Cytogenet.*, 1:9–14.

205. Van Furth, R., Gorter, H., Nadkarni, J. S., Klein, E., and Clifford, P. (1972): Synthesis of

immunoglobulins by biopsied tissues and cell lines from Burkitt's lymphoma. *Immunology*, 22:847–857.

206. Vestergaard, B. F., Hesse, J., Norrild, B., and Klein, G. (1978): Production of rabbit antibodies against the viral capsid antigen (VCA) of the Epstein-Barr virus (EBV). *Int. J. Cancer*, 21:323–328.

207. Volsky, D. J., Shapiro, I. M., and Klein, G. (1980): Transfer of Epstein-Barr virus receptors to receptor-negative cells permits virus penetration and antigen expression. *Proc. Natl. Acad. Sci. USA*, 77:5453–5457.

208. Volsky, D. J., Klein, G., Volsky, B., and Shapiro, I. M. (1981): Production of infectious Epstein-Barr virus in mouse lymphocytes. *Nature*, 293:399–401.

209. Wallace, L. E., Moss, D. J., Rickinson, A. B., McMichael, A. J., and Epstein, M. A. (1981): Cytotoxic T cell recognition of Epstein-Barr virus-infected B cells. II. Blocking studies with monoclonal antibodies to HLA determinants. *Eur. J. Immunol.*, 11:694–699.

210. Wallace, L. E., Rickinson, A. B., Rowe, M., and Epstein, M. A. (1982): Epstein-Barr virus-specific cytotoxic T-cell clones restricted through a single HLA antigen. *Nature*, 297:413–415.

211. Wells, A., Koide, N., and Klein, G. (1981): Difference in viral binding between two Epstein-Barr virus substrains to a spectrum of receptor-positive target cells. *Int. J. Cancer*, 27:303–309.

212. Wells, A., Koide, N., and Klein, G. (1982): Two large virion envelope glycoproteins mediate Epstein-Barr virus binding to receptor positive cells. *J. Virol.*, 41:286–297.

213. Wiels, J., Fellous, M., and Tursz, T. (1981): Monoclonal antibody against a Burkitt lymphoma-associated antigen. *Proc. Natl. Acad. Sci. USA*, 78:6485–6488.

214. Yamamoto, N., and Hinuma, Y. (1976): Clonal transformation of human leukocytes by Epstein-Barr virus in soft agar. *Int. J. Cancer*, 17:191–196.

215. Yefenof, E., and Klein, G. (1976): Difference in antibody induced redistribution of membrane IgM in EBV-genome free and EBV-carrying human lymphoma lines. *Exp. Cell Res.*, 99:175–178.

216. Yefenof, E., and Klein, G. (1977): Membrane receptor stripping confirms the association between EBV receptors and complement receptors on the surface of human B lymphoma lines. *Int. J. Cancer*, 20:347–352.

217. Yefenof, E., Klein, G., Jondal, M., and Oldstone, M. B. A. (1976): Surface markers on human B- and T-lymphocytes. IX: Two-color immunofluorescence studies on the association between EBV receptors and complement receptors on the surface of human lymphoid cell lines. *Int. J. Cancer*, 17:693–700.

218. Yefenof, E., Klein, G., and Kvarnung, K. (1977): Relationships between complement activation complement binding, and EBV absorption by human hematopoietic cell lines. *Cell. Immunol.*, 31:225–233.

219. Zech, L., Haglund, U., Nilsson, K., and Klein, G. (1976): Characteristic chromosomal abnormalities in biopsies and lymphoid-cell lines from patients with Burkitt and non-Burkitt lymphomas. *Int. J. Cancer*, 17:47–56.

220. Zerbini, M., and Ernberg, I. (1983): Can Epstein-Barr virus infect and transform all the B-lymphocytes of human cord blood? *J. Gen. Virol.*, 64:539–547.

221. Zeuthen, J., and Nilsson, K. (1976): Hybridization of a human myeloma permanent cell line with mouse cells. *Cell Differentiation*, 4:355–368.

222. Zeuthen, J., Friedrich, U., Rosén, A., and Klein, E. (1977): Structural abnormalities in chromosome 15 in cell lines with reduced expression of beta-2 microglobulin. *Immunogenetics*, 4:567–580.

223. Zeuthen, J., Stenman, S., Fabricius, H. Å., and Nilsson, K. (1976): Expression of immunoglobulin synthesis in human myeloma × non-lymphoid cell heterokaryons: Evidence for negative control. *Cell Differentiation*, 4:369–383.

224. Zeuthen, J., and Klein, G. (1981): Some recent trends in studies of human lymphoid cells: B-cells, Epstein-Barr virus, and transformation. In: *Haematology and Blood Transfusion 26, Modern Trends in Human Leukemia IV*, edited by R. Neth, R. C. Gallo, T. Graf, K. Mannwieler, and K. Winkler, pp. 179–190. Springer-Verlag, Berlin.

225. Zeuthen, J., Klein, G., Ber, R., Masucci, G., Bisballe, S., Povey, S., Terasaki, P., and Ralph, P. (1982): Human lymphoma-lymphoma hybrids and lymphoma-leukemia hybrids. I. Isolation characterization, cell surface markers, and B-cell markers. *J. Natl. Cancer Inst.*, 68:179–195.

226. Ziegler, A., Laudien, D., Heinrichs, H., Müller, C., Uchanska-Ziegler, B., and Wernet, P.

(1981): K562 cells express human major histocompatibility antigens. *Immunogenetics*, 13:359–365.

227. Ziegler, A., Uchanska-Ziegler, B., Zeuthen, J., and Wernet, P. (1982): HLA antigens expression at the single cell level on a K562 × B cell hybrid: An analysis with monoclonal antibodies. *Somatic Cell Genet.*, 8:775–789.

228. Zimmermann, J. E., Glaser, R., and Rapp, F. (1973): Effect of dibutyryl cyclic AMP on the induction of Epstein-Barr virus in hybrid cells. *J. Virol.*, 12:1442–1445.

229. zur Hausen, H., Schulte-Holthausen, H., Klein, G., Henle, W., Henle, G., Clifford, P., and Santesson, L. (1979): EBV DNA in biopsies of Burkitt tumours and anaplastic carcinomas of the nasopharynx. *Nature*, 228:1056–1058.

230. zur Hausen, H., Bornkamm, G. W., Schmidt, R., and Hecker, E. (1979): Tumor initiators and promoters in the induction of Epstein-Barr virus. *Proc. Natl. Acad. Sci. USA*, 76:782–785.

Advances in Viral Oncology, Volume 3, edited by
George Klein. Raven Press, New York © 1983.

Epstein-Barr Virus-Induced Transformation: Immunological Aspects

*A. B. Rickinson and **D. J. Moss

*Department of Pathology, The Medical School, University of Bristol,
Bristol BS8 1TD, United Kingdom; and **Queensland Institute of Medical Research,
Bramston Terrace, Herston, Queensland 4006, Australia

Despite its well-documented association with particular forms of malignant disease (15,41,43), Epstein-Barr virus (EBV) exists as a widespread and largely asymptomatic infection in all human communities (29). Clearly, a long period of coevolution of the virus with its host species has established a finely balanced relationship that guarantees persistence of this potentially pathogenic agent within the population without endangering host survival. The recent demonstration that certain other Old World primate species also carry their own EBV-like agents in a precisely analogous fashion (16,47,72) bears witness to the antiquity and to the evolutionary success of this particular type of virus–host relationship.

In most communities, primary infection with EBV occurs naturally during the first few years of life and is almost always subclinical. In contrast, when infection is delayed until the second decade or later, as happens increasingly in the Western world, it is accompanied in a significant proportion of cases by the clinical symptoms of infectious mononucleosis (IM) (27). It should be remembered, therefore, that our knowledge of the cellular events of the primary infection is derived almost entirely from the study of a clinical condition, IM, which because it is an accompaniment of materially improved living conditions, must be regarded in evolutionary terms as a novelty. It remains to be seen if the acute phase of IM presents a true magnification of events as they occur during subclinical infection or if the two situations are qualitatively as well as quantitatively distinct. However, all primary infections in whatever form induce permanent seroconversion to antiviral antibody positivity (29) and the establishment of a lifelong carrier state whereby the virus persists in some as yet unidentified form in the lymphoid tissue of the immune host. The mechanisms by which the virus–host balance is maintained in the longer term are only now beginning to be understood, and this chapter seeks to describe recent contributions to our knowledge in this area that have come from the experimental analysis of EBV–host-cell interactions in vitro.

EBV–B-CELL INTERACTIONS IN VITRO

The properties that distinguish EBV from virtually all other infectious agents are its strict tropism for B lymphocytes (24,33,65) and its capacity to transform or "immortalize" these cells *in vitro* into immunoglobulin-secreting permanent lymphoblastoid cell lines (28,68). These activities have been described in accompanying chapters of this volume, and it only remains to emphasize here those particular aspects of the virus-induced transformation system that are salient to the ensuing discussion of regulatory control by non-B cells.

First, the efficiency of transformation is unusually high when compared with that seen in other *in vitro* viral transformation systems. Most, though it is now clear not all (109), human circulating B cells possess EBV receptors, and recent results would suggest that at least 30%, and probably the majority, of such cells can go on, within a few days of exposure to a potent virus preparation, to synthesize the virus-associated nuclear antigen EBNA (8,60,117), a DNA-binding protein through which the virus is thought to exercise its proliferative influence on the infected cell (42,50). Cellular DNA synthesis is thus initiated (13), and morphological transformation of the cells to lymphoblasts is accompanied by a variety of cell surface changes (86), followed, in some cells at least, by activation of immunoglobulin synthesis and secretion to an easily detectable level within 7 days of infection (8,37,85). At this stage, foci of proliferating cells are apparent within the culture, and when allowances are made for the relatively low colony-forming ability that even well-established cell lines display in the *in vitro* environment, kinetic studies would suggest that at least 10%, and probably more, of the original virus-infected B cell population does indeed acquire a capacity for unlimited growth that is the hallmark of the transformed state (26,35,55,117).

Second, it must not be forgotten that the proportion of B cells in a virus-infected culture that sustain active infection, and as a result the times post infection at which the various parameters of transformation reach detectable levels within the cultured population as a whole, will be critically dependent on the input virus dose (116). In this context, most studies concerned with the regulatory control of transformation have used relatively potent virus preparations capable of inducing microscopically visible foci of transformed cells within 7 to 14 days *(vide infra)*. It is, of course, more difficult, though perhaps no less important, to examine regulation in cultures where much lower threshold values of input virus induce the appearance of isolated foci only after a much longer incubation time.

Third, it should be stressed that the virologist's view of the virus as an immortalizing agent and the immunologist's view of it as a polyclonal B cell activator are really two different interpretations of the same viral activity. The two effects are irrevocably linked, because both depend on the viability of the virus preparation, initiation of the infectious cycle, and synthesis of EBNA (8,37,90). Thus, the activation of immunoglobulin synthesis in B cells following EBV infection stands in marked contrast to conventional antigen- or mitogen-induced activation (4,30) in being helper-T-cell-independent and in being sustained at a high level for at least several weeks post infection with serial passage of the emerging B cell line (67). Indeed, using limiting dilutions, it is possible to select out from the parent population cloned sublines that retain high immunoglobulin secretor status for much longer periods (44), thus offering a potential method for effective human monoclonal antibody production.

The unique ability of EBV to transform human B cells therefore provides a highly efficient, reproducible, and quantifiable *in vitro* system that is particularly amenable to experimental analysis. This has, in recent years, been turned to advantage by a number of groups who have sought to identify those host-cell-mediated mechanisms that are capable of regulating the process of virus-induced transformation *in vitro* and that therefore may play an analogous role *in vivo*.

REGULATION OF EBV–HOST INTERACTIONS *IN VITRO*: ENDOGENOUS CONTROLS

Delayed Transformation: The Interferon Response

One of the first indications that T cells present in EBV-infected blood mono-nuclear cell cultures could influence the kinetics of B cell transformation came from the work of Thorley-Lawson and colleagues (103). Using a virus dose that induced foci of transformed cells to appear in cultures of purified adult donor B cells within 14 days of infection, these workers showed that the time of appearance of such foci was significantly delayed in corresponding cultures reconstituted with autolo-gous T cells; such T-cell-mediated delay was not observed in parallel cultures of cells from fetal cord blood. Although there are certain problems inherent in using a morphological assay of this kind, these differences in time to outgrowth were observable over a range of initial cell concentrations of seeding as well as in cultures reconstituted at known B:T ratios; indeed, the results were later confirmed using both EBNA induction and ^{3}H-thymidine labeling as alternative parameters of the course of the virus–B-cell interaction (101).

Further studies revealed that adult T cells could delay transformation only if they were added to autologous B cells within the first 24 hr postinfection. This did not reflect any disturbance of the adsorption and/or penetration of the virus *per se*, but it did suggest that T cells were responding to residual viral envelope (or other virion-associated) material that is known to persist for some hours on the surface of infected B cells (13). As to the mechanism of this effect, if these authors' attempts to reisolate B cells from mononuclear cell cultures by positive selection on an anti-human-F(ab)′ immunoabsorbent column did indeed remove all accompanying T cells, then the results would suggest that the T cell effector phase was complete within a few hours, even though it was made manifest only much later by delays in the appearance of EBNA-positive cells, of virus-induced cell proliferation, and of transformed foci (101). The later demonstration that even mitomycin-C-treated T cells could delay transformation (12) supported the view of an immediate effector phase that was not dependent on T cell proliferation *in vitro*.

One important point that the initial studies left unresolved was the possible relationship between an individual's immune status with respect to EBV and the capacity to effect delayed transformation. It was left to two other groups to demonstrate that the phenomenon could be observed in EBV-infected lymphocyte cultures from seronegative donors as well as from seropositive donors (5,95). Clearly, delay was not mediated by "immune" cells in the accepted sense, and recently, in what must be regarded as an important advance, Thorley-Lawson has presented evidence favoring the view that adult donor T cells achieve their effect by causing, either directly or indirectly, the synthesis and release into culture medium of leukocyte α-interferon (102). Thus, in double-chamber experiments it was found that the transformation of virus-infected B cells cultured alone could be significantly delayed through the influence of a culture of virus-infected B + T cells on the other side of a 0.2-μ filter; this diffusible influence could be completely and specifically abrogated by anti-α-interferon antiserum. Moreover, the delayed transformation of EBV-infected adult B cells could be reproduced in the complete absence of T cells by experimental addition of an α-interferon preparation to the medium; in these same experiments the transformation of fetal B cells proved quite insensitive to α-interferon treatment, thus offering a ready and most interesting explanation of the contrasting results obtained in the original work with adult and fetal lymphocyte cultures (103).

Certainly, further work needs to be carried out in order to define more precisely the mechanism of delayed transformation. Identification of the soluble factor as α-interferon must at present be regarded as preliminary, particularly because more recent studies indicate that not all anti-α-interferon antisera will negate the phenomenon (D. Thorley-Lawson, *personal communication*), thus raising the possibility that a particular subtype of α-interferon or even some other factor contaminating certain α-interferon preparations may be the true effector molecule. Indeed, another group has recently presented evidence indicating a role for γ-interferon in this same phenomenon (63). It is also questionable to what extent interferon might mediate delay directly through its well-documented antiviral activity and to what extent it might function indirectly through a capacity to activate natural killer (NK) cells *in vitro* (107). Thorley-Lawson's work would favor a direct antiviral effect as the major mechanism (102), but it does not exclude some contribution from NK cells, a possibility already apparent from the observation of Shope and Kaplan that the capacity to delay EBV-induced B cell transformation *in vitro* was an exclusive property of the NK-cell-enriched Fc γ-receptor-positive T (Tg) cell subpopulation (95).

Immune Inhibition of Transformation on Fibroblast Feeder Layers

A substantial body of earlier work on the virus-induced transformation system clearly established that adherent cells (mainly monocytes) within the mononuclear cell pool provide an *in vitro* feeder layer that, though not essential for the establishment of virus-transformed cell lines (21), is certainly necessary for optimal outgrowth (70,89). Fibroblast feeder layers can substitute for monocytes in this situation, and it was during an investigation into this effect that another mechanism for regulating EBV–B-cell interactions was revealed. Thus, virus-induced transformation of nonadherent mononuclear cell (lymphocyte) preparations from adult donors, which occurred successfully when the cells were seeded either onto a fetal fibroblast underlay (Fig. 1A) or even into culture wells alone, was completely inhibited on a feeder layer of adult fibroblasts (Fig. 1B) (56). Although EBNA was expressed in at least a proportion of the infected cells in such cultures, and the cells remained viable for extended periods, there was no evidence of virus-induced cell proliferation or focus formation up to 3 months post infection. Yet successful outgrowth could be initiated from cultures at 1 month either by the addition of phytohemagglutinin or by transferring the virus-infected cells off the feeder layer. This reversibility strongly suggested that regulation was not being exercised through some cytotoxic mechanism.

Further experiments clearly showed that this inhibition of transformation had an immunological basis, for the effect was seen only if the adult mononuclear cell donor (though not the donor of the fibroblast feeder layer) had serological indication of a prior EBV infection (57). Unfortunately, further work on this potentially interesting system has been hampered by the extreme sensitivity of immune inhibition to very small, often ill-defined changes in culture conditions. This may well reflect the fact that maintenance of inhibition requires a complex combination of cellular interactions, any one of which might be broken by changes in the *in vitro* environment.

The possibility remains that this effect is mediated through some soluble factor whose *in vitro* synthesis and release are dependent on an immune recognition event. Certainly there is now strong independent evidence that antigenic components within virus preparations themselves (i.e., within virus-producing cell extracts) can induce the synthesis of a variety of lymphokines (10,22,45) and that one *in vitro* action of such lymphokines could be impairment of EBV-induced transformation (46). More recent work by Szigeti and colleagues has shown conclusively that lymphokine release can also be induced in immune donor leukocytes by stimulation either with partially purified EBNA preparations (98) or with plasma membrane preparations from EBV-transformed cells that do not express seriologically defined viral structural antigens (99). It remains to determine the nature of these lymphokines, their relationship (if any) to immune γ-interferon, and their possible contribution to the immune inhibition of transformation on fibroblast feeder layers described earlier.

Regression of Transformation: The Cytotoxic T Cell Response

The search for a bona fide EBV-specific T cell activity, exclusive to previously infected (seropositive) individuals, was initiated in several laboratories on the grounds that T-cell-dependent mechanisms, perhaps akin to those implicated in the response to the primary infection in IM patients (88,94,97), were likely to be important in long-term control of EBV persistence (38). The existence of just such a memory T cell system was first demonstrated through its capacity to regulate the course of *in vitro* virus-induced transformation (58,59,78,79). When blood mononuclear cells from seronegative adult donors (or from cord blood) were exposed to EBV and

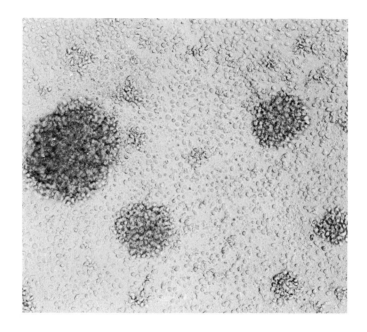

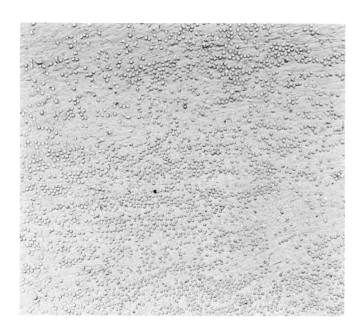

FIG. 1. Nonadherent mononuclear cells from seropostive donor D.M. were exposed to EBV *in vitro* and then seeded at 5 × 10⁴ cells per Microtest plate well onto a fibroblast feeder layer. **Top:** Virus-induced transformation after 5 weeks in cultures containing fetal fibroblasts. **Bottom:** Immune inhibition of transformation after 5 weeks in cultures containing adult fibroblasts (× 110).

cultured over a range of initial cell concentrations, foci of EBNA-positive B cells appeared regularly within the first 8 to 10 days post infection and thereafter continued to expand, undisturbed by T cells coresident in the culture, so that subcultures made at 28 days always gave rise to EBNA-positive B lymphoblastoid cell lines. In the corresponding cultures from seropositive donors, proliferation of EBNA-positive B cells was again observed during the first 8 to 10 days (Fig. 2A) but was followed by a regression of growth, seen preferentially in those cultures seeded at the higher initial cell concentrations and often apparent by day 14 (Fig. 2B), that culminated by day 28 in degeneration of the culture (Fig. 2C), destruction of EBNA-positive cells, and complete abrogation of cell line establishment (58).

Mechanism of Regression

The results from double-chamber experiments argued against any involvement of soluble factors (such as interferons or antiviral antibodies produced endogenously within the seropositive donor cultures) as mediators of regression (78), whereas very strong independent evidence was forthcoming to indicate an effector role for immune T cells. Thus, the appearance of regression was absolutely dependent on the inclusion of T cells in the initial cultures and was preceded by a T cell proliferative response occurring within the first 14 days of culture (59). Regression occurred across a wide range of virus doses and was particularly well displayed following exposure of the cells to very potent virus preparations, where the phenomenon of delayed transformation appears to be completely overridden (103). The distinction between these two *in vitro* phenomena was further emphasized in subsequent, hitherto unpublished, experiments involving the reconstitution of EBV-infected T -depleted (TD) cell cultures with various preparations of autologous T cells. The results in Table 1 show that the effector cells for regression are drawn largely, if not exclusively, from the Tg-depleted and not the Tg-enriched T cell subpopulation and that prior mitomycin C treatment of the T cells abrogates their effect. This was quite different from the results in corresponding studies on delayed transformation in reconstituted cultures (12,95).

When T cells were prepared from regressing cultures by E rosetting followed by NH_4Cl lysis of erythrocytes, such preparations were demonstrably cytotoxic to autologous EBV-transformed target cells in growth-inhibition assays (59,80) and in chromium-relase assays (52,61). Parallel T cell preparations from seronegative donor cultures did not show this activity. In subsequent studies, the effector function of these cytotoxic T cells (61,110), and, more recently, effector cell lines derived from them using T cell growth factor (TCGF) (111,112), has been rigorously analyzed with respect to antigen specificity and the possible restriction of target cell recognition by histocompatibility antigens.

First, strong lysis of the autologous EBV-transformed cell line by T cells from regressing cultures was consistently observed irrespective of whether or not the target cells expressed serologically defined virus-envelope-related membrane antigens on their surfaces. Moreover, as the specimen results obtained from sero-

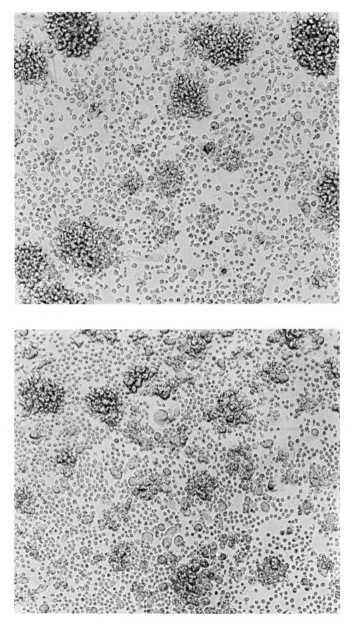

FIG. 2. Mononuclear cells from seropositive donor D.M. were exposed to EBV *in vitro* and then seeded at 1.5 × 10⁵ cells per Microtest plate well. **Top:** Virus-induced foci of proliferating cells apparent by day 8 p.i. **Bottom:** Onset of regression by day 14 p.i.

positive donor S.G. (Fig. 3) illustrate, this lysis of the autologous line was not accompanied by any killing of autologous mitogen-stimulated lymphoblasts or of any of a range of EBV-genome-negative human leukemia/lymphoma cell lines (61),

FIG. 2. *(continued)* Culmination of regression by day 28 p.i. (×110).

included as indicators of the various activated NK-like responses that can under other circumstances be readily induced *in vitro* (1,34,39,92). This would suggest T cell recognition of a B cell surface change that is induced specifically by EBV infection, rather than some other target structure either introduced as an artifact of the culture environment (for instance, fetal calf serum proteins) or associated with the lymphoproliferative state *per se*. Under certain conditions, some fetal-calf-serum-related cytotoxicity can be detected in such cultures (53,54), but this is always at a low level, and its appearance in cultures from both seropositive and seronegative donors discounts any involvement in regression.

Within the limits of the target cells tested to date, the T cell response underlying regression appears to be directed specifically to an EBV-associated lymphocyte-detected membrane antigen, LYDMA, whose existence was first invoked in an attempt to explain the apparently EBV-selective cytotoxicity shown by effector T cells isolated directly from the blood of IM patients (88,97). LYDMA was therefore conceived as a virus-induced transformation-associated cell surface change with immunogenicity for the T cell system (38). Now that the EBV antigen specificity of IM T cell cytotoxicity is in doubt *(vide infra)*, it seems sensible to adopt *in-vitro*-reactivated virus-specific T cell cytotoxicity as the current operational test for LYDMA. This is not to deny the possible virus specificity of IM T cells, but solely to establish a solid experimental base for current terminology; certainly the antigenic change detected by *in-vitro*-reactivated effector T cells fulfills exactly all the criteria originally invoked for LYDMA (38,81).

TABLE 1. Regression in cultures reconstituted with T cell subpopulations

Donor (status)	Treatment of culture	TD alone	TD + mmC-T at 1:3	TD + total T at 1:1	1:2	1:3	TD + Tg-depleted T at 1:1	1:2	1:3	TD + Tg-enriched T at 1:1	1:2	1:3
146	—	0/4	0/6	0/4	0/4	0/4	0/4	0/4	0/4	0/4	0/4	0/4
(+)	+EBV	6/6	6/6	6/6	6/6	6/6	6/6	6/6	6/6	4/4	4/4	1/4
147	—	0/4	0/6	0/4	0/4	0/4	0/4	0/4	0/4	0/4	0/4	0/4
(+)	+EBV	6/6	6/6	1/6	0/6	0/6	1/6	1/6	0/6	6/6	5/6	4/6
169	—	0/5	0/5	0/5	0/5	0/5	0/5	0/5	0/5	0/5	0/5	0/5
(+)	+EBV	5/5	5/5	5/5	4/5	0/5	4/5	3/5	0/5	5/5	5/5	4/5
168	—	0/5	0/5	0/5	0/5	0/5	0/5	0/5	0/5	0/5	0/5	0/5
(−)	+EBV	5/5	5/5	5/5	5/5	5/5	5/5	5/5	5/5	5/5	5/5	5/5

TD cells freshly prepared from seropositive (+) and seronegative (−) donors were cultured at 4×10^4 cells per 0.3-ml Microtest plate flat well after incubation either in culture medium (RPMI-1640 + 10% fetal calf serum) alone or in the presence of an EBV preparation. To some of these cultures were then added known numbers of autologous T cells of one of the following kinds: viable cells of the circulating T cell pool (total T); mitomycin-C-treated (40 µg/ml for 30 min at 37°C followed by extensive washing) cells of the circulating T cell pool (mmC-T); circulating T cells exhaustively depleted of Tg cells by two successive cycles of EA rosetting and centrifugation over Ficoll-Hypaque (Tg-depleted T); Tg cells obtained from the first cycle of EA rosetting above, resuspended in rosetted form and recentrifuged through Ficoll-Hypaque before NH$_4$Cl lysis of the erythrocytes (Tg-enriched T). The TD:T ratio of seeding was 1:1, 1:2, or 1:3. All cultures were maintained for 4 weeks and were observed regularly to assess the incidence of successful transformation and/or regression.

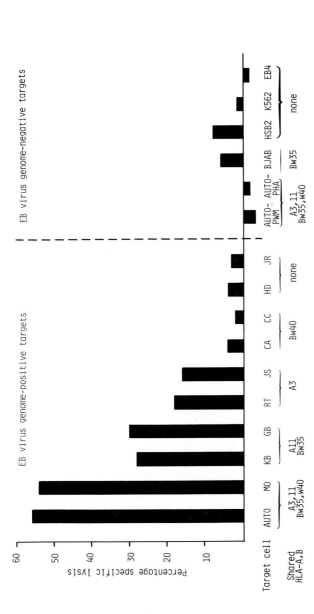

FIG. 3. Target cells specificity of effector T cells prepared from regressing cultures of EBV-infected mononuclear cells from seropositive donor S.G. (day 10 p.i.). The results of a 5-hr chromium release assay, at an effector:target ratio of 10:1, are expressed as percentages specific lysis of the autologous EBV-transformed cell line, of allogeneic EBV-transformed cell lines from donors M.O., K.B., G.B., R.T., J.S., C.A., C.C., H.D., and J.R., of autologous pokeweed-mitogen(PWM)- and phytohemagglutinin(PHA)-stimulated lymphoblasts, and of the EBV-genome-negative human hemopoietic cell lines BJAB, HSB2, K562, and EB4 included as sensitive indicators of nonspecific NK-like cytotoxicity. The degree of HLA-A and -B antigen sharing between effector and target cells is indicated in each case.

The molecular nature of LYDMA is uncertain, because the antigen has not been unequivocally defined by serological means. No antibodies to such a determinant can be detected in human sera (110), and attempts to raise specific antisera by conventional xenogeneic immunizations have failed. More recently, however, in at least three different laboratories, mouse monoclonal antibodies have been raised that bind to a 45K protein or proteins whose expression appears, on tests performed to date, to be exclusive to the EBV-transformed state (36,86,96). Independent proof that these antibodies are actually detecting LYDMA, for instance a demonstrated ability to protect target cells from EBV-specific cytolysis, has not been forthcoming (86,96), although in the light of experience from other viral systems this kind of negative result in blocking assays still does not preclude the possibility that such antibodies do indeed bind to the relevant virus-induced target antigen (2,17,23).

The 45K protein appears on the surface of EBV-infected B cells within 24 hr of EBNA expression and coincident with the initiation of cellular DNA synthesis (86), kinetics that precisely match those already revealed by cytotoxicity testing for the induction of LYDMA (60). The coordinate appearance of EBNA, a DNA-binding mitogenic protein, and of LYDMA, a cell surface change consistently associated with the virus-transformed state, is reminiscent of the situation in SV40-induced transformation, where the large T antigen and the T-cell-detected surface change TSTA are not only simultaneously expressed (71) but also would appear to be antigenically related products coded from a common region of the viral genome (48,114). There is as yet no evidence that EBNA and LYDMA have a similar relationship; indeed, we cannot yet say with certainty that LYDMA is a virally coded protein and not, for instance, some derepressed or virally altered product of the host cell genome.

As regards the existence of genetic controls governing the LYDMA-specific response, experiments in several independent laboratories have now clearly shown that the recognition of allogeneic EBV-transformed cell lines by *in-vitro*-reactivated effector T cells is restricted through HLA-A and -B antigens on the target cell surface (18,52,61,80,82,100,108,112,113). In general, as illustrated again by the specimen results in Fig. 3, the level of recognition is proportional to the extent of HLA-A and-B antigen matching between effector and target cells (61), reflecting the existence within the effector population of discrete clones each recognizing LYDMA in association with one particular HLA determinant (87,111). The restricted nature of the cytotoxic response underlying regression was independently confirmed by experiments showing that lysis was specifically reduced following pretreatment of the target cells with saturating concentrations of monoclonal antibodies binding framework determinants of the HLA-A,B,C/β_2-microglobulin complex (110,111). Likewise, regression can be averted by including such monoclonal antibodies in the medium of EBV-infected lymphocyte cultures (A. Rickinson and D. Moss, *unpublished observations*).

Quantitative Aspects of Regression

One of the earliest recognizable features of regression was its preferential appearance in more densely seeded cultures (58). Thus, in the standard Microtest plate assay where EBV-infected cells were seeded over a range of dilutions into flat-bottom wells, the "strength" of regression shown by any one individual could be quantified in terms of the minimum cell input required for a 50% incidence of the effect among replicate culture wells. Individual donors gave remarkably reproducible results when repeatedly tested in this assay, and healthy seropositive donors as a group showed a range of end points (2×10^4 to 2×10^5 mononuclear cells per culture) that was reduced more than 10-fold down to 1.5×10^3 to 1.5×10^4 mononuclear cells per culture when the assays were repeated in round-bottom wells under conditions allowing better *in vitro* survival at these very low cell seedings (81). These values demonstrate just how prevalent EBV-specific memory T cells are in the peripheral blood of individuals long after the primary infection, that is, at least one memory cell per 10^3 to 10^4 circulating T cells.

Such values may again be an underestimate of the true cytotoxic precursor cell frequency, because recent work has suggested that efficient regression actually requires collaboration between two separate T cell subpopulations. Thus, the ability of the immunosuppressive drug cyclosporin A (CSA) to prevent regression (7,11) and allow successful outgrowth of virus-transformed cell lines from the cultures, can be completely overridden by exogenous addition of lectin-depleted TCGF preparations to the drug-containing medium (84). This and other experiments suggest that a CSA-sensitive T helper cell (whose antigen specificity and restriction are presently unknown) is required to magnify the *in vitro* response of EBV-specific cytotoxic T cell precursors through secretion of TCGF into the culture medium. These recent indications of a T-T collaboration serve to emphasize that even in the regression system, which represents perhaps the best analyzed of all regulatory controls governing EBV transformation, our knowledge of the cellular interactions effecting such control is woefully thin.

Late Suppression of Transformation: An Immune T Cell Response

In a recent paper, Tosato and colleagues reported experiments in which the course of an EBV infection of adult-donor mononuclear cells was monitored in terms of the total number of immunoglobulin-secreting cells per culture, as detected in a reverse hemolytic plaque assay (106). Cultures from seronegative donors yielded increasing numbers of plaque-forming cells throughout the course of the 2-week observation, whereas cultures from seropositive donors showed increasing yields up to 8 or 10 days post infection, followed by a dramatic downturn. In B + T cell reconstitution experiments, this downturn was seen only if autologous T cells had been added back to the cultured B cells within 3 days of the latters' exposure to EBV; here again, as in the regression system (Table 1), reconstitution with inactivated (X-irradiated) T cells did not reproduce the effect.

These results were interpreted by these authors as indicating an activation of a "late suppressor T cell" activity that is exclusive to EBV-antibody-positive donors. They considered the alternative explanation (namely, that the decreasing yield of plaque-forming cells in such cultures merely reflects cytotoxic-T-cell-mediated destruction of the virus-transformed B cell population) less attractive, principally on the basis of one further type of experiment. Here T cells from late-suppressed cultures were unable to display any suppressive effect when subsequently transferred (at a suppressor:target ratio of 4:1) onto a target population of autologous B cells already activated to immunoglobulin synthesis by EBV infection 14 days earlier.

Relationships Between Endogenous Controls

There are therefore at least four different ways in which the regulatory control of EBV-induced B cell transformation can be recognized in experimentally infected mononuclear cell cultures. The culture conditions necessary for *in vitro* expression of these controls are ostensibly so similar that the general reader of the literature might well be forgiven for assuming that all four phenomena are in fact different manifestations of a single mechanism. This impression has no doubt been reinforced by the misuse of such terms as "suppression" and "inhibition," whose general connotations inevitably blur any specific meaning they may have assumed in the context of EBV transformation work. For this reason we have attempted here to assign a particular descriptive term to each of the reported phenomena so that a discussion of the possible relationships between them might be more easily conducted.

Table 2 presents the essential information for such a discussion. It is clear from the general characteristics of the four systems that the phenomenon of "delay," in which the usual sequence of detectable transformation-related events is not altered but is simply initiated at a later time post infection, is distinct from that of "immune inhibition," where a complete barrier is introduced between the expression of EBNA and the initiation of cell proliferation. Both, in turn, are different from "regression" and "late suppression," where control is not exercised until after the virus-infected B cell pool has begun to expand, but is then remarkably effective.

Such distinctions are made clearer when one considers the mechanisms of these effects. Thus, "delay" is a nonimmune phenomenon that involves T cells, perhaps the NK-cell-enriched Tg population selectively, and that is mediated through the release into culture medium of α-interferon (or some related factor) with antiviral and/or NK-cell-activating properties. "Immune inhibition" may well also be mediated through soluble factors, but here the response, which is confined to seropositive donors, clearly has an immunological basis. "Regression," on the other hand, is dependent on *in vitro* activation and expansion of a pool of EBV-specific cytotoxic T cell precursors present exclusively in the blood of seropositive individuals. Thorley-Lawson has speculated that this late reversal of B cell outgrowth, sometimes seen following delayed transformation in his experiments, may be due to an NK-like cytotoxicity that is activated in the cultures (101). This cannot be the case, however, because this kind of broad-ranging cytotoxicity, detectable in unfractionated but not in E-rosetting cell populations, appears transiently in both seropositive and seronegative donor cultures (52,112); in contrast, the virus-specific cytotoxic T cell response is seen only in EBV-infected cultures from seropositive

TABLE 2. Regulatory controls over EBV-induced B cell transformation

Term	General characteristics	Donor type	Effector population	Mechanism
Delay	Delayed appearance of EBNA-positive cells, cell proliferation, and cell line outgrowth	Seropositive and seronegative adults	T cells (? Tg)	? α-interferon
Immune inhibition	Inhibition of cell proliferation and cell line outgrowth *after* appearance of EBNA-positive cells	Seropositive adults	Nonadherent mononuclear cells in adult fibroblast feeder layer	?
Regression	Late reversal of EBNA-positive cell proliferation; no cell line establishment	Seropositive adults	T cells (non-Tg)	EBV-specific cytotoxic T cells
Late suppression	Late reversal of virus-induced immunoglobulin synthesis	Seropositive adults	T cells	EBV-specific cytotoxic or suppressor T cells

donors, and, most important, the magnitude of this response is directly related to the "strength" of the subsequent regression (61). It is, in fact, most significant that transformation is *not* demonstrably disturbed by *in vitro* activation of NK-like cytotoxicity, perhaps reflecting not just the transient nature of this response but also its well-documented selectivity for long-established tissue culture lines rather than for newly transformed populations (93).

Perhaps the one remaining issue of contention concerns the relationship between "regression" and "late suppression." The kinetics of these phenomena are so very similar as to suggest that the two systems are merely employing different methods of detecting the same course of events, i.e., cytotoxic T-cell-mediated destruction of EBV-infected B cells. Indeed, as a recent independent study has shown, one can follow this process just as well by monitoring cell proliferation (91) as one can by EBNA staining and/or morphological observation (i.e., the parameter of "regression") or by the numbers of immunoglobulin-secreting cells (i.e., the parameter of "late suppression"). In our view, the evidence that Tosato and colleagues have advanced to date in support of a noncytotoxic mechanism for late suppression (106) is not at all persuasive. Thus, the fact that T cells transferred from late-suppressed cultures were unable to control ongoing immunoglobulin synthesis by autologous B cells infected with EBV 14 days earlier is reminiscent of our frequent experience with the cytotoxic assay system, namely, that the success of such T cell transfer experiments not only requires testing over a range of B:T ratios but also depends critically on preparing T cells from cultures at the very initial stages of regression, before the reversal in growth is obvious and before cytotoxic T cell activity has waned (61).

There are, fortunately, a number of ways in which this interesting question of the nature of late suppression might be resolved. If the phenomenon is really a reflection of EBV-specific cytotoxic activity, then one would predict that late suppression should (a) be preferentially seen in cultures seeded at high initial cell concentrations, (b) vary in intensity within a group of healthy seropositive donors in a way that matches these donors' relative "strengths" of regression, (c) be inhibited by those concentrations of monoclonal antibodies to the HLA/β_2-microglobulin complex that are known to block regression (110), (d) in properly conducted T cell transfer experiments, be transferable to cultures of EBV-infected B cells in an HLA-A- and -B-antigen-restricted fashion but show no equivalent suppressive activity in mitogen-induced B cell activation systems.

In order to sustain the concept of an EBV-induced late-suppressor T cell whose activation in virus-infected cultures accompanies that of the cytotoxic T cell response but is separate from it, it would be necessary to show that at least some of these predictions were wrong. Resolution of this question may ultimately depend on the availability of monoclonal antibodies that distinguish the cytotoxic and the suppressor T cell subsets.

REGULATION OF EBV–B-CELL INTERACTIONS *IN VITRO*: EXOGENOUS CONTROLS

Neutralizing Antibody

EBV-induced transformation, like all virus–host-cell interactions *in vitro*, can be blocked at the outset by experimental addition of virus-neutralizing antibody (69). Sensitivity of this control can be demonstrated during the initial stages of the infection until such time as viral adsorption and penetration are complete. Almost all studies of this kind in the EBV system have used as the antibody source sera from previously infected individuals, each containing a spectrum of anti-EBV activities, but more recently it has been shown that neutralizing activity is specifically associated with antibodies to the two high-molecular-weight viral envelope glycoproteins of the membrane antigen (MA) complex (63,104), that is, to those glycoproteins that are involved in virus binding to the B cell surface (115). Either the same or a closely related family of anti-MA antibodies of IgG class are also capable of mediating antibody-dependent cellular cytotoxicity (ADCC) against MA-positive target cells (32,66).

Addition of EBV-antibody-positive serum to cultures of lymphocytes immediately after the infection has been successfully initiated has had no demonstrable effect on the subsequent efficiency of transformation (75). This negative result is important in that it argues against any further role for antibody-dependent mechanisms such as ADCC in the control of EBNA expression and/or proliferation and/or outgrowth of virus-infected B cells. It is worth noting in this context that the transformation process, though always associated with EBNA and LYDMA expression, does not usually involve the *de novo* appearance of MA components on the cell membrane and so would be unlikely to render the cells sensitive to such antibody-dependent recognition.

T Cells from IM Patients

The acute phase of IM is characterized by a vigorous polyclonal T cell proliferation, not just in the blood but also infiltrating many of the tissues (9,94). This population of T cells is heterogeneous, perhaps more so than is currently realized, and would appear to contain at least two types of activity demonstrable *in vitro*: (a) a potent suppressor cell activity first revealed in the T-helper-cell-dependent pokeweed-mitogen(PWM)-induced B cell activation system (25,31,105) but now also found to suppress the proliferative responses of T cells to mitogenic and antigenic stimuli (73), and (b) an apparently EBV-selective cytotoxicity that is best revealed in rather long (12-hr) chromium-release assays at high effector:target ratios, usually using, as a source of effectors, not T cell preparations *per se* but mononuclear cell populations depleted of conventional NK activity by removal of Fcγ-receptor-positive cells (3,88,97). In contrast to the *in-vitro*-reactivated memory T cell response, this primary response to the viral infection shows no obvious HLA restriction (49,93). Indeed, there is now a strong body of opinion holding that the IM effector cell population is dominated by a particular type of activated NK cell that is induced by the primary EBV infection but that is not truly EBV-specific (39,40).

Continuing uncertainties as to the true nature of the cellular response in IM patients make it difficult to interpret the results of experiments in which IM T cells have been added as exogenous effectors to EBV-infected lymphocyte cultures. This is certainly the case for those early studies where the efficiency of transformation in cord blood lymphocyte cultures was impaired by additions of IM T cells much more than by additions of T cells from healthy adult donors (77). Discussion is best centered on more recent work using *autologous* combinations of effector and target cells, because at least in such cases the results are free from the possible influence of spurious allogeneic effects. Clearly, IM T cells do suppress the responses of autologous B cells to PWM (105) in a manner that appears to mirror that of suppressor T cells stimulated by concanavalin A (con-A), i.e., by interfering with an early helper T cell function essential for the B cell response (6). EBV-induced B cell activation, on the other hand, is independent of helper T cells, and it is an interesting point whether or not such a system could ever be sensitive to conventional suppressor T cell activity. When this question has been approached using autologous con-A-stimulated suppressor T cells, one group has reported active suppression (90), whereas two other laboratories have found no such effect (6; S. Finerty and A. Rickinson, *unpublished data*).

Against this background, the recent report that virus-induced activation of IM B cells to immunoglobulin synthesis can be suppressed in cultures containing autologous IM T cells (105,106) is most interesting, but it requires confirmation and a careful appraisal of the possible mechanisms involved. Is this a specific suppression of virus-induced immunoglobulin synthesis or a secondary consequence of delayed B cell transformation? In any case, it is clear that in this type of autologous coculture, experimentally infected B cells do grow out to yield cell lines, reflecting the failure of the IM T cells to mount an *in vitro* cytotoxic response of the kind that could bring about regression of the culture (79,91). Thus, any immediate effect that IM T cells might have on virus-induced immunoglobulin synthesis does not seem to disturb the ultimate course of the virus–B-cell interaction. It is indeed something of a paradox that IM T cells, which would appear on the basis of chromium-release assays to be preferentially cytotoxic to established EBV-transformed cell lines, should prove to be so inefficient at regulating the virus-induced transformation of newly infected autologous B cells *(vide infra)*.

REGULATION OF EBV–B-CELL INTERACTIONS *IN VIVO*

The unique interaction of EBV with human B lymphocytes provides an ideal *in vitro* system with which to examine the various controls that other mononuclear leukocytes might exercise over the viral transformation process. The prime aim of this review has been to summarize the evidence that has come from this type of *in vitro* work and, in so doing, to highlight the multiplicity of routes by which such control can occur. To set this work in a broader perspective, we must consider what contributions it can make to our understanding of the EBV–host interaction *in vivo*, both during the acute infection and in the longer term. At the outset it must be emphasized that these are major questions that we can but touch on in the present context. Many of the issues raised here are to be discussed much more fully elsewhere (74,83).

Primary Infection

By the time of onset of the clinical symptoms of IM, virus-neutralizing (and anti-MA) antibodies are already present in the serum (27). Their appearance during the incubation period of the disease must obviously curtail any further hematogenous spread of the virus by classic viremia (76), although, as *in vitro* studies have made clear (75), this will not completely prevent the intercellular passage of infectious virus from a productively infected cell to a susceptible cell in contact with it. Full virus replication occurs in some as yet unidentified (perhaps epithelial) cell type within the region of the oropharynx, and this not only forms the reservoir of infectious virus found in buccal fluid (20,51) but also must serve to infect those circulating B lymphocytes that happen to make close contact with productively infected cells during B cell transit through the oropharynx. *In vitro* studies would suggest that the subsequent course of the virus–B-cell interaction is largely beyond antibody-mediated control, particularly because those IgG antibodies capable of mediating ADCC do not even develop until after the symptoms of IM have resolved (32).

As already discussed, the circulating lymphocyte pool in IM patients is dominated by a functionally heterogeneous population of T lymphoblasts, and these reactive cells are widely, and probably rightly, believed to play an important role in curtailing the acute viral infection. The recent evidence from *in vitro* studies, however, must call into question the efficiency of this cellular response. Certainly suppressor T cells, whose influence is clearly demonstrable *in vitro* over T-helper-cell-dependent mitogenic stimulations, are activated during the acute phase of IM, perhaps as a homeostatic response to the enhanced immunoglobulin production (with many heterophile and autoimmune reactivities) that characterizes this disease. Whether or not these same suppressor cells can mediate similar control over EBV-induced *in vitro* activation of B cells to immunoglobulin synthesis is still open to debate; this is an important point to resolve, because it will indicate whether or not the suppressor T cell response in IM patients can make any positive contribution to the control of the viral infection.

Likewise, although IM T cells may display cytotoxicity against established virus-genome-positive target cell lines in chromium-release assays, they are nevertheless unable to influence successful virus-induced *in vitro* transformation of autologous B cells. This result may simply reflect the fact that the cytotoxic effector cells, already activated *in vivo*, survive poorly *in vitro*; however, there remains the suspicion that the antigen against which they are directed is not truly EBV-specific and hence might not be expressed on B cells during the early stages of virus-infected transformation *in vitro*.

It is arguable, therefore, that a large part of the cellular response to primary EBV infection that is seen in IM patients is either misdirected or else relatively inefficient in its attempt to control virus–B-cell interactions. This reappraisal of IM T cell activity, which *in vitro* studies have forced on us, might indeed help to explain an obvious though frequently underemphasized aspect of the disease, namely, that its clinical course can be so prolonged despite the unusually large T cell response that the viral infection evokes.

Persistent Infection

The various mechanisms whereby virus-induced transformation can be regulated in experimentally infected mononuclear cell cultures (Table 2) indicate the multiplicity of host cell responses that might play roles in long-term control of EBV infection. Thus, nonimmune interferonlike factors could serve to delay the induction of EBNA and hence the initiation of proliferation in virus-infected B cells; this might constitute an auxiliary rather than a prime effector mechanism *in vivo*, because it cannot itself prevent the subsequent outgrowth of transformed cells. Likewise, the phenomenon of immune inhibition suggests that immune control, perhaps mediated via lymphokine release, can be exercised at the onset of virus-induced cell proliferation. If this *in vitro* phenomenon, which requires such a precise set of conditions for its expression, has an *in vivo* correlate, this could provide a means of maintaining virus-infected B cells in a nonproliferative state, although it would never eliminate the possibility of their subsequent escape and outgrowth.

Control exercised by suppressor T cells, particularly by those cells that have been invoked as the mediators of late suppression *in vitro*, would by definition be directed against virus-induced immunoglobulin synthesis, and it is difficult to envisage this forming an effective *in vivo* defense against the viral infection as a whole unless suppression were accompanied by some secondary effect on virus-induced cell proliferation *per se*. Somewhat in contrast, LYDMA-specific cytotoxic T cell precursors, present at high frequency in the peripheral blood of all healthy seropositive individuals and responsible for the regression of cell line outgrowth in virus-infected mononuclear cell cultures, could form an extremely powerful surveillance system *in vivo* by virtue of their ability to recognize and kill virus-infected B cells at the very onset of virus-induced cell proliferation (60). Indeed, the existence of this virus-specific cytotoxic T cell system has given fresh impetus to the question as to how the virus carrier status of host B lymphoid tissues is maintained at all (74,83).

To conclude this discussion, it would be naive to suppose that the *in vitro* transformation system, on which so much of the work described here is based, can reveal all or even most facets of the host response to EBV infection. Clearly, elimination of virus-infected cells from the body can also occur through ADCC and NK-like mechanisms, directed against cell surface changes preferentially expressed at later stages of the infectious cycle (64), and indeed such mechanisms may be crucially important in individuals with impaired immune T cell function (11,19,43). One of the most interesting aspects of the EBV–host relationship is the development, in rare individuals, of virus-genome-positive malignancies (15,41,43), and the sensitivity of these malignant cells to the various host-cell-mediated controls discussed here remains an exciting but unresolved question.

ACKNOWLEDGMENTS

The authors are most grateful to many colleagues who have, through discussion, helped to formulate the content of this review. Work in our laboratories is supported by the Cancer Research Campaign, London, by the Medical Research Council, London (A.B.R.), and by the Australian National Health and Medical Research Council (D.J.M.).

REFERENCES

1. Allen, D. J., Rickinson, A. B., Wallace, L. E., Rowe, M., Moss, D. J., and Epstein, M. A. (1982): Stimulation of human lymphocytes with irradiated cells of the autologous Epstein-Barr virus-transformed cell line. II. Cytotoxic response to repeated stimulation. *Cell. Immunol.*, 67:141–151.
2. Askonas, B. A., and Webster, R. G. (1980): Monoclonal antibodies to hemagglutinin and to H-2 inhibit the cross-reactive cytotoxic T cell populations induced by influenza. *Eur. J. Immunol.*, 10:151–156.
3. Bakacs, T., Svedmyr, E., and Klein, E. (1978): EBV-related cytotoxicity of Fc-receptor negative T lymphocytes separated from the blood of infectious mononucleosis patients. *Cancer Letters*, 4:185–189.
4. Ballieux, R. E., Heijnen, C. J., Uytdehaag, F., and Zegers, B. J. M. (1979): Regulation of B cell activity in man: Role of T cells. *Immunol. Rev.*, 45:3–39.
5. Bardwick, P. A., Bluestein, H. G., Zvaifler, N. J., Depper, J. M., and Seegmiller, J. E. (1980): Altered regulation of Epstein-Barr virus-induced lymphoblast proliferation in rheumatoid arthritis lymphoid cells. *Arthritis Rheum.*, 23:626–632.
6. Bird, A. G., and Britton, S. (1979): A new approach to the study of human B lymphocyte function using an indirect plaque assay and a direct B cell activator. *Immunol. Rev.*, 45:41–67.
7. Bird, A. G., McLachlan, S. M., and Britton, S. (1981): Cyclosporin A promotes spontaneous outgrowth *in vitro* of Epstein-Barr virus-induced B cell lines. *Nature*, 289:300–301.
8. Bird, A. G., Britton, S., Ernberg, I., and Nilsson, K. (1981): Characteristics of Epstein-Barr virus activation of human B lymphocytes. *J. Exp. Med.*, 154:832–839.
9. Carter, R. L. (1975): Infectious mononucleosis: Model for self-limiting lymphoproliferation. *Lancet*, 1:846–849.
10. Chan, S. H., Wallen, W. C., Levine, P. H., Periman, P., and Perlin, E. (1977): Lymphocyte responses to EBV-associated antigens in infectious mononucleosis, and Hodgkin's and non-Hodgkin's patients, with the leukocyte adherence inhibition assay. *Int. J. Cancer*, 19:356–363.
11. Crawford, D. H., Sweny, P., Edwards, J., Janossy, G., and Hoffbrand, A. V. (1981): Long-term T cell-mediated immunity to Epstein-Barr virus in renal allograft recipients receiving cyclosporin A. *Lancet*, 1:10–12.
12. Depper, J. M., Bluestein, H. G., and Zvaifler, N. J. (1981): Impaired regulation of Epstein-Barr virus-induced lymphocyte proliferation in rheumatoid arthritis is due to a T cell defect. *J. Immunol.*, 127:1899–1902.
13. Dölken, G., and Klein, G. (1976): Expression of Epstein-Barr virus-associated membrane antigen in Raji cells superinfected with two different virus strains. *Virology*, 70:210–213.
14. Einhorn, L., and Ernberg, I. (1978): Induction of EBNA precedes the first cellular S-phase after EBV-infection of human lymphocytes. *Int. J. Cancer*, 21:157–160.
15. Epstein, M. A., and Achong, B. G. (1979): The relationship of the virus to Burkitt's lymphoma. In: *The Epstein-Barr Virus*, edited by M. Epstein and B. Achong, pp. 321–337. Springer-Verlag, Berlin.
16. Falk, L., Deinhardt, F., Nonoyama, M., Wolfe, L. G., and Bergholz, C. (1976): Properties of a baboon lymphotropic herpesvirus related to Epstein-Barr virus. *Int. J. Cancer*, 18:798–807.

17. Frankel, M. E., Effros, R. B., Doherty, P. C., and Gerhard, W. U. (1979): A monoclonal antibody to viral glycoprotein blocks virus-immune effector T cells operating at H-2D^d but not at H-2K^d. *J. Immunol.*, 123:2438–2440.

18. Fukukawa, T., Hirano, T., Sakaguchi, N., Teranishi, T., Tsuyuguchi, I., Nagao, N., Yoshimura, K., Okuba, Y., Tohda, H., and Oikawa, A. (1981): In vitro induction of HLA-restricted cytotoxic T lymphocytes against autologous Epstein-Barr virus transformed B lymphoblastoid cell line. *J. Immunol.*, 126:1697–1701.

19. Gaston, J. S. H., Rickinson, A. B., and Epstein, M. A. (1982): Epstein-Barr virus-specific T cell memory in renal-allograft recipients under long-term immunosuppression. *Lancet*, 1:923–925.

20. Gerber, P., Nonoyama, M., Lucas, S., Perlin, E., and Goldstein, L. I. (1972): Oral excretion of Epstein-Barr virus by healthy subjects and patients with infectious mononucleosis. *Lancet*, 2:988–989.

21. Gergely, P., and Ernberg, I. (1977): Blastogenic response and EBNA induction in human lymphocytes by Epstein-Barr virus only requires B cells but not macrophages. *Cancer Letters*, 2:217–220.

22. Gergely, P., Ernberg, I., Klein, G., and Steinitz, M. (1977): Blastogenic response of purified human T-lymphocyte populations to Epstein-Barr virus (EBV). *Clin. Exp. Immunol.*, 30:347–353.

23. Gooding, L. R. (1979): Antibody blockade of lysis by T lymphocyte effectors generated against syngeneic SV40 transformed cells. *J. Immunol.*, 122:2328–2336.

24. Greaves, M. F., Brown, G., and Rickinson, A. B. (1975): Epstein-Barr virus binding sites on lymphocyte subpopulations and the origin of lymphoblasts in cultured lymphoid cell lines and in the blood of patients with infectious mononucleosis. *Clin. Immunol. Immunopathol.*, 3:514–524.

25. Haynes, B. F., Schooley, R. T., Payling-Wright, C. R., Grouse, J. E., Dolin, R., and Fauci, A. S. (1979): Emergence of suppressor cells of immunoglobulin synthesis during acute Epstein-Barr virus-induced mononucleosis. *J. Immunol.*, 123:2095–2101.

26. Henderson, E., Miller, G., Robinson, J., and Heston, L. (1977): Efficiency of transformation of lymphocytes by Epstein-Barr virus. *Virology*, 76:152–163.

27. Henle, G., and Henle, W. (1979): The virus as the etiologic agent of infectious mononucleosis. In: *The Epstein-Barr Virus*, edited by M. Epstein and B. Achong, pp. 297–320. Springer-Verlag, Berlin.

28. Henle, W., Diehl, V., Kohn, G., zur Hausen, H., and Henle, G. (1967): Herpes-type virus and chromosome marker in normal leukocytes after growth with irradiated Burkitt cells. *Science*, 157:1064–1065.

29. Henle, W., and Henle, G. (1979): Seroepidemiology of the virus. In: *The Epstein Barr Virus*, edited by M. Epstein and B. Achong, pp. 61–78. Springer-Verlag, Berlin.

30. Janossy, G., and Greaves, M. F. (1975): Functional analysis of murine and human B lymphocytes subsets. *Transplant. Rev.*, 24:177–236.

31. Johnson, H. E., Madsen, M., and Kristensen, T. (1979): Lymphocyte subpopulations in man: Suppression of PWM-induced B cell proliferation by infectious mononucleosis T cells. *Scand. J. Immunol.*, 10:251–255.

32. Jondal, M. (1976): Antibody-dependent cellular cytotoxicity (ADCC) against Epstein-Barr virus-determined membrane antigens. I. Reactivity in sera from normal persons and from patients with acute infectious mononucleosis. *Clin. Exp. Immunol.*, 25:1–5.

33. Jondal, M., and Klein, G. (1973): Surface markers on human B and T lymphocytes. II. Presence of Epstein-Barr virus receptor on B lymphocytes. *J. Exp. Med.*, 138:1365–1378.

34. Jondal, M., and Targan, S. (1978): In vitro induction of cytotoxic effector cells with spontaneous killer activity. *J. Exp. Med.*, 147:1621–1636.

35. Katsuki, T., Hinuma, Y., Yamamoto, N., Abo, T., and Kumagai, K. (1977): Identification of the target cells in human B lymphocytes for transformation by Epstein-Barr virus. *Virology*, 83:287–294.

36. Kinter, C., and Sugden, B. (1981): Identification of antigenic determinants unique to the surfaces of cells transformed by Epstein-Barr virus. *Nature*, 294:458–460.

37. Kirchner, H., Tosato, G., Blaese, R. M., Broder, S., and Magrath, I. T. (1979): Polyclonal immunoglobulin secretion by human B lymphocytes exposed to Epstein-Barr virus in vitro. *J. Immunol.*, 122:1310–1313.

38. Klein, E., Klein, G., and Levine, P. H. (1976): Immunoglobulin control of human lymphoma: Discussion. *Cancer Res.*, 36:724–727.

39. Klein, E., Masucci, M. G., Berthold, W., and Blazar, B. A. (1980): Lymphocyte-mediated cytotoxicity towards virus-induced tumor cells; natural and activated killer lymphocytes in man. *Cold Spring Harbor Conference on Cell Proliferation*, 7:1187–1197.
40. Klein, E., Ernberg, I., Masucci, M. G., Szigeti, R., Wu, Y. T., Masucci, G., and Svedmyr, E. (1981): T-cell response to B-cells and Epstein-Barr virus antigens in infectious mononucleosis. *Cancer Res.*, 41:4210–4215.
41. Klein, G. (1979): The relationship of the virus to nasopharyngeal carcinoma. In: *The Epstein-Barr Virus*, edited by M. Epstein and B. Achong, pp. 339–350. Springer-Verlag, Berlin.
42. Klein, G., Luka, J., and Zeuthen, J. (1979): Transformation induced by Epstein-Barr virus and the role of the nuclear antigen. *Cold Spring Harbor Symp. Quant. Biol.*, 44:253–261.
43. Klein, G., and Purtilo, D. T. (editors) (1981): Symposium on Epstein-Barr virus-induced lymphoproliferative diseases in immunodeficient patients. *Cancer Res.*, 41:4209–4304.
44. Kozbor, D., and Roder, J. C. (1981): Requirements for the establishement of high-titred human monoclonal antibodies against tetanus toxoid using the Epstein-Barr virus technique. *J. Immunol.*, 127:1275–1280.
45. Lai, P. K., Mackay-Scollay, E. M., Fimmel, P. J., Alpers, M. P., and Keast, D. (1974): Cell-mediated immunity to Epstein-Barr virus and a blocking factor in patients with infectious mononucleosis. *Nature*, 252:608–609.
46. Lai, P. K., Alpers, M. P., and Mackay-Scollay, E. M. (1977): Epstein-Barr herpesvirus infection: Inhibition by immunologically induced mediators with interferon-like properties. *Int. J. Cancer*, 20:21–29.
47. Landon, J. C., Ellis, L. B., Zeve, V. H., and Fabrizio, D. P. (1968): Herpes-type virus in cultured leukocytes from chimpanzees. *J. Natl. Cancer Inst.*, 40:181–192.
48. Lewis, A., and Rowe, W. (1973): Studies of non-defective adenovirus-2-simian virus 40 hybrid viruses. VIII. Association of simian virus 40 transplantation antigen with a specified region of the early viral genome. *J. Virol.*, 12:836–840.
49. Lipinski, M., Fridman, W. H., Tursz, T., Vincent, C., Pious, D., and Fellous, M. (1979): Absence of allogeneic restriction in human T cell-mediated cytotoxicity to Epstein-Barr virus-infected target cells. Demonstration of an HLA-linked control at the effector level. *J. Exp. Med.*, 150:1310–1322.
50. Luka, J., Jörnvall, H., and Klein, G. (1980): Purification and biochemical characterisation of the Epstein-Barr virus (EBV), determined nuclear antigen (EBNA) and an associated protein with a 53K subunit. *J. Virol.*, 35:592–602.
51. Miller, G., Niederman, J. C., and Andrews, L. (1973): Prolonged oropharyngeal excretion of EB virus following infectious mononucleosis. *N. Engl. J. Med.*, 288:229–232.
52. Misko, I. S., Moss, D. J., and Pope, J. H. (1980): HLA antigen-related restriction of T lymphocyte cytotoxicity to Epstein-Barr virus. *Proc. Natl. Acad. Sci. USA*, 77:4247–4250.
53. Misko, I. S., Kane, R. G., and Pope, J. H. (1982): Generation in vitro of HLA-restricted EB virus-specific cytotoxic human T cells by autologous lymphoblastoid cell lines: The roles of previous EB virus infection and foetal calf serum. *Int. J. Cancer*, 29:41–48.
54. Misko, I. S., Pope, J. H., Kane, R. G., Bashir, H., and Doran, T. (1982): Evidence for the involvement of HLA-DR antigens in restricted cytotoxicity by foetal calf serum-specific human T cells. *Human Immunol., (in press)*.
55. Moss, D. J., and Pope, J. H. (1975): EB virus-associated nuclear antigen production and cell proliferation in adult peripheral blood leukocytes inoculated with the QIMR-WIL strain of EB virus. *Int. J. Cancer*, 15:503–511.
56. Moss, D. J., Pope, J. H., and Scott, W. (1976): Inhibition of EB virus transformation of non-adherent human lymphocytes by co-cultivation with adult fibroblasts. *Med. Microbiol. Immunol.*, 162:159–167.
57. Moss, D. J., Scott, W., and Pope, J. H. (1977): An immunological basis for the inhibition of transformation of human lymphocytes by EB virus. *Nature*, 268:735–736.
58. Moss, D. J., Rickinson, A. B., and Pope, J. H. (1978): Long-term T-cell mediated immunity to Epstein-Barr virus in man. I. Complete regression of virus-induced transformation in cultures of seropositive donor leukocytes. *Int. J. Cancer*, 22:662–668.
59. Moss, D. J., Rickinson, A. B., and Pope, J. H. (1979): Long-term T cell-mediated immunity to Epstein-Barr virus in man. III. Activation of cytotoxic T cells in virus-infected leukocyte cultures. *Int. J. Cancer*, 23:618–625.
60. Moss, D. J., Rickinson, A. B., Wallace, L. E., and Epstein, M. A. (1981): Sequential appearance

of Epstein-Barr virus nuclear and lymphocyte-detected membrane antigens in B cell transformation. *Nature*, 291:664–666.

61. Moss, D. J., Wallace, L. E., Rickinson, A. B., and Epstein, M. A. (1981): Cytotoxic T cell recognition of Epstein-Barr virus-infected B cells. I. Specificity and HLA-restriction of effector cells reactivated *in vitro. Eur. J. Immunol.*, 11:686–693.

62. North, J. R., Morgan, A. J., and Epstein, M. A. (1980): Observations on the EB virus envelope and virus-determined membrane antigen polypeptides. *Int. J. Cancer*, 26:231–240.

63. Palacios, R., Andersson, U., and Britton, S. (1982): OKT4$^+$ T lymphocytes suppress Epstein-Barr virus-induced activation of B lymphocytes. *Immunobiology, (in press)*.

64. Patarroyo, M., Blazar, B., Pearson, G., Klein, E., and Klein, G. (1980): Induction of the EBV cycle in B-lymphocyte-derived lines is accompanied by increased natural killer (NK) sensitivity and the expression of EBV-related antigen(s) detected by the ADCC reaction. *Int. J. Cancer*, 26:365–375.

65. Pattengale, P. K., Smith, R. W., and Gerber, P. (1973): Selective transformation of B lymphocytes by EB virus. *Lancet*, 2:93.

66. Pearson, G. R., and Orr, T. W. (1976): Antibody-dependent lymphocyte cytotoxicity against cells expressing Epstein-Barr virus antigens. *J. Natl. Cancer Inst.*, 56:485–488.

67. Pereira, R. S., Webster, A. D. B., and Platts-Mills, T. A. E. (1982): Immature B cells in foetal development and immunodeficiency: Studies of IgM, IgG, IgA and IgD production *in vitro* using EB virus activation. *Eur. J. Immunol.*, 12:540–546.

68. Pope, J. H., Horne, M. K., and Scott, W. (1968): Transformation of foetal human leukocytes *in vitro* by filtrates of a human leukaemic cell line containing herpes-like virus. *Int. J. Cancer*, 3:857–866.

69. Pope, J. H., Horne, M. K., and Scott, W. (1969): Identification of the filtrable leukocyte-transforming factor of QIMR-WIL cells as herpes-like virus. *Int. J. Cancer*, 4:255–260.

70. Pope, J. H., Scott, W., and Moss, D. J. (1973): Human lymphoid cell transformation by Epstein-Barr virus. *Nature [New Biol.]*, 246:140–141.

71. Pretell, J., Greenfield, R. S., and Tevethia, S. S. (1979): Biology of simian virus 40 (SV40) transplantation antigen (TrAg). V. In vitro demonstration of SV40 TrAg in SV40 infected non-permissive mouse cells by the lymphocyte mediated cytotoxicity assay. *Virology*, 97:32–41.

72. Rasheed, S., Rongey, R. W., Bruszweski, J., Nelson-Rees, W. A., Rabin, H., Neubauer, R. H., Esra, G., and Gardner, M. B. (1977): Establishment of a cell line with associated Epstein-Barr-like virus from a leukaemic orangutan. *Science*, 198:407–409.

73. Reinhertz, E. L., O'Brien, C., Rosenthal, P., and Schlossman, S. F. (1980): The cellular basis for viral-induced immunodeficiency: analysis by monoclonal antibodies. *J. Immunol.*, 125:1269–1274.

74. Rickinson, A. B. (1983): T cell control of herpesvirus infections: Lessons from the Epstein-Barr virus. *Prog. Brain Res., (in press)*.

75. Rickinson, A. B., Jarvis, J. E., Crawford, D. H., and Epstein, M. A. (1974): Observations on the type of infection by Epstein-Barr virus in peripheral lymphoid cells of patients with infectious mononucleosis. *Int. J. Cancer*, 14:704–715.

76. Rickinson, A. B., Epstein, M. A., and Crawford, D. H. (1975): Absence of infectious Epstein-Barr virus in blood in acute infectious mononucleosis. *Nature*, 258:236–238.

77. Rickinson, A. B., Crawford, D. H., and Epstein, M. A. (1977): Inhibition of the in vitro outgrowth of Epstein-Barr virus-transformed lymphocytes by thymus-dependent lymphocytes from infectious mononucleosis patients. *Clin. Exp. Immunol.*, 28:72–79.

78. Rickinson, A. B., Moss, D. J., and Pope, J. H. (1979): Long-term T cell-mediated immunity to Epstein-Barr virus in man. II. Components necessary for regression in virus-infected leukocyte cultures. *Int. J. Cancer*, 23:610–617.

79. Rickinson, A. B., Moss, D. J., Pope, J. H., and Ahlberg, N. (1980): Long-term T cell-mediated immunity to Epstein-Barr virus in man. IV. Development of T cell memory in convalescent infectious mononucleosis patients. *Int. J. Cancer*, 25:59–65.

80. Rickinson, A. B., Wallace, L. E., and Epstein, M. A. (1980): HLA-restricted T cell recognition of Epstein-Barr virus-infected B cells. *Nature*, 283:865–867.

81. Rickinson, A. B., Moss, D. J., Wallace, L. E., Rowe, M., Misko, I. S., Epstein, M. A., and Pope, J. H. (1981): Long-term T cell-mediated immunity to Epstein-Barr virus. *Cancer Res.*, 41:4216–4221.

82. Rickinson, A. B., Moss, D. J., Allen, D. J., Wallace, L. E., Rowe, M., and Epstein, M. A.

(1981): Reactivation of Epstein-Barr virus-specific cytotoxic T cells by in vitro stimulation with the autologous lymphoblastoid cell line. *Int. J. Cancer*, 27:593–601.

83. Rickinson, A. B., and Moss, D. J. (1983): The Epstein-Barr virus–host interaction: Viral persistence and pathogenicity. *Adv. Cancer Res., (in press)*.

84. Rickinson, A. B., Hart, I., Rowe, M., and Epstein, M. A. (1982): A role for helper T cells in the Epstein-Barr virus-specific in vitro cytotoxic T cell response. *(in preparation)*.

85. Rosen, A., Gergely, P., Jondal, M., Klein, G., and Britton, S. (1977): Polyclonal Ig production after Epstein-Barr virus infection of human lymphocytes *in vitro*. *Nature*, 267:52–54.

86. Rowe, M., Hildreth, J. E. K., Rickinson, A. B., and Epstein, M. A. (1982): Monoclonal antibodies to Epstein-Barr virus-induced, transformation-associated cell surface antigens: Binding patterns and effect upon virus-specific T cell cytotoxicity. *Int. J. Cancer*, 29:373–381.

87. Rowe, M., Rickinson, A. B., Beer, S., Epstein, M. A., and Bradley, B. A. (1982): Selective reactivation of Epstein-Barr virus-specific cytotoxic T cells by stimulation *in vitro* with allogeneic virus-transformed HLA-homozygous typing cells. *Human Immunol., (in press)*.

88. Royston, I., Sullivan, J. L., Periman, P. O., and Perlin, E. (1975): Cell-mediated immunity to Epstein-Barr virus-transformed lymphoblastoid cells in acute infectious mononucleosis. *N. Engl. J. Med.*, 293:1159–1163.

89. Schneider, U., and zur Hausen, H. (1975): Epstein-Barr virus-induced transformation of human leukocytes after cell fractionation. *Int. J. Cancer*, 15:59–66.

90. Schooley, R. T., Haynes, B. F., Payling-Wright, C. R., Grouse, J. E., Dolin, R., and Fauci, A. S. (1980): Mechanism of Epstein-Barr virus-induced human B-lymphocyte activation. *Cell. Immunol.*, 56:518–525.

91. Schooley, R. T., Haynes, B. F., Grouse, J., Payling-Wright, C., Fauci, A. S., and Dolin, R. (1981): Development of suppressor T lymphocytes for Epstein-Barr virus-induced B-lymphocyte outgrowth during acute infectious mononucleosis: Assessment by two quantitative systems. *Blood*, 57:510–517.

92. Seeley, J. K., and Golub, S. H. (1978): Studies on cytotoxicity generated in human mixed lymphocyte cultures. I. Time course and target spectrum of several distinct concomitant cytotoxic activities. *J. Immunol.*, 120:1415–1422.

93. Seeley, J., Svedmyr, E., Weiland, O., Klein, G., Muller, E., Ericksson, E., Andersson, K., and Van der Waal, L. (1981): Epstein-Barr virus-selective T cells in infectious mononucleosis are not restricted to HLA-A and B antigens. *J. Immunol.*, 127:293–300.

94. Sheldon, P. J., Papamichail, M., Hemsted, E. H., and Holborow, E. J. (1973): Thymic origin of atypical lymphoid cells in infectious mononucleosis. *Lancet*, 1:1153–1155.

95. Shope, T. C., and Kaplan, J. (1979): Inhibition of the in vitro outgrowth of Epstein-Barr virus-infected lymphocytes by Tg lymphocytes. *J. Immunol.*, 123:2150–2155.

96. Slovin, S. F., Frisman, D. M., Tsoukas, C. D., Royston, I., Bird, S. M., Wormsley, S. B., Carson, D. A., and Vaughan, J. H. (1982): Membrane antigen on Epstein-Barr virus-infected human B cells recognised by a monoclonal antibody. *Proc. Natl. Acad. Sci. USA*, 79:2649–2653.

97. Svedmyr, E., and Jondal, M. (1975): Cytotoxic effectors cells specific for B cell lines transformed by Epstein-Barr virus are present in patients with infectious mononucleosis. *Proc. Natl. Acad. Sci. USA*, 72:1622–1626.

98. Szigeti, R., Luka, J., and Klein, G. (1981): Leukocyte migration inhibition studies with Epstein-Barr virus (EBV) determined nuclear antigen (EBNA) in relation to the EBV-carrier status of the donor. *Cell. Immunol.*, 58:269–276.

99. Szigeti, R., Volsky, D. J., Luka, J., and Klein, G. (1981): Membranes of EBV-carrying virus non-producer cells inhibit leukocyte migration of EBV seropositive but not seronegative donors. *J. Immunol.*, 126:1676–1679.

100. Tanaka, Y., Sugamura, K., Hinuma, Y., Sato, H., and Okochi, K. (1980): Memory of Epstein-Barr virus-specific cytotoxic T cells in normal seropositive adults as revealed by an in vitro restimulation method. *J. Immunol.*, 125:1426–1431.

101. Thorley-Lawson, D. A. (1980): The suppression of Epstein-Barr virus infection *in vitro* occurs after infection but before transformation of the cell. *J. Immunol.*, 124:745–751.

102. Thorley-Lawson, D. A. (1981): The transformation of adult but not newborn human lymphocytes by Epstein-Barr virus and phytohaemagglutinin is inhibited by interferon: The early suppression of T cells by Epstein-Barr virus infection is mediated by interferon. *J. Immunol.*, 102:829–833.

103. Thorley-Lawson, D. A., Chess, L., and Strominger, J. L. (1977): Suppression of in vitro Epstein-Barr virus infection. A new role for adult human T lymphocytes. *J. Exp. Med.*, 146:495–508.

104. Thorley-Lawson, D. A., and Geilinger, K. (1980): Monoclonal antibodies against the major gly-coprotein (gp 350/220) of Epstein-Barr virus neutralise infectivity. *Proc. Natl. Acad. Sci. USA*, 77:5307–5311.
105. Tosato, G., Magrath, I., Koski, I., Dooley, N., and Blaese, M. (1979): Activation of suppressor T cells during Epstein-Barr virus-induced infectious mononucleosis. *N. Engl. J. Med.*, 301:1133–1137.
106. Tosato, G., Magrath, I., and Blaese, R. M. (1982): T cell-mediated immunoregulation of Epstein-Barr virus (EBV)-induced B lymphocyte activation in EBV-seropositive and EBV-seronegative individuals. *J. Immunol.*, 128:575–579.
107. Trinchieri, G., and Santoli, D. (1978): Anti-viral activity induced by culturing lymphocytes with tumour-derived or virus-transformed cells. Enhancement of human natural killer cell activity by interferon and antagonistic inhibition of susceptibility of target cells to lysis. *J. Exp. Med.*, 147:1314–1333.
108. Tsoukas, C. D., Fox, R. I., Slovin, S. F., Carson, D. A., Pellegrino, M., Fong, S., Pasquali, J.-L., Ferrone, S., Kung, P., and Vaughan, J. H. (1981): T lymphocyte-mediated cytotoxicity against autologous EBV genome-bearing B cells. *J. Immunol.*, 126:1742–1746.
109. Tsukuda, K., Volsky, D. J., Shapiro, I. M., and Klein, G. (1982): Epstein-Barr virus (EBV) receptor implantation onto human B lymphocytes changes immunoglobulin secretion patterns induced by EBV infection. *Eur. J. Immunol.*, 12:87–90.
110. Wallace, L. E., Moss, D. J., Rickinson, A. B., McMichael, A. J., and Epstein, M. A. (1981): Cytotoxic T cell recognition of Epstein-Barr virus-infected B cells. II. Blocking studies with monoclonal antibodies to HLA determinants. *Eur. J. Immunol.*, 11:694–699.
111. Wallace, L. E., Rickinson, A. B., Rowe, M., and Epstein, M. A. (1982): Epstein-Barr virus-specific cytotoxic T cell clones restricted through a single HLA antigen. *Nature*, 297:413–415.
112. Wallace, L. E., Rickinson, A. B., Rowe, M., Moss, D. J., Allen, D. J., and Epstein, M. A. (1982): Stimulation of human lymphocytes with irradiated cells of the autologous Epstein-Barr virus-transformed cell line. I. Virus-specific and non-specific components of the cytotoxic response. *Cell. Immunol.*, 67:129–140.
113. Wallace, L. E., Rowe, M., Gaston, J. S. H., Rickinson, A. B., and Epstein, M. A. (1982): Cytotoxic T cell recognition of Epstein-Barr virus infected B cells. III. Establishment of HLA-restricted cytotoxic T cell lines using interleukin 2. *Eur. J. Immunol.*, 12:1012–1018.
114. Weil, R. (1978): Viral "tumor antigens." A novel type of mammalian regulator protein. *Biochim. Biophys. Acta*, 516:301–388.
115. Wells, A., Koide, N., and Klein, G. (1982): Two large virion envelope glycoproteins mediate Epstein-Barr virus binding to receptor-positive cells. *J. Virol.*, 41:286–297.
116. Yamamoto, N., and Hinuma, Y. (1976): Clonal transformation of human leukocytes by Epstein-Barr virus in soft agar. *Int. J. Cancer*, 17:191–196.
117. Zerbini, M., and Ernberg, I. (1983): Can Epstein-Barr virus infect and transform all the B lymphocytes of human cord blood? *J. Gen. Virol.*, 64:539–547.

Advances in Viral Oncology, Volume 3, edited by
George Klein. Raven Press, New York © 1983.

Transcription Patterns in HSV Infections

Edward K. Wagner

*Department of Molecular Biology and Biochemistry, University of California, Irvine,
Irvine, California 92717*

An increasingly detailed picture of the phenomenology of animal virus gene
expression during productive infection is being achieved. In the case of herpesvirus
(particularly herpes simplex virus type 1, HSV-1), this is entirely dependent on the
revolution in molecular biology resulting from restriction enzyme analysis of viral
DNA (106) and, more recently, from the use of recombinant DNA technology for
the construction and analysis of fine probes of HSV-1 DNA transcription. Workers
in the United States and Great Britain have been able to use fine restriction and
polypeptide analysis of HSV-1 and HSV-2 intertypic recombinants to locate many
HSV marker proteins on the viral genome, as reviewed by Halliburton (64). Marker
rescue will have an increasing role in defining specific HSV genes (110,147).
Hybridization of viral RNA present at specific stages of infection to separated
restriction fragments of HSV DNA has allowed workers in our laboratory, along
with those working in other laboratories, to locate specific viral transcripts on the
viral genome. *In vitro* translation of resolvable viral mRNA species, notably by
Preston in Glasgow, Cremer and Summers at Yale, and Anderson and Holland in
our laboratory, has allowed some correlation of these mRNAs with viral gene
products seen *in vivo*; for reviews, see Spear and Roizman (142) and Wagner et
al. (159). A moderate-resolution map of HSV-1 mRNAs present at various stages
of infection, along with some of the biological markers correlated with these regions
of the genome, is shown in Fig. 1, which combines the specific contributions of
many workers.

Most recently, techniques for high-resolution mapping of viral transcripts using
hybrid selection and nuclease mapping have allowed those working in our laboratory, as well as others, to locate HSV transcripts to the precision necessary for
nucleotide sequence analysis. As will be outlined later, one can now describe a
"typical" HSV-1 gene and begin to understand those factors involved in regulation
of viral gene expression. Other workers are in the midst of similar studies on other
herpesviruses, and a picture of those aspects of HSV-1 transcription that are general
and those that are particular to HSV is emerging.

BASIC PATTERNS OF HSV-1 GENE EXPRESSION

HSV and Its Genome

HSV occurs in two distinct subtypes: type 1 (HSV-1), associated with facial
lesions, and type 2 (HSV-2), associated with genital infection. The two types can

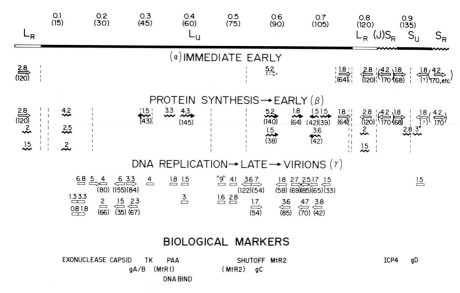

FIG. 1. Location of HSV-1 mRNA species abundant at the three stages of replication. This figure summarizes studies in our laboratory described in detail elsewhere (4,7,34,54,55,67,68,159) and described briefly here. Also included are results of experiments currently in progress. Individual mRNA species are localized to the nearest restriction fragment or junction of two fragments found to have significant homology with them. The size of RNA (in kb) is indicated above the location. The direction of transcription, where known, is indicated by arrows pointing toward the 3′ end in the P arrangement of HSV-1. The sizes of polypeptides encoded (where determined) are shown in thousands of daltons below the mRNA species in question. Locations of other markers were determined from data described elsewhere (21,23,24,27,38,39, 41,42,49,58,74,77,91,94,98,101,109,119,123,131,134,161,166,167,169).

cross-react antigenically, and their genomes are partially homologous (105,170). The HSV virion comprises as many as 50 distinct polypeptides (69,93) arranged in a defined series of layers and shells. The viral DNA is encapsulated in the core of the virion associated with one or several proteins. These probably are involved in binding the viral DNA to facilitate the encapsulation process (12,59). The viral capsid is surrounded by a glycoprotein inner envelope and a lipid-rich membrane. The viral DNA itself is infectious (138); therefore, none of the virion proteins and derivatives is absolutely essential for replication.

Characteristics of the viral DNA have been reviewed by Roizman (133). Briefly, the DNA has a molecular mass of 95 to 100 $\times$ 10^6 daltons (d) (62,155). The KOS strain, which is used in our laboratory, is 150,000 base pairs in length, based on the ratio of its contour length to that of ϕX174 RFII (149). As mentioned by Holland et al. (68), earlier lower values reported from this laboratory were based on low values for both ϕXRFII DNA and T4 DNA used as size standards.

Like all the herpesviruses, HSV-1 is characterized by an unusual arrangement of its genome. The linear HSV-1 genome is segmented into a long unique region (U_L, ca. 105 kb) and a short unique region (U_S, ca. a5 kb), each bounded by different-length inversely reiterated sequences (R_L, 9 kb; R_S, 6 kb). Such a structure results in four equimolar populations of the viral DNA differing in the relative orientation of the long and short segments (66,141,155,171). In view of this fact, one arrangement is, by convention, chosen as the prototypical (P) configuration (101,133). A representation of this arrangement, with specific restriction endonuclease cleavage sites, is shown in Fig. 2.

Gene Expression during HSV-1 Infection

HSV-1 mRNA shares general properties with host cell mRNA; i.e., it is synthesized in the nucleus, is polyadenylated on the 3' end and capped on the 5' end, and is internally methylated (8,11,102,139,140,148,158).

It is interesting to note that although HSV-1 mRNA is in many ways like its host cell mRNA, it differs in one respect—its degree of splicing. RNA splicing appears to be a common feature of mammalian mRNA biogenesis, where unneeded internal sequences are removed by an as yet uncharacterized mechanism and the resulting mRNA sequences are spliced back together (65,137). Although some HSV-1 mRNAs are spliced during this biogenesis (54,167,168), many others do not appear to be (5,34,54,55,63). Whether or not this is a reflection of the unusual natural history of the virus is as yet unclear.

Although HSV-1 is the most extensively studied of the herpesviruses, many of the general features of gene expression during the HSV-1 replication cycle were first described in other herpesviruses. Workers with Kaplan and Ben-Porat demonstrated a requirement for protein synthesis for full early gene expression and for transition from early phase to late phase of gene expression in pseudorabies virus (16,48,129). Randall, O'Callaghan, and associates (30,31,72) clearly demonstrated early and late phases of gene expression of equine abortion (herpes) virus, and recent work on cytomegalovirus (40,163) has shown that the limited, immediate-early transcription patterns seen for HSV-1 also are seen with this virus. Therefore, patterns of HSV-1 gene expression should be considered general for the herpesviruses.

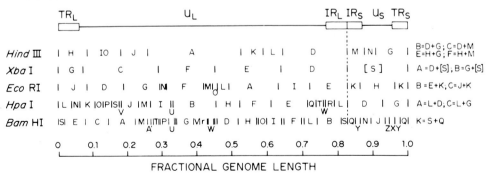

FIG. 2. Restriction endonuclease cleavage sites for HSV-1 DNA. The prototypical (P) arrangement of the HSV-1 genome is shown, and restriction cleavage sites for *Hind*III, *Xba*I, *Hpa*I, *Bam*HI, and *Eco*RI digests are shown. The whole genome is 150 kb pairs in length. There are three other arrangements possible; these are reviewed by Roizman (133).

The viral proteins seen in infected cells can be differentiated into three groups: α, β, and γ, based on their kinetics of synthesis (70,71). This general "cascade" pattern of HSV protein expression mirrors the stages of expression of HSV mRNA. Each stage is characterized by an increasing complexity of viral mRNA expressed (142,159). In the first stage, α or immediate-early mRNA species are seen. These can be expressed abundantly without *de novo* protein synthesis, i.e., in an unmodified host cell nucleus (75,81). Abundant members of this class of mRNA are quite limited; they map in regions of the HSV-1 genome at or near the R_L and R_S regions and encode only a limited number of polypeptides *in vivo* and *in vitro* (4,26, 27,68,71,77,93,94,122,126,164,166). Two α mRNAs encoding different polypeptides are chimeric in that their 5' ends map in the R_S region, but their 3' ends map in different ends of the U_S region (4,26,166). The coding sequence for their identical 5' ends contains the currently best characterized HSV-1 intron, which is about 150 bases in length and occurs approximately 260 bases from the 5' ends of the mRNAs (167,168).

Following expression of one or several HSV-1 α proteins, a more complex population of viral mRNA becomes abundant prior to viral DNA replication (72,104, 150,151,156,160). Those mRNAs expressed after the α mRNAs, but prior to viral DNA replication, compose the β or early class. These β viral mRNAs map throughout the HSV-1 genome in noncontiguous regions, but only a limited number of readily resolvable species are found (68,76,149). As will be described in a later section, a number of β mRNAs have been rigorously mapped. None of these mRNAs appears to be spliced.

Many β mRNAs are involved with priming the cell for viral DNA replication. Workers in our laboratory, as well as in others, have found that without viral DNA replication, the β viral mRNA and protein population appears to persist (120, 148,150,151,156,162). In spite of this, there has been controversy over whether or not DNA replication does, in fact, have a role in γ gene expression. Honess and Roizman (70) found reduced but significant γ protein synthesis occurring in the absence of readily detectable viral DNA replication. They suggested that β proteins alone are sufficient for γ gene expression. Ward and Stevens (162), however, examined total infected cell polypeptides from normal cells and from cells in which DNA synthesis was rigorously inhibited and suggested a requirement for viral DNA replication for expression of certain viral functions, as suggested by Swanstrom et al. (151). Also, Powell et al. (120) showed that certain late (γ) viral polypeptides were missing in cells in the absence of DNA synthesis. Holland, working in our laboratory, examined the role of viral DNA replication in the normal expression of late viral mRNA (67,68). He found that inhibition of HSV-1 DNA synthesis with ara-A or ara-T showed a viral mRNA population identical with that seen early by the criteria of quantitative hybridization, specific mRNA species identifiable by Southern blot hybridization of size-fractionated RNA, or the size of polypeptides resolved by *in vitro* translation of purified viral mRNA. We concluded that normal late mRNA expression requires viral DNA replication in addition to β polypeptides.

This conclusion is in general agreement with more recent data presented by Jones and Roizman (76) and Pedersen et al. (112).

Concomitant with viral DNA replication is the appearance of late HSV-1 mRNA (52,156,160). Two subclasses of late mRNA are readily distinguishable. These are a group that is detectable in the absence of viral DNA replication, the "leaky-late" or βγ mRNAs, and a group that cannot be seen at all in the cytoplasm in the absence of viral DNA replication, the "true-late" or γ mRNAs. Both groups of mRNA species encode a large number of polypeptides (67), many of which presumably are structural proteins of the virion. As will be described in the next section, workers in our laboratory have precisely mapped a number of βγ and γ mRNAs. At least one HSV-1 γ mRNA family appears to contain spliced members (54).

Effect of HSV Infection on Host Cell Function

Studies on the inhibition of host cell macromolecular synthesis following HSV infection go back at least 20 years, well into the "dark ages" prior to the availability of more modern molcular biological techniques. Host cell polysomes are dispersed and stable RNA synthesis is rapidly inhibited after infection (152,157). Stringer et al. (148) showed that viral mRNA on polyribosomes becomes a major class early after infection, so that by late times, as much as 90% of newly synthesized polyribosomal mRNA in infected cells is viral. Studies on specific cellular mRNAs have shown a rapid shutoff of synthesis and apparent degradation of cellular mRNA (107,115,143).

Although specific mechanisms for this shutoff are not known, it is clear that a definable viral function is involved (49), and the fact that there are rapid- and slow-shutoff strains of HSV may mean that more than one viral function is operating. In view of the fact that most HSV mRNA seems to be unspliced, the idea that the virus might inhibit cellular mRNA synthesis by inhibiting splicing had a vogue, but the fact that HSV is an effective helper for adeno-associated virus, which requires splicing for its replication, makes this model questionable.

DETAILED ANALYSIS OF SPECIFIC HSV-1 TRANSCRIPTS

Isolation, Localization, and Translation of Specific HSV-1 mRNA Species

The data reviewed in the preceding section indicate that the general patterns of HSV mRNA expression are clear. It also is clear that detailed information concerning HSV-1 gene function and mechanisms of control of gene expression must come from analysis of specific viral genes and the mRNAs and proteins they encode. The use of hybrid selection and size fractionation, coupled with *in vitro* translation, to isolate and characterize viral mRNA was pioneered by workers using somewhat more tractable viruses, such as adenovirus (3,87). In theory, recombinant DNA technology is not a requirement for such studies, and some of the earliest results from our laboratory were obtained using purified restriction fragments from viral

DNA (6). However, the purity and large quantities of recombinant DNA available make its use a practical necessity. Our procedures for specific viral mRNA isolation and characterization have been described (159). Variations on these methods are used in many laboratories, but for simplicity's sake, I shall use our general procedures as a guide.

The first report of cloning HSV-1 DNA was by Enquist et al. (47), using a λ phage vector (WES·B). Such vectors are convenient for cloning large DNA fragments, and thanks to the generosity of Enquist and Vande Woude at NIH, the phage λ clones were immediately available to workers in the HSV field. Cloning in the plasmid vector pBR322 is useful for *Bam*HI, *Sal*I, and *Hin*dIII fragments ranging from less than 1 kilobase (kb) pair up to 15 kb pairs. Recently, Goldin et al. (61) reported cloning *Eco*RI fragments of HSV-1 DNA in pBR325; therefore, a number of vehicles and clones covering essentially the whole genome are available. We concentrate on *Hin*dIII fragments cloned in pBR322 as our primary clones and subclone from these as needed (5).

Our laboratory finds hybrid selection of HSV-1 mRNA species to be conveniently carried out using DNA fragments bound to diazotized cellulose powder (7,108). Hybridization near the T_m of the DNA in high (80%) formamide concentration (22) minimizes background. Following preparative hybridization of fragment-specific mRNA, it can be translated directly or size-fractionated using methylmercury-containing agarose gels for electrophoresis (9). These gels have the advantage that specific viral mRNA species can be eluted and then translated (6,34,54,63). We find oligo-dT reselection of mRNA after elution from gels to be valuable. Similar procedures using DNA bound to nitrocellulose or diazotized paper have been reported (32,125).

An example of the selection of HSV-1 mRNA species encoded by different regions of the viral genome is shown in Fig. 3. Here, ^{32}P-labeled total infected cell polysomal poly(A) mRNA yields a large number of resolvable bands, whereas the use of *Bgl*II fragment N (0.23–0.27), *Hin*dIII fragment K (0.53–0.59), or *Xho*I fragment W (0.69–0.71) to select mRNAs yields a small number of well-resolved individual species.

RNA or Northern blots (1) were used to good effect for the localization of HSV-1 mRNA species using radioactive probes made to cloned DNA fragments. The method is so convenient that fairly detailed localization of transcripts of many refractory herpesviruses, such as Epstein-Barr virus, have been reported (73,154). Published studies from our laboratory have all used the original diazotized paper method for RNA blotting, but good results have been reported using nitrocellulose blots (153). Recently, we used RNA immobilized in agarose with excellent results (63).

Generally, the complexity of the HSV-1 mRNA encoded by large (>4–5 kb) HSV-1 DNA fragments makes it important to use smaller DNA fragments as reagents for isolation or localization of specific viral mRNA species. However, the fact that α (immediate-early) and β (early) stages of gene expression yield a simpler pattern of transcripts means that in some cases a large piece of DNA can be used

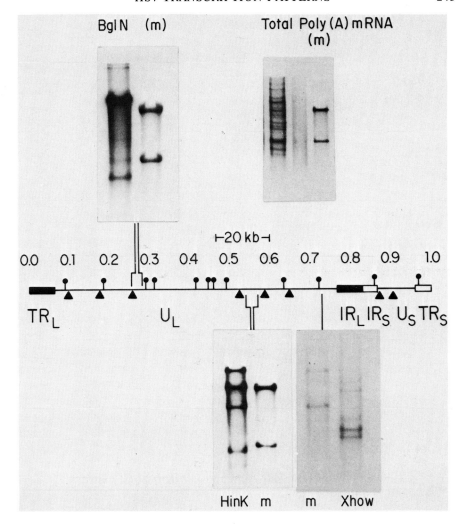

FIG. 3. Use of hybrid selection to isolate region-specific HSV-1 mRNA. Shown are methyl-mercury agarose gels (9) of total HSV-1 mRNA from infected cell polyribosomes or those isolated by hybrid selection using the restriction fragments indicated. *Bgl*II fragment N maps between 0.23 and 0.27, *Hin*dIII fragment K maps between 0.53 and 0.59, and *Xho*I fragment W maps between 0.69 and 0.71 on the prototypical arrangement of the HSV-1 genome. The tracks indicated (m) are 5.2-kb and 2.0-kb HeLa cell rRNA markers.

to gain definite information about a single mRNA, or at least a limited number of mRNAs. The general mapping of the immediate-early HSV-1 mRNAs described in the preceding section is an example of the use of a metabolically blocked replication stage to limit mRNA complexity. Another example is shown in the Northern blot of Fig. 4, where, under early conditions, only 5.2 kb and 1.5 kb mRNAs are seen as major products encoded by the 9.8-kb-pair *Hin*dIII fragment K (0.527–0.592), whereas a 3.8-kb species is seen in low amounts. *In vitro* translation of

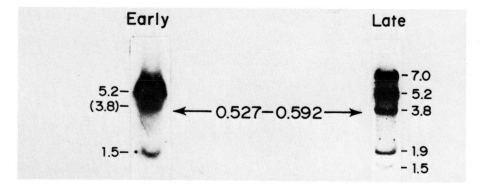

FIG. 4. Effect of temporal stage of infection on complexity of viral mRNA seen in a specific region of the viral genome. The data are based on experiments described by Anderson et al. (5). In the absence of viral DNA synthesis **(Early)**, two major (5.2 kb and 1.5 kb) and one minor (3.8 kb) HSV mRNA species are homologous to HindIII fragment K. Following viral DNA replication **(Late)**, major species include 7-kb, 5.2-kb, 3.8-kb, and 1.9-kb members; the 1.5-kb species is not amplified and thus is considered a minor early species. Experimental details of Northern blotting are described in the original reference.

*Hin*dIII fragment K hybrid-selected early mRNA has indicated that the 5.2-kb mRNA encodes a 140,000-d polypeptide (6). This has been confirmed by translation of size-fractionated *Hin*dIII-fragment-K-specific mRNA (5). Late mRNA gives a much more complex pattern, with mRNAs of 7 kb, 3.8 kb, and 1.9 kb becoming abundant, in addition to the 5.2 kb mRNA. Translation of such a mixture of mRNAs cannot yield a specific assignment of polypeptide to each mRNA species.

Cloned DNA fragments ranging from 1 to 3 kb pairs are the most suitable sizes of probes for "walking down" a region of the viral genome; the use of limited areas of overlap in these probes tends to minimize error. An example is shown in Fig. 5, based on recent data (63). Figure 5 shows Northern blots of mRNA homologous to the region mapping between the *Hin*dIII site at 0.65 and the *Eco*RI site at 0.72. In this region, nine resolvable mRNA species are seen, and such a complex pattern is relatively common for HSV-1. Northern blots using early HSV mRNA allow temporal-class assignment of individual species. Some of these mRNAs overlap, and some translate into the same-size polypeptides and thus appear to be "redundant." Mechanisms for generation of overlapping mRNA will be discussed in the next section. Overlapping mRNAs often are not of the same temporal class; examples of this abound in the HSV genome. We have described several in our recent experimental publications.

Translation of specific HSV-1 mRNAs has been efficiently carried out either using reticulocyte lysates (37,38,67,121) or by microinjecting amphibian oocytes (33,99). The latter method is laborious, but it has been well suited for assays of biological activity. Further it can be used as a coupled transcription-translation system if the proper DNA fragment is injected. As discussed earlier, translation of total mRNA from a region is feasible and can be used to generally locate viral genes. In general, however, such techniques are most useful when biological activity

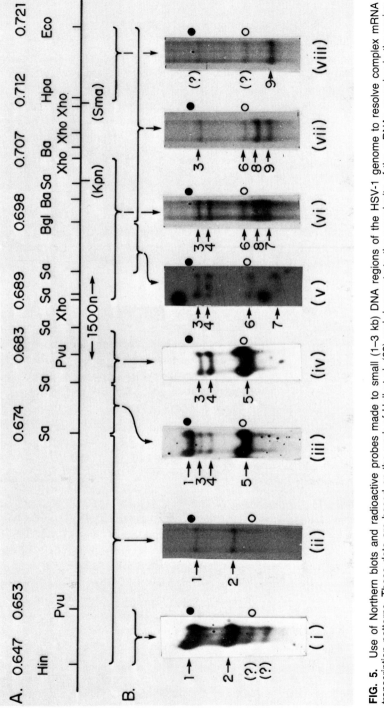

FIG. 5. Use of Northern blots and radioactive probes made to small (1–3 kb) DNA regions of the HSV-1 genome to resolve complex mRNA transcription patterns. These data are based on the work of Hall et al. (63) and demonstrate the complexity of the mRNAs mapping in the region between 0.65 and 0.72. A minimum of nine specific mRNAs can be identified and are numbered in panel B. Some of these mRNAs appear to be redundant, as described in the primary reference.

can be measured, such as for thymidine kinase (tk) or the alkaline exonuclease (124,125). Translation of size-fractionated region-specific mRNAs affords both the most unambiguous assignment of polypeptide products to mRNA and a good check on possible mRNA redundancy. Denaturing methylmercury agarose gel electrophoresis gives excellent resolution of even small mRNAs, as shown in Fig. 6, where the translation of separated 1.9-kb and 1.5-kb mRNAs mapping in the region between the *Hin*dIII site at 0.59 and the *Bam*HI site at 0.60 (*Hin*dIII-*Bam*HI fragment L-O) shows that the latter mRNA encodes a 40,000-d polypeptide, whereas the former encodes a 58,000-d polypeptide. However, even translation of size-fractionated mRNA does not always yield completely unambiguous results, as witnessed by our consistent finding that the 3.8-kb mRNA mapping in the left half of *Hin*dIII fragment K encodes both a 122,000-d polypeptide and an 86,000-d polypeptide (5). Preston and McGeoch (125) found that purified mRNA from *Bam*HI fragment P, which encodes tk, also encodes a 39,000-d polypeptide, and sequence analysis indicates that both polypeptides are from the same mRNA. It is unknown whether such findings are due to an artifact of the *in vitro* translating systems not discriminating between a real initiation AUG codon and an internal one or whether there is a biological function to such degeneracy. However, it will be seen later that even more complex patterns can be detected.

Despite these ambiguities, the ability to isolate, locate, and translate HSV mRNAs generally leads to readily interpretable map locations for viral transcripts and the polypeptides they encode. This type of information was used to construct the moderate-resolution map of Fig. 1, and it allows the construction of high-resolution maps of individual HSV mRNAs to be described later.

High-Resolution Mapping of HSV-1 mRNA

The use of the S1 nuclease and exonuclease VII to digest hybrids between viral RNA and defined fragments of DNA was developed by Berk and Sharp to provide a reliable and (fairly) rapid means of precisely locating viral transcripts and locating splices in them (18–20). Provided the proper standards and separation techniques are used, resolution can be taken to the nucleotide level *(vide infra)*. A good basic outline of the method was recently presented by Flint and Broker (51). Although the size of the HSV genome is so large as to necessitate, at best, "deliberate" progress, the general lack of splicing makes things somewhat easier. The highest-level resolution of S1 digests of hybrids of HSV-1 mRNA species was used to locate the tk gene on its DNA sequence (98,161), to precisely locate splices in the two 1.8-kb (immediate-early) genes (168), and to locate the 5' ends of model early and late mRNAs for comparative purposes (55) *(vide infra)*. We used this method to locate (± 50 bases) more than 20 mRNAs on the HSV-1 genome. Such resolution is sufficient to allow one to see detailed overlap and to begin sequence studies on mRNAs of interest. Such a map is shown in Fig. 7.

Our procedures have been published (5,63), and several examples follow. The general lack of interior splices in HSV-1 mRNAs was readily seen by hybridizing ^{32}P-labeled *Hin*dIII fragment K DNA with the four major viral mRNA species

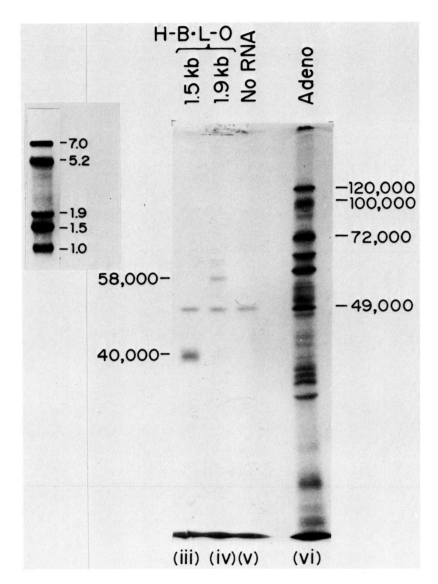

FIG. 6. Translation of hybrid-selected HSV-1 mRNAs size-fractionated on methylmercury agarose gels. The Northern blot (**left**) indicates the resolution of the 1.9-kb and 1.5-kb mRNAs mapping in the region of 0.59 to 0.6 of the HSV-1 genome. Other mRNAs (7, 5.2, and 1 kb) also are seen. The left side shows the products of *in vitro* translation of the 1.5-kb and 1.9-kb mRNAs. As described in the original report (5), the translation products of adenovirus mRNA serve as good size markers, and the no-RNA control shows that the 50,000-d band is an endogenous product of the system.

encoded by this region. The hybrids then were digested with S1 nuclease and size-fractionated on a neutral agarose gel. The gel then was turned 90 degrees, and the fragments were separated under alkaline conditions. The strict diagonal of the four

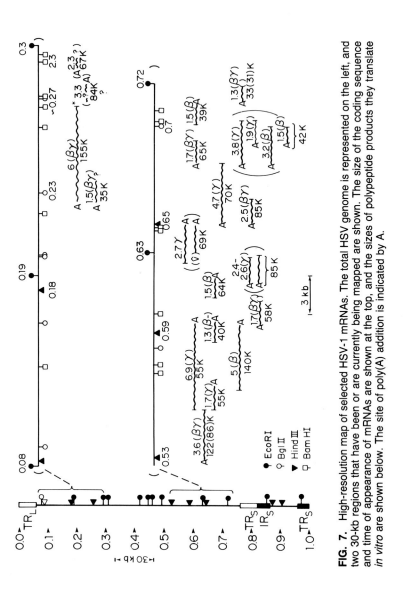

FIG. 7. High-resolution map of selected HSV-1 mRNAs. The total HSV genome is represented on the left, and two 30-kb regions that have been or are currently being mapped are shown. The size of the coding sequence and time of appearance of mRNAs are shown at the top, and the sizes of polypeptide products they translate in vitro are shown below. The site of poly(A) addition is indicated by A.

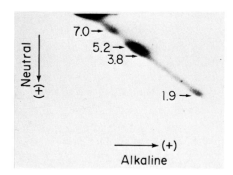

FIG. 8. Lack of splices of HSV-1 mRNA mapping in *Hind*III fragment K. An S1 digest of late poly(A) mRNA hybridized to *Hind*III fragment K was first subjected to agarose gel electrophoresis at neutral pH; then the gel was turned 90 degrees and subjected to electrophoresis at alkaline pH. The arrows indicate the four major bands corresponding to mRNA encoded by the fragment. The material at the top of the gel is undigested material. Data are from Anderson et al. (5).

DNA replicas of the mRNAs is seen in Fig. 8. As discussed by Anderson et al. (5), this is possible only if there are no interruptions (introns) in the DNA sequence encoding the viral RNA.

We used 5'- and 3'-end-labeled HSV-1 DNA probes for hybridization to define the direction of transcription of transcripts, and these also allow very precise characterization of overlapping mRNA sequences. Although many overlapping mRNA "families" are seen (Fig. 7), only a few species show any evidence of splices. These include the 1.7-kb βγ mRNA mapping through the *Bam*HI site at 0.602 and the 1.3-kb βγ mRNA mapping near the *Eco*RI site at 0.72. Both have regions of about 50 to 100 bases on their 5' ends that could be noncontiguous and may define a "leader." More strikingly, the mRNA family mapping from the left of the *Eco*RI site at 0.63 to the *Hind*III site at 0.65 contains members that appear to have splices in them (54). Recent work has suggested that these spliced members are in the minority (R. Frink and E. Wagner, *unpublished data*). Some of the details concerning this family will be described in the next section, but it is clear that most readily resolvable HSV-1 mRNA species lack splices down to this resolution.

Correlation of HSV-1 Biological Markers with Specific Viral mRNAs

One goal of the precise localization of HSV transcripts on the viral genome is to identify them with biological functions. Some information for such correlation can be inferred from intertypic recombination data (64), and other information can be obtained from studies on biological markers. Such markers include the location of drug resistance, assays of enzymatic activity, and so forth.

It is very clear that the 4.2 α mRNA mapping wholly in the short repeat region encodes an important regulatory protein of nominal molecular weight 172,000 (ICP4). This identification comes from direct *in vitro* translation of 4.2-kb α mRNA size-fractionated from cells held at the immediate-early stage of replication by cycloheximide block (26,166) and from *in vitro* translation of such mRNA hybrid-selected using DNA from the short repeat region (4). Both Schaffer and associates and workers with Subak-Sharpe (36,94,127) have described mutants mapping in the region encoding the 4.2-kb mRNA. In both cases it has been shown that at the nonpermissive temperatures (39°C) the immediate-early transcription pattern persists in spite of available *de novo* protein synthesis (68,122,164). Further, Watson and Clements (165) found that the immediate-early transcription pattern can be reestablished on temperature upshift. Such a result suggests that ICP4 is a protein required continuously throughout infection.

Other immediate-early proteins appear to be candidates for regulatory roles; however, mutants mapping in these genes have not been described, and recent work from Roizman's laboratory (116) indicates that the 68,000-d gene product (VP22) encoded by the 1.8-kb mRNA mapping around 0.85 is not required for lytic infection in cultured cells.

Three types of glycoproteins, gA/B, gC, and gD, are mapped on the viral genome (Fig. 1). The glycosylated character of these glycoproteins makes measurement of the precise size of the primary translation product of any of these uncertain (29). This uncertainty makes for difficulty in correlating purified mRNA translation products with the glycoprotein precursor. On the basis of two-dimensional O'Farrell gels and glycosylation inhibitors, Marsden *(personal communication)* in Glasgow has suggested that the precursor for glycoprotein C is of the size range of 69,000 to 72,000 d. Because the HSV-1 glycoprotein C maps in the *Hin*dIII fragment L (0.597–0.645) region, there is only a limited number of candidate mRNAs for encoding it.

Tremendous excitement has been generated by the finding that HSV-1 and HSV-2 genes can cause morphological transformation (Mtr) (44,45,130). Such transformation is a convenient and fashionable biological marker, especially in view of early and recently confirmed reports that HSV gene products can be seen in cervical cancer tissue (53,97). Interestingly, it is one of the few that does not appear to map in the same region in HSV-1 and HSV-2. The HSV-1 Mtr (Mtr-1) region maps in the left part of the U_L region (Fig. 1) (21), and no demonstration of a viral gene product is at hand. It would appear that the Mtr-1 gene product is not required for maintenance of the transformed phenotype. The situation in HSV-2 is no less complex. A major Mtr-2 region lies in the HSV-2 *Bgl*II fragment N (42,58,131). This region corresponds to the right-hand portion of *Hin*dIII fragment K and the left portion of *Hin*dIII fragment L of HSV-1. Two research groups have detected a 38,000- to 40,000-d polypeptide in some HSV-2-transformed cells (42,58). This corresponds to the same size polypeptide encoded by the 1.5-kb β mRNA mapping at the *Hin*dIII site at 0.592 in HSV-1 (5). Further, Galloway et al. (58) have found that this region of HSV-2 also has sequences homologous to a 138,000-d polypeptide and a 58,000-d polypeptide, both homologous to similar size polypeptides seen in HSV-1 infection (5,54). It is natural to suggest, as do Docherty et al. (42), that the 38,000-d polypeptide seen in HSV-2-transformed cells is somehow involved with the action of the Mtr-2 region. However, Galloway has found that even though the left-hand region of HSV-2 DNA *Bgl*II fragment N that encodes this polypeptide is able to induce transformation, it is not necessarily maintained in transformed cells. If this be the case, then this putative "transforming" protein is not required for maintenance of this phenotype. It is clear, then, that this polypeptide is an interesting one, and although it appears to map colinearly with a similar polypeptide in HSV-1, it also is clear there are important differences. The HSV-1 mRNA encoding the polypeptide is not highly abundant (5), and there are no reports to date that this region is an Mtr in HSV-1. It is tempting to speculate that the differences between the polypeptides from HSV-1 and HSV-2 will have impact on studies on the mechanism of viral transformation.

To add to the confusion, it is clear that HSV-2 DNA encoded in *Bgl*II fragment C (just to the left of the Mtr-2 discussed earlier) also can transform cells (74). No particular viral polypeptide or mRNA involved with this Mtr-2 has yet been identified, and, again, there is no evidence that the region from HSV-1 DNA induces transformation. From this it is clear that despite the readily identifiable biological marker for transformation, full identification of an HSV "transforming" gene is not yet at hand.

The latency phase of HSV infection is another biologically interesting marker. It is well established that latent HSV is harbored in nerve cells (144–146). Further, it is clear that herpes genes are required to induce latency (88). Recently, Galloway, McDougall, and associates have found that RNA mapping in the left 30% of the U_L region of HSV-1 can be detected in sections of human autopsy neurons that can reasonably be assumed to contain latent virus (56,57). Interpretation is complicated by the possibility of reactivation, especially in light of the fact that the most abundant mRNA in HSV-infected cells maps in this region (34). HSV nucleic acid can be detected in persistently infected cultured neural cells (60,84,85), and the recently described cultured cell models for herpesvirus latency (46,172) should have an impact in assigning the latency function to a specific gene product.

The fact that HSV encodes so much of its own machinery for DNA replication, which must be β functions, means that a number of enzymological and DNA-associating functions involved in DNA replication are potentially identifiable. Four specific DNA replication functions are carefully mapped, and the mRNA encoding two of them is at least partially characterized. The HSV DNA polymerase marker was mapped, by virtue of the association of phosphonoacetic acid sensitivity with it, to the region around *Eco*RI fragment M (24,39). HSV DNA polymerase is a single polypeptide of about 145,000 d (118) with two functional domains (28). The general map location of the enzymatic function led us to suggest that a 4.5-kb β mRNA found isolable using *Eco*RI fragment M might encode the HSV-1 DNA polyermase, because it could encode a polypeptide of about that size (159). However, Powell et al. (119) also found a major early DNA binding protein of this same size mapping in this region of HSV-1; so it is clear that the situation is more complex than originally envisioned. Certainly, careful mRNA isolation and translation, perhaps coupled with immune precipitation and/or biological assay, will lead to definitive identification of both these mRNAs.

The tk gene of HSV-1 is a favorite subject for study by virtue of its tremendous utility as a selectable marker (78,91,103,113,169). Its mRNA has been identified by biological assay of size-fractionated infected cell mRNA (37,38,121), assay of hybrid-selected mRNA translation products (125), and assay of coupled transcription-translation products synthesized in amphibian oocytes microinjected with cloned *Bam*HI fragment P (33,99). This enzyme is encoded by a 1,200-base coding sequence mapping in this *Bam*HI fragment, and as will be discussed later, the expression of the gene in transfected cells has allowed some careful analyses of HSV promoters.

Recently, Preston and associates used enzymatic assay and hybrid-arrested translation to locate the coding region for the alkaline exonuclease encoded by HSV-1 in the region 0.15 to 0.2 (124). Several early mRNAs were located in that region (Fig. 1), although none exactly corresponded to the size of the exonuclease mRNA reported (3.6 kb).

Such enzymatic assays are ideal subjects for use of hybrid-arrested translation techniques, because one is assaying a single entity–activity. In principle, any identifiable translation product can be mapped by hybrid arrest (111); however, with HSV the complexity of the total translation products makes this difficult, unless careful two-dimensional gel analysis is carried out, or unless a hybrid-selected mRNA population is used first. We did use it to confirm the fact that *Hin*dIII fragment J (34) is homologous to an mRNA encoding the only major 155,000-d polypeptide translated from total late mRNA. This experiment is shown in Fig. 9. This information, along with the close correspondence between the map location of the 6-kb mRNA encoding this polypeptide and the location of the 155,000-d major HSV-1 capsid protein by intertypic recombinant mapping, allows us to be relatively sure that this very abundant mRNA does, indeed, encode this protein. It also is clear, however, that immune precipitation will be the best evidence.

Most of the *in vitro* translation products determined for the precisely located mRNAs shown in Fig. 7 correspond to infected cell viral proteins seen mapping in the same region by intertypic recombinant studies (94,101). For example, there is a major 140,000-d polypeptide mapping at about 0.56 in infected cells, several small phosphoproteins mapping between 0.7 and 0.72, and so forth. Until the

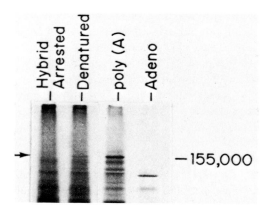

FIG. 9. Hybrid-arrested translation to locate the mRNA encoding the major 155,000-d polypeptide in HSV-1. This experiment is based on the technique of Paterson et al. (111) and is described by Costa et al. (34). Total late infected cell poly(A) mRNA encodes a 155,000-d polypeptide. Its translation is arrested when the RNA is hybridized to *Hin*dIII fragment J DNA, but is recovered when the hybrids are denatured.

biological function of these proteins is known, however, we can only tentatively identify them with specific mRNAs.

DESCRIPTION OF A "TYPICAL" HSV-1 GENE

Control Regions

The lack of splices in most HSV-1 mRNAs and the fact that a very small segment of viral DNA (*Bam*HI fragment P) can transduce expressible tk activity (91,169) suggested that HSV genes have control regions (promoters) rather near the structural gene. Full nucleotide sequence analysis of the HSV-1 tk gene has shown that there are recognizable "TATA" (14,15) and "CAT" box (95) sequences within 100 bases of the 5' end of the mRNA (98,161). Controlled deletion experiments by McKnight and collaborators have demonstrated that sequences beyond 120 bases upstream of the 5' end of the viral mRNA are not required for expression of the tk in amphibian oocytes (99,100). This allows one to define a promoter region in the 120 bases directly upstream of the 5' end of the viral mRNA. One thus can describe a typical HSV-1 gene as shown in Fig. 10. The rather elegant experiments of Post et al. (117), in which an α promoter was made to control the normally β tk gene, have demonstrated that α promoters also are closely linked to the 5' end of the mRNA. We are carrying out comparative sequence analysis around the 5' ends of several models of early and late viral mRNAs. Such experiments require precise positioning of the 5' end of the mRNA by S1 nuclease or exonuclease VII digestion of a hybrid formed between the mRNA and a DNA fragment 5'-labeled very near the position of the 5' end of the mRNA. Such a hybrid-protected DNA fragment, run on a sequencing gel, provides a direct location of the 5' end of the mRNA (Fig. 11). We did such analysis on the 5' end region of the 5.2-kb β mRNA in *Hind*III fragment K and the 6-kb βγ mRNA in *Bgl*II fragment N (55), as well as the 1.5 β mRNA mapping in the 3' region of the 5.2-kb early mRNA (43) and the 2.7-kb γ mRNA mapping through the *Eco*RI site at 0.63 (R. Frink and E. Wagner, *unpublished data*). Comparisons of the nucleotide sequences from the 5' ends of the mRNAs to 35 bases upstream, and from 75 to 115 bases upstream, are shown in Fig. 12, along with data for the HSV-1 tk gene (98,161) and for the α 4.7-kb

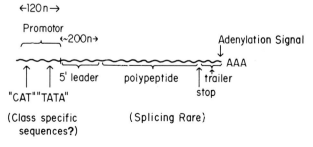

FIG. 10. A "typical" HSV-1 gene. The data used to arrive at the parameters are discussed in the text.

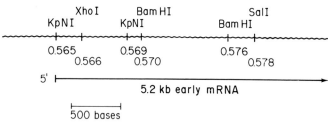

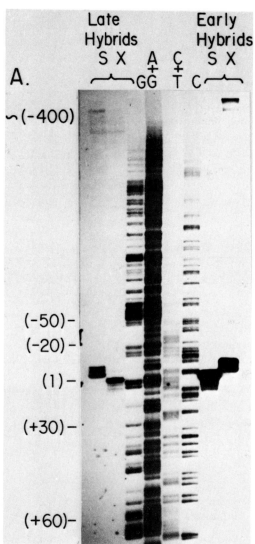

FIG. 11. Precise localization of the 5′ end of the 5.2-kb early mRNA mapping in *Hind*III fragment K. The left-hand portion shows the fine-structure restriction map of the region near the 5′ end of this mRNA. This has been described by Frink et al. (55). RNA was 5′-end-labeled at the *Xho*I site at 0.566 and hybridized to early or late viral mRNA. Exonuclease-VII- or S1-nuclease-protected fragments were run against a Maxam-Gilbert (96) sequencing gel from the same 5′-labeled DNA to locate the end of the mRNA.

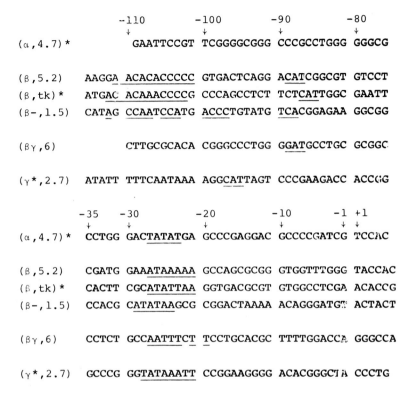

```
                   -110         -100        -90          -80
                    ↓            ↓           ↓            ↓
(α,4.7)*                  GAATTCCGT TCGGGGCGGG CCCGCCTGGG GGGCG


(β,5.2)     AAGGA ACACACCCCC GTGACTCAGG ACATCGGCGT GTCCT
(β,tk)*     ATGAC ACAAACCCCG CCCAGCCTCT TCTCATTGGC GAATT
(β-,1.5)    CATAG CCAATCCATG ACCCTGTATG TCACGGAGAA GGCGG


(βγ,6)            CTTGCGCACA CGGGCCCTGG GGATGCCTGC GCGGC


(γ*,2.7)    ATATT TTTCAATAAA AGGCATTAGT CCCGAAGACC ACCGG


            -35   -30         -20          -10        -1  +1
             ↓     ↓           ↓            ↓          ↓  ↓
(α,4.7)*    CCTGG GACTATATGA GCCCGAGGAC GCCCCGATCG TCCAC


(β,5.2)     CGATG GAAATAAAAA GCCAGCGCGG GTGGTTTGGG TACCAC
(β,tk)*     CACTT CGCATATTAA GGTGACGCGT GTGGCCTCGA ACACCG
(β-,1.5)    CCACG CATATAAGCG CGGACTAAAA ACAGGGATGT ACTACT


(βγ,6)      CCTCT GCCAATTTCT TCCTGCACGC TTTTGGACCA GGGCCA


(γ*,2.7)    GCCCG GGTATAAATT CCGGAAGGGG ACACGGGCTA CCCTG
```

FIG. 12. Comparative DNA sequences upstream of the 5′ ends of the 4.2-kb (α), 5.2-kb tk and 1.5-kb (β), 6-kb (βγ), and 2.7-kb (γ) mRNAs discussed in the text. The sequence of the mRNA "sense" strand is shown.

mRNA encoding ICP4 mapping in the short repeat region (89). All 5′ ends of the mRNAs have an AC at or very near the start; all have TATA boxes around 28 to 30 bases upstream. The β, βγ, and γ mRNAs have a CAT sequence or variant of it (GAT or TCA) 85 to 95 bases upstream, but no such sequence is seen for the α gene. Finally, all three β mRNAs have a region containing only A's and C's between 100 and 110 bases upstream. Only further comparative and sequence-modification studies will yield data on precisely which elements (if any) in the 120-base control region define HSV mRNAs as early or late. Such studies also may reveal other sequences removed from this 120-base region that influence viral gene expression. In spite of such caveats, it is tempting to speculate that sequences within these HSV promoters do have a role in temporal expression. As will be discussed later, it is clear that many, if not all, early viral genes can be recognized by unmodified host polymerase and thus have promoters recognizable as open to RNA polymerase II.

Properties of "Typical" HSV-1 Structural Genes

At the time of writing, full sequence data on only tk (98,161) and the 1.5-kb early mRNA mapping through the *Hind*III site at 0.59 (43) are available to me.

However, other partial sequence data can be used to fill in a picture of the structure of a typical HSV gene. In the case of both tk and the 1.5-kb β mRNA, the initiation codon (AUG) occurs about 150 bases downstream of the 5' end of the mRNA. A similar-length leader is seen to the first open reading in the 2.7-kb late mRNA (R. Frink and E. Wagner, *unpublished data*), and leaders at least 240 bases and 320 bases long are seen for reading frames for the 5.2-kb (β) and 6-kb (βγ) mRNAs (55). It is clear, then, that a leader on the order of 200 bases is a reasonable choice for the typical gene shown in Fig. 10.

The factors that determine whether or not a given AUG sequence near the 5' end of an mRNA molecule will act as a translation initiator are unknown. Kozak (80) identified the sequence Pu-base-base-A-U-G-G as a very common one for an initiator. This sequence G-C-C-A-U-G-G initiates the 40,000-d polypeptide encoded by the 1.5-kb β mRNA sequenced by Draper et al. (43), but the relatively rarely used sequence C-G-U-A-U-G-G is found for HSV-1 tk.

Because HSV-1 mRNA generally lacks splices, one would expect the reading frame to stay open between initiation and termination codons. The length of sequence following the terminator codon (trailer) and the actual end of the mRNA is about 80 bases for HSV-1 tk and 50 bases for the 1.5-kb β mRNA. In certain cases, to be discussed in the next section, the trailer sequence can be extremely long. Such length arises if an mRNA initiates in the interior of another mRNA beyond the translation terminator of the latter. An example is the 5.2-kb β mRNA that overlies the 1.5-kb mRNA. Our sequence analysis shows chain terminators in all three reading frames upstream of the 5' end of the 1.5-kb mRNA. Therefore, the trailer for the 5.2-kb mRNA is over 1,000 bases. Similar findings have been reported by Clements and McLauchlan (25). Of course, if the overlapping mRNA is quite long, very long trailers can occur. The 7-kb γ mRNA, whose 5' end is upstream of the 5.2-kb (5) mRNA, would appear to have a trailer of 5 kb length.

The sequence A-A-T-A-A-A-A appears to be a nominal transcription terminator signal for eukaryotic mRNAs (128). This sequence ends HSV-1 tk mRNA and is found near the 3' ends of the colinear 7-kb, 5.2-kb, and 1.5-kb mRNAs of *Hin*dIII fragment K (43) and near the 3' ends of several other HSV-1 mRNAs, including the 2.7 γ mRNA in *Hin*dIII fragment L (R. Frink and E. Wagner, *unpublished data*).

Generation of HSV mRNA Families

The simple model for a typical HSV-1 gene shown in Fig. 10 suggests that the virus is aptly named in terms of mRNA packaging, if not in terms of biology, genome arrangment, or other parameters. In spite of this simple picture, it is clear from the high-resolution maps of Fig. 7 that overlapping HSV-1 mRNA families encoding the same or different polypeptides are common. Results from our laboratory indicate that a number of mechanisms for the generation of these families are operating in HSV transcription (Fig. 13).

One method of generating overlapping mRNAs is by having a second promoter nearby upstream or downstream of the principal one. Such a promoter could have

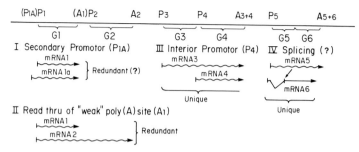

FIG. 13. Schematic representation of the generation of overlapping HSV-1 mRNA families. As described in the text, all the illustrated precursors have been observed with HSV-1.

the same or different temporal regulation. If the promoter affected the length of leader sequence, the two mRNAs would encode the same polypeptide products and would be redundant. An example of such mRNAs includes two minor colinear mRNAs seen mapping in *Hind*III fragment L (0.592–0.647) (54). A second example is found where a minor promoter appears to lie about 450 bases upstream of the major one for the abundant β mRNA mapping in *Hind*III fragment K (0.527–0.592) (55). A potentially very interesting example is found with colinear mRNAs mapping with their 5′ ends near the *Bgl*II site at 0.7 (63). Here, the upstream promoter appears to be late, whereas the downstream principal promoter is a β. Such a region will be very useful in studies of structural differences between promoter classes.

There is no *a priori* reason why such multiple promoters need generate redundant mRNAs, and situations may be found where an upstream promoter leads to an mRNA molecule with additional encoded amino acids or an altered reading frame. Such phenomena are seen in other virus systems (10), and their analysis requires sophisticated genetic and molecular techniques. On the basis of *in vitro* translation, none of the multiple mRNAs mentioned earlier falls into such a category, but *in vitro* translation can lead to artifacts because of lack of precision in initiation, and so forth. Full sequence analysis of multiple promoters can at least suggest whether or not complex patterns of gene packaging are possible.

Another mechanism for the generation of multiple mRNAs is found when an mRNA species is inefficiently terminated at a given polyadenylation site. Then, transcription proceeds downstream to the next polyadenylation site. Here, two resolvable mRNA species are found that are colinear on their 5′ ends and encode the same polypeptide and translation termination signals, but the largest mRNA contains nontranslated sequences beyond the nominal polyadenylation sites. An example is seen with 1.9-kb and 7-kb γ mRNA species mapping in *Hind*III fragment K (0.527–0.592) (5). A second example is seen at the 3′ end of the colinear mRNAs mapping near the *Bgl*II site at 0.7 (63). Here, the inefficient polyadenylation signal, along with secondary promoters, leads to the rather bizarre situation of having four colinear and apparently redundant mRNAs.

There are several cases where the promoter for an HSV mRNA lies in the interior of another mRNA, but there is no evidence for transcription termination of the latter. The best characterized example is the 1.5-kb β mRNA underlying the 3′ region of the 5.2-kb β and 7-kb γ mRNAs in HindIII fragment K. Other potential examples are seen with the colinear 4.7-kb and 2.5-kb mRNAs mapping to the right of the HindIII site at 0.65 and with the 1.5-kb mRNA underlying the 3′ end of the 6-kb mRNA mapping in BglII fragment N (0.23–0.27). Until it is rigorously established that such mRNAs are not spliced near their 5′ ends, the possibility of a shared promoter remains, but I regard this possibility as rather remote.

The reason for inefficient polyadenylation near the 5′ end of certain mRNAs may lie in the precise sequence of the TATA box of the downstream mRNA. Because the polyadenylation signal appears to be A-A-T-A-A-A-A or its complement, a TATA box resembling this could lead to polyadenylation. Such speculation requires comparative sequence data for confirmation, but the fact that the TATA box for the 5.2-kb β mRNA mapping in HindIII fragment K is A-A-A-T-A-A-A-A-A and maps near the 3′ end of the inefficiently terminated 1.9-kb γ mRNA is at least suggestive evidence.

Splicing of mRNA in the generation of mRNA families, which is so ubiquitous in adenovirus and papovaviruses, must be regarded as relatively infrequent in HSV. There is one apparent case of a family of spliced HSV-1 mRNAs, those mapping between the EcoRI site at 0.63 and the HindIII site at 0.65 (54). Others may be found later. We are carefully analyzing via sequence analysis the information encoded by the 2.7-kb γ mRNA family (R. Frink and E. Wagner, *unpublished data*). The following facts are clear: (a) The unspliced member is the most abundant in infected HeLa cells. (b) This mRNA contains at least two open reading regions, one 525 bases long lying in the 3′ region of the unspliced mRNA and encoding a polypeptide of molecular weight 17,800, based on amino acid composition, and a second reading frame upstream of this and presumably encoding the 69,000-d polypeptide encoded by the 2.7-kb mRNA. (c) When unspliced 2.7-kb mRNA is translated *in vitro*, the polypeptide products seen include both 69,000-d and 17,800-d products (Fig. 14). (d) Two potential leader sequences, one 25 bases long and ending in the sequence T-G-G-T, and one 75 bases long and ending in A-G-G-T, have been identified. Further, three splice acceptor sites, beginning with the sequence A-G, have been located. These sequences are the nominal donor and acceptor sequences for eukaryotic mRNA splices (86,137). (e) The location of the splices is such as to remove the initiator sequence for the open frame seen in the unspliced mRNA; so splicing could potentially play a role in the differential expression of the 69,000-d and 17,800-d polypeptides. This must be regarded as a very tentative conclusion, particularly because of the observed low frequency of splices. Hopefully, further experiments now in progress and projected will clarify the significance of the observed splices in this mRNA family.

Possible Mechanisms Controlling HSV Gene Expression

The search for the factors that control the temporal regulation of DNA virus gene expression is an active field of research. It has long been known that RNA poly-

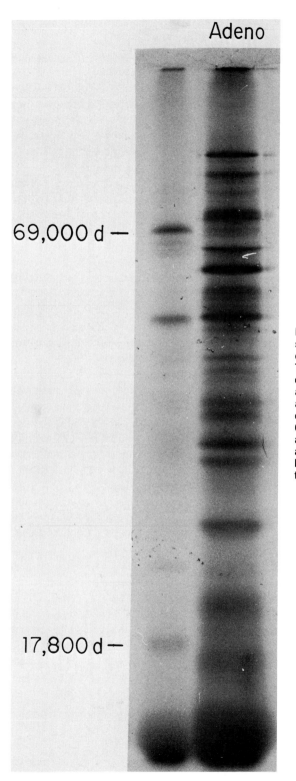

FIG. 14. Translation of unspliced 2.7-kb HSV-1 mRNA encoded in the region 0.63 to 0.65. The *in vitro* translation was carried out as described by Frink et al. (54), and products were size-fractionated next to the translation product of adenovirus mRNA. Both the 69,000-d and 17,800-d products are clearly seen. The bands at around 60,000 d and the major band at 50,000 d are endogenous to the system.

merase II can use HSV DNA as a template, but the question remains as to specific recognition of viral genes (2,17,35,135). The development of faithful uninfected cell transcription systems (92), as well as other techniques, has led to the following observations concerning this regulation in the smaller DNA viruses. In the papovaviruses (132), the uninfected cell polymerase system favors the recognition of promoters for early genes. However, this preference is not absolute, and at relatively high template DNA concentrations the late promoters are efficiently recognized. In adenovirus, the situation is somewhat different, in that the major late promoter appears to be readily recognized during the early phases of adenovirus gene expression. Here, the appearance of abundant late mRNA involves changes in processing patterns of mRNA precursors, although some adenovirus promoters may require viral functions for recognition (50).

We have examined the ability of an uninfected cell "Manley" (92) polymerase system to recognize HSV-1 promoters (43,55). We have found, using transcription "run-off" and, more recently, S1 nuclease protection analysis, that accurate (± 20 bases) transcription initiation occurs at regions corresponding to the 5' ends of the 5.2-kb, 1.5-kb, and 1.8-kb β mRNAs mapping in *Hin*dIII fragments K and L. It also is clear that the HSV-1 tk gene is recognizable by RNA polymerase II, because accurate expression of this gene is seen in amphibian oocytes and biochemically transformed cells. *In vitro* studies using the HSV-1 tk gene and RNA polymerase II systems have yielded more complex results than we found with our early mRNAs, because a number of transcription initiations have been seen (13,136).

This latter case, and the fact that the Manley polymerase system can recognize transcription initiation signals in pBR322 and other DNA sequences not normally functioning as promoters, makes it imperative that *in vitro* transcription studies be interpreted very conservatively. However, it is clear that some aspects of the structure of the promoters for these β HSV-1 genes must share features with those of cellular ones. In spite of this inferred similarity between HSV-1 early promoters and cellular promoters, there are important differences between the structures of early HSV-1 and cellular genes. First, many of the HSV-1 mRNAs are not spliced; therefore, any requirements for splicing in the expression of cellular genes cannot be present here. Second, the HSV-1 β genes are not efficiently expressed in cells in which the α genes are not expressed or are not functional.

The mechanism of modulation of HSV gene expression by the α gene ICP4 is unknown, but certain facts are clear. First, HSV DNA is not packaged as cellular chromatin in infected cells (83), and HSV uncoating in the infected cell appears to be a regulated process (79). It is consistent with known data to speculate that HSV early gene promoters are blocked in the infected cell and that the α gene product serves to open or activate them. The mechanism of the blocking is unknown; however, it cannot be purely physical, because α promoters can be linked to β genes and cause their expression as α genes (117). The blocking is very efficient, because no tk transcription can be seen at all under α conditions (84). Further, superinfection of cells carrying the HSV tk gene results in increased gene activity (82).

We have not seen efficient transcription of βγ or γ HSV-1 genes using uninfected cell polymerase (55). This does not mean that there is no low-level transcription, but it must be of considerably lower efficiency than early transcription. The lack of efficient recognition of late HSV-1 genes by the polymerase may be due to unique features of the DNA sequence around late HSV-1 promoters, as compared with cellular and early promoters, as well as to the action of viral or cellular modulators during normal infection. Unique structural elements of late HSV-1 promoters may define them as "late" and may become apparent when further comparative sequence studies are carried out and the data are compared with the growing amount of information concerning similar areas for cellular genes. Studies using infected cell polymerase preparations also will be of value. The data so far suggest, however, that differential promoter recognition has a definite role in the temporal regulation of HSV transcription.

It is important to conclude this section with a strong caution in that the mechanistic interpretation of control of HSV gene function is based on the very simple three-phase cascade described in an earlier section. In fact, the situation is much more complex. Certain β genes are marginally expressed under nominal α conditions (4,68). Other β genes are delayed beyond normal time of β expression. We have found that α mRNAs continue to be synthesized as translatable mRNA throughout infection, but are not amplified (4). Although there does not appear to be a hierarchy of α genes based on stringency of inhibition of protein synthesis (90), it is possible that different α genes regulate the expression of different groups of β genes (114,122). Finally, certain late genes are expressed in the absence of DNA replication, although they do not become abundant, and other late genes are delayed. This complex pattern suggests the control mechanisms will be complex, and the approaches toward studies described here will serve as only a very general outline of the detailed processes.

ACKNOWLEDGMENTS

Work described in this review was performed using funds from the National Institutes of Health (CA-11861), the National Institute of Alcoholism and Alcohol Abuse (AA-03506), and a University of California, Irvine, institutional grant from the American Cancer Society to Dr. R. Frink. I wish to thank current workers in our laboratory (R. Costa, K. Draper, R. Frink, and L. Hall) for allowing me to quote their work in progress. I am grateful to J. Wagner for manuscript editing.

REFERENCES

1. Alwine, J., Kemp, D., and Stark, G. (1977): Method for detection of specific RNAs in agarose gels by transfer to diazobenzyloxymethyl-paper and hybridization with DNA probes. *Proc. Natl. Acad. Sci. USA*, 74:5350–5354.
2. Alwine, J., Steinhart, W., and Hill, C. (1974): Transcription of herpes simplex type 1 DNA in nuclei isolated from infected HEp-2 and KB cells. *Virology*, 60:302–307.
3. Anderson, C., Lewis, J., Atkins, J., and Gesteland, R. (1974): Cell free synthesis of adenovirus 2 proteins programmed by fractionated messenger RNA: A comparison of polypeptide products and messenger RNA lengths. *Proc. Natl. Acad. Sci. USA*, 71:2756–2760.

4. Anderson, K., Costa, R., Holland, L., and Wagner, E. (1980): Characterization and translation of HSV-1 mRNA abundant in the absence of *de novo* protein synthesis. *J. Virol.*, 34:9–27.
5. Anderson, K., Frink, R., Devi, G., Gaylord, B., Costa, R., and Wagner, E. (1981): Detailed characterization of the mRNA mapping in the *Hin*dIII fragment K region of the HSV-1 genome. *J. Virol.*, 37:1011–1027.
6. Anderson, K., Holland, L., Gaylord, B., and Wagner, E. (1980): Isolation and translation of mRNA encoded by a specific region of the herpes simplex virus type 1 genome. *J. Virol.*, 33:749–759.
7. Anderson, K., Stringer, J., Holland, L., and Wagner, E. (1979): Isolation and localization of HSV-1 mRNA. *J. Virol.*, 30:805–820.
8. Bachenheimer, S., and Roizman, B. (1972): Ribonucleic acid synthesis in cells infected with herpes simplex virus. VI: Polyadenylic acid sequences in viral messenger ribonucleic acid. *J. Virol.*, 10:875–879.
9. Bailey, J., and Davison, N. (1976): Methylmercury as a reversible denaturing agent for agarose gel electrophoresis. *Anal. Biochem.*, 70:75–85.
10. Barrell, B., Air, G., and Hutchison, C., III (1976): Overlapping genes in bacteriophage. *Nature*, 264:34–41.
11. Bartkoski, M., and Roizman, B. (1976): RNA synthesis in cells infected with herpes simplex virus. XIII: Differences in the methylation patterns of viral RNA during the reproductive cycle. *J. Virol.*, 20:583–588.
12. Bayliss, G., Marsden, H., and Hay, J. (1975): Herpes simplex virus proteins: DNA-binding proteins in infected cells and in the virus structure. *Virology*, 68:124–134.
13. Beck, T., and Millette, R. (1981): *In vitro* transcription of HSV-1 DNA by RNA polymerase II from HEp-2 cells. In: *International Workshop on Herpesviruses*, edited by A. S. Kaplan, M. La Placa, F. Rapp, and B. Roizman, p. 62. Esculapio Publishing, Bologna.
14. Benoist, C., and Chambon, P. (1981): *In vivo* sequence requirements of the SV40 early promoter region. *Nature*, 290:304–310.
15. Benoist, C., O'Hare, K., Breathnach, R., and Chambon, P. (1980): The ovalbumin gene—sequence of putative control regions. *Nucleic Acids Res.*, 8:127–142.
16. Ben-Porat, T., Jean, J.-H., and Kaplan, A. (1974): Early functions of the genome of herpesvirus. IV. Fate and translation of immediate-early viral RNA. *Virology*, 59:524–531.
17. Ben-Zeev, A., and Becker, Y. (1977): Requirement of host cell RNA polymerase II in the replication of herpes simplex virus in α-amantin-sensitive and -resistant cell lines. *Virology*, 76:246–253.
18. Berk, A., and Sharp, P. (1977): Sizing and mapping of early adenovirus mRNAs by gel electrophoresis of S1 endonuclease-digested hybrids. *Cell*, 12:721–732.
19. Berk, A., and Sharp, P. (1978): Spliced early mRNAs of simian virus 40. *Proc. Natl. Acad. Sci. USA*, 75:1274–1278.
20. Berk, A., and Sharp, P. (1978): Structure of the adenovirus 2 early mRNAs. *Cell*, 14:695–711.
21. Camacho, A., and Spear, P. (1978): Transformation of hamster embryo fibroblasts by a specific fragment of the herpes simplex virus genome. *Cell*, 15:993–1002.
22. Casey, J., and Davidson, N. (1977): Rate of formation and thermal stabilities of RNA:DNA and DNA:DNA duplexes at high concentrations of formamide. *Nucleic Acids Res.*, 4:1539–1552.
23. Chartrand, P., Crumpacker, C., Schaffer, P., and Wilkie, N. (1980): Physical and genetic analysis of the herpes simplex virus DNA polymerase locus. *Virology*, 103:311–326.
24. Chartrand, P., Stow, N., Timbury, M., and Wilkie, N. (1979): Physical mapping of *paa* mutations of herpes simplex virus type 1 and type 2 by intertypic marker rescue. *J. Virol.*, 31:265–276.
25. Clements, J., and McLauchlan, J. (1981): Control regions involved in the expression of two 3' co-terminal early mRNAs. In: *International Workshop on Herpesviruses*, edited by A. S. Kaplan, M. La Placa, F. Rapp, and B. Roizman, p. 57. Esculapio Publishing, Bologna.
26. Clements, J., McLauchlan, J., and McGeoch, D. (1979): Orientation of herpes simplex virus type 1 immediate-early mRNAs. *Nucleic Acids Res.*, 7:77–91.
27. Clements, J., Watson, R., and Wilkie, N. (1977): Temporal regulation of herpes simplex virus type 1 transcription: Location of transcripts on the viral genome. *Cell*, 12:275–285.
28. Coen, D., and Schaffer, P. (1980): Two distinct loci confer resistance to acycloguanosine in herpes simplex virus type 1. *Proc. Natl. Acad. Sci. USA*, 77:2265–2269.
29. Cohen, G., Long, D., and Eisenberg, R. (1980): Synthesis and processing of glycoproteins gD and gC of herpes simplex virus type 1. *J. Virol.*, 36:429–439.

30. Cohen, J., Perdue, M., Randall, C., and O'Callaghan, D. (1977): Herpesvirus transcription: Altered regulation induced by FUdR. *Virology*, 76:621–633.
31. Cohen, J., Randall, C., and O'Callaghan, D. (1975): Transcription of equine herpesvirus type 1: Evidence for classes of transcripts differing in abundance. *Virology*, 68:561–565.
32. Conley, A., Knipe, D., Jones, P., and Roizman, B. (1981): Molecular genetics of herpes simplex virus. VII. Characterization of a temperature-sensitive mutant produced by *in vitro* mutagenesis and defective in DNA synthesis and accumulation of γ polypeptides. *J. Virol.*, 37:191–206.
33. Cordingly, M., and Preston, C. (1981): Transcription and translation of the herpes simplex virus type 1 thymidine kinase gene after microinjection into *Xenopus laevis* oocytes. *J. Gen. Virol.*, 54:409–414.
34. Costa, R., Devi, G., Anderson, K., Gaylord, B., and Wagner, E. (1981): Characterization of a major late HSV-1 mRNA. *J. Virol.*, 38:483–496.
35. Costanzo, F., Campadelli-Fiume, G., Foa-Tomasi, L., and Cassai, E. (1977): Evidence that herpes simplex virus DNA is transcribed by cellular RNA polymerase B. *J. Virol.*, 21:996–1001.
36. Courtney, R., Schaffer, P., and Powell, K. (1976): Synthesis of virus-specific polypeptides by temperature-sensitive mutants of herpes simplex virus type 1. *Virology*, 75:306–318.
37. Cremer, K., Bodemer, M., and Summers, W. (1978): Characterization of the mRNA for herpes simplex virus thymidine kinase by cell-free synthesis of active enzyme. *Nucleic Acids Res.*, 5:2333–2344.
38. Cremer, K., Summers, W., and Gesteland, R. (1977): Cell-free synthesis of herpes simplex virus proteins. *J. Virol.*, 22:750–757.
39. Crumpacker, C., Chartrand, P., Subak-Sharpe, J., and Wilkie, N. (1980): Resistance of herpes simplex virus to acycloguanosine—genetic and physical analysis. *Virology*, 105:171–184.
40. DeMarchi, J., Schmidt, C., and Kaplan, A. (1980): Patterns of transcription of human cytomeg alovirus in permissively infected cells. *J. Virol.*, 35:277–286.
41. Dixon, R., and Schaffer, P. (1980): Fine-structure mapping and functional analysis of temperature-sensitive mutants in the gene encoding the herpes simplex virus type 1 immediate-early protein VP175. *J. Virol.*, 36:189–203.
42. Docherty, J., Subak-Sharpe, J., and Preston, C. (1981): Identification of a virus-specific poly-peptide associated with a transforming fragment (*Bgl*II-N) of herpes simplex virus type 2 DNA. *J. Virol.*, 40:126–132.
43. Draper, K., Frink, R., and Wagner, E. (1982): Detailed characterization of an unspliced β HSV-1 gene mapping in the interior of another. *J. Virol.*, 43:1123–1128.
44. Duff, R., and Rapp, F. (1971): Oncogenic transformation of hamster cells after exposure to herpes simplex virus type 2. *Nature [New Biol.]*, 233:48–50.
45. Duff, R., and Rapp, F. (1973): Oncogenic transformation of hamster embryo cells after exposure to inactivated herpes simplex virus type 1. *J. Virol.*, 12:209–217.
46. Dutko, F., and Oldstone, M. (1981): Cytomegalovirus causes a latent infection in undifferentiated cells and is activated by induction of cell differentiation. *J. Exp. Med.*, 154:1636–1640.
47. Enquist, L., Madden, M., Schiop-Stansly, P., and Vande Woude, G. (1979): Cloning of herpes simplex type 1 DNA fragments in a bacteriophage lambda vector. *Science*, 203:541–544.
48. Feldman, L., Rixon, F., Jean, J.-H., Ben-Porat, T., and Kaplan, A. (1979): Transcription of the genome of pseudorabies virus (a herpesvirus) is strictly controlled. *Virology*, 97:316–327.
49. Fenwick, M., Morse, L., and Roizman, B. (1979): Anatomy of herpes simplex virus DNA. XI. Apparent clustering of functions effecting rapid inhibition of host DNA and protein synthesis. *J. Virol.*, 29:825–827.
50. Fire, A., Baker, C., Manley, J., Ziff, E., and Sharp, P. (1981): In vitro transcription of adenovirus. *J. Virol.*, 40:703–719.
51. Flint, S., and Broker, T. (1981): Lytic infection by adenoviruses. In: *Molecular Biology of Tumor Viruses. Part II: DNA Tumor Viruses*, edited by J. Tooze, pp. 443–546. Cold Spring Harbor Laboratory, Cold Spring Harbor, N.Y.
52. Frenkel, N., and Roizman, B. (1972): Ribonucleic acid synthesis in cells infected with herpes simplex virus. VI. Control of transcription and of RNA abundance. *Proc. Natl. Acad. Sci. USA*, 69:2654–2658.
53. Frenkel, N., Roizman, B., Cassai, E., and Nahmias, A. (1972): A herpes simplex 2 DNA fragment and its transcription in human cervical cancer tissue. *Proc. Natl. Acad. Sci. USA*, 69:3784–3789.
54. Frink, R., Anderson, K., and Wagner, E. (1981): Herpes simplex virus type 1 *Hind*III fragment L encodes spliced and complementary mRNA species. *J. Virol.*, 39:559–572.

55. Frink, R., Draper, K., and Wagner, E. (1981): Uninfected cell polymerase efficiently transcribes early not not late herpes simplex virus type 1 mRNA. *Proc. Natl. Acad. Sci. USA*, 78:6139–6143.

56. Galloway, D., Fenoglio, C., and McDougall, J. (1982): Limited transcription of the herpes simplex virus genome when latent in human sensory ganglia. *J. Virol.*, 41:686–691.

57. Galloway, D., Fenoglio, C., Shevchuk, M., and McDougall, J. (1979): Detection of herpes simplex RNA in human sensory ganglia. *Virology*, 95:265–268.

58. Galloway, D., Goldstein, L., and Lewis, J. (1982): The identification of proteins encoded by a fragment of HSV-2 DNA that has transforming activity. *J. Virol.*, 42:530–537.

59. Gibson, W., and Roizman, B. (1972): Proteins specified by herpes simplex virus. VIII. Characterization and composition of multiple capsid forms of subtypes 1 and 2. *J. Virol.*, 10:1044–1052.

60. Goldin, A., Sandri-Goldin, R., and Levine, M. (1981): Persistence of viral sequences from the short region of the HSV-1 genome in neuronal cells. In: *International Workshop on Herpesviruses*, edited by A. S. Kaplan, M. La Placa, F. Rapp, and B. Roizman, p. 143. Esculapio Publishing, Bologna.

61. Goldin, A., Sandri-Goldin, R., Levine, M., and Glorioso, J. (1981): Cloning of herpes simplex virus type 1 sequences representing the whole genome. *J. Virol.*, 38:50–58.

62. Grafstrom, R., Alwine, J., Steinhart, W., Hill, C., and Hyman, R. (1975): The terminal repetition of herpes simplex virus DNA. *Virology*, 67:144–157.

63. Hall, L., Draper, K., Frink, R., Costa, R., and Wagner, E. (1982): HSV mRNA species mapping in EcoRI fragment I. *J. Virol.*, 43:594–607.

64. Halliburton, I. (1980): Review article: Intertypic recombinants of herpes simplex viruses. *J. Gen. Virol.*, 48:1–23.

65. Hamer, D., and Leder, P. (1979): Splicing and the formation of stable RNA. *Cell*, 18:1299–1302.

66. Hayward, G., Jacob, R., Wadsworth, S., and Roizman, B. (1975): Anatomy of herpes simplex virus DNA: Evidence for four populations of molecules that differ in the relative orientations of their long and short components. *Proc. Natl. Acad. Sci. USA*, 72:4243–4247.

67. Holland, L., Anderson, K., Shipman, C., Jr., and Wagner, E. (1980): Viral DNA synthesis is required for the efficient expression of specific herpes simplex virus type 1 mRNA species. *Virology*, 101:10–24.

68. Holland, L. Anderson, K., Stringer, J., and Wagner, E. (1979): Isolation and localization of HSV-1 mRNA abundant prior to viral DNA synthesis. *J. Virol.*, 31:447–462.

69. Honess, R., and Roizman, B. (1973): Proteins specified by herpes simplex virus. XI. Identification and relative molar rates of synthesis of structural and nonstructural herpes virus polypeptides in the infected cell. *J. Virol.*, 12:1347–1365.

70. Honess, R., and Roizman, B. (1974): Regulation of herpesvirus macromolecular synthesis. I. Cascade regulation of the synthesis of three groups of viral proteins. *J. Virol.*, 14:8–19.

71. Honess, R., and Roizman, B. (1975): Regulation of herpesvirus macromolecular synthesis: Sequential transition of polypeptide synthesis requires functional viral polypeptides. *Proc. Natl. Acad. Sci. USA*, 72:1276–1280.

72. Huang, H., Szabocsik, J., Randall, C., and Gentry, G. (1971): Equine abortion (herpes) virus-specific RNA. *Virology*, 45:381–389.

73. Hummel, M., and Kieff, E. (1982): Epstein-Barr virus RNA. VII. Viral RNA in permissively infected B95-8 cells. *J. Virol.*, 43:262–272.

74. Jariwalla, R., Aurelian, L., and Tso, P. (1980): Tumorigenic transformation induced by a specific fragment of DNA from HSV-2. *Proc. Natl. Acad. Sci. USA*, 77:2279–2283.

75. Jean, J.-H., Ben-Porat, T., and Kaplan, A. (1974): Early functions of the genome of herpesvirus. III. Inhibition of the transcription of the viral genome in cells treated with cycloheximide early during the infective process. *Virology*, 59:516–523.

76. Jones, P., and Roizman, B. (1979): Regulation of herpesvirus macromolecular synthesis. VIII. The transcription program consists of three phases during which both extent of transcription and accumulation of RNA in the cytoplasm are regulated. *J. Virol.*, 31:299–314.

77. Jones, P., Hayward, G., and Roizman, B. (1977): Anatomy of herpes simplex virus DNA. VII. α RNA is homologous to noncontiguous sites in both the L and S components of viral DNA. *J. Virol.*, 21:268–276.

78. Kit, S., and Dubbs, D. (1963): Acquisition of thymidine kinase activity by herpes simplex infected mouse fibroblast cells. *Biochem. Biophys. Res.Commun.*, 11:55–59.

79. Knipe, D., Batterson, W., Nosal, C., Roizman, B., and Buchan, A. (1981): Molecular genetics of herpes simplex virus. VI. Characterization of a temperature-sensitive mutant defective in the expression of all early viral gene products. *J. Virol.*, 38:539–547.
80. Kozak, M. (1981): Possible role of flanking nucleotides in recognition of the AUG initiator codon by eukaryotic ribosomes. *Nucleic Acids Res.*, 9:5233–5252.
81. Kozak, M., and Roizman, B. (1974): Regulation of herpesvirus macromolecular synthesis: Nuclear retention of nontranslated viral RNA sequences. *Proc. Natl. Acad. Sci. USA*, 71:4322–4326.
82. Leiden, J., Buttyan, R., and Spear, P. (1976): Herpes simplex virus gene expression in transformed cells. I. Regulation of the viral thymidine kinase gene in transformed L cells by products of superinfecting virus. *J. Virol.*, 20:413–424.
83. Leinbach, S., and Summers, W. (1980): The structure of HSV-1 DNA as probed by micrococcal nuclease digestion. *J. Gen. Virol.*, 51:45–59.
84. Leung, W.-C., Dimock, K., Smiley, J., and Bacchetti, S. (1980): Herpes simplex virus thymidine kinase transcripts are absent from both nucleus and cytoplasm during infection in the presence of cycloheximide. *J. Virol.*, 36:361–365.
85. Levine, M., Goldin, A., and Glorioso, J. (1980): Persistence of herpes simplex virus genes in cells of neuronal origin. *J. Virol.*, 35:203–210.
86. Lewin, B. (1980): Alternatives for splicing: Recognizing the ends of introns. *Cell*, 22:324–326.
87. Lewis, J., Atkins, J., Anderson, C., Baum, P., and Gesteland, R. (1975): Mapping of late adenovirus genes by cell-free translation of RNA selected by hybridization to specific DNA fragments. *Proc. Natl. Acad. Sci. USA*, 72:1344–1348.
88. Lofgren, K., Stevens, J., Marsden, H., and Subak-Sharpe, J. (1977): Temperature-sensitive mutants of herpes simplex virus differ in the capacity to establish latent infections in mice. *Virology*, 76:440–443.
89. Mackem, S. (1981): Coordinate expression and fine structures of HSV-1 α genes. In: *International Workshop on Herpesvirus*, edited by A. S. Kaplan, M. La Placa, F. Rapp, and B. Roizman, pp. 80–81. Esculapio Publishing, Bologna.
90. Mackem, S., and Roizman, B. (1981): Regulation of herpesvirus macromolecular synthesis: Temporal order of transcription of α genes is not dependent on the stringency of inhibition of protein synthesis. *J. Virol.*, 40:319–322.
91. Maitland, N., and McDougall, J. (1977): Biochemical transformation of mouse cells by fragments of herpes simplex virus DNA. *Cell*, 11:233–241.
92. Manley, J., Fire, A., Cano, A., Sharp, P., and Gefter, M. (1980): DNA-dependent transcription of adenovirus genes in a soluble whole cell extract. *Proc. Natl. Acad. Sci. USA*, 77:3855–3859.
93. Marsden, H., Crombie, I., and Subak-Sharpe, J. (1976): Control of protein synthesis in herpesvirus-infected cells; analysis of the polypeptides induced by wild-type and 16 temperature-sensitive mutants of HSV strain 17. *J. Gen. Virol.*, 31:347–372.
94. Marsden, H., Stow, N., Preston, V., Timbury, M., and Wilkie, N. (1978): Physical mapping of herpes simplex virus-induced polypeptides. *J. Virol.*, 28:624–642.
95. Mathis, D., and Chambon, P. (1981): The SV40 early region TATA box is required for accurate *in vitro* initiation of transcription. *Nature*, 290:310–315.
96. Maxam, A., and Gilbert, W. (1980): Sequencing end labeled DNA with base-specific chemical cleavages. *Methods Enzymol.*, 65:499–559.
97. McDougall, J., Galloway, D., Purifoy, D., Powell, K., Richart, R., and Fenoglio, C. (1980): Herpes simplex virus expression in latently infected ganglion cells and in cervical neoplasia. In: *Viruses in Naturally Occurring Cancers*, edited by M. Essex, G. Todaro, and H. zur Hausen, pp. 101–116. Cold Spring Harbor Laboratory, Cold Spring Harbor, N.Y.
98. McKnight, S. (1980): The nucleotide sequence and transcript map of the herpes simplex virus thymidine kinase gene. *Nucleic Acids Res.*, 8:5949–5964.
99. McKnight, S., and Gavis, E. (1980): Expression of the herpes thymidine kinase gene in *Xenopus laevis* oocytes: An assay for the study of deletion mutants constructed *in vitro*. *Nucleic Acids Res.*, 8:5931–5948.
100. McKnight, S., Gavis, E., Kingsbury, R., and Axel, R. (1981): Analysis of transcriptional regulatory signals of the HSV thymidine kinase gene: Identification of an upstream control region. *Cell*, 25:385–398.
101. Morse, L., Pereira, L., Roizman, B., and Schaffer, P. (1978): Anatomy of herpes simplex virus (HSV) DNA. X. Mapping of viral genes by analysis of polypeptides and functions specified by HSV-1 × HSV-2 recombinants. *J. Virol.*, 26:389–410.

102. Moss, B., Gershowitz, A., Stringer, J., Holland, L., and Wagner, E. (1977): 5'-terminal and internal methylated nucleosides in herpes simplex virus type 1 mRNA. *J. Virol.*, 23:234–239.
103. Munyon, W., Kraiselburd, E., Davis, D., and Mann, J. (1971): Transfer of thymidine kinase to thymidine kinaseless L cells by infection with ultraviolet-irradiated herpes simplex virus. *J. Virol.*, 7:813–820.
104. Murray, B., Benyesh-Melnick, M., and Biswal, N. (1974): Early and late viral-specific polyribosomal RNA in herpes virus-1 and -2-infected rabbit kidney cells. *Biochem. Biophys. Acta*, 361:209–220.
105. Nahmias, A., and Roziman, B. (1973): Infection with herpes simplex viruses 1 and 2. *N. Engl. J. Med.*, 289:667–674, 719–725, 781–789.
106. Nathans, D., and Smith, H. O. (1975): Restriction endonucleases in the analysis and restructuring of DNA molecules. *Annu. Rev. Biochem.*, 44:273–293.
107. Nishioka, Y., and Silverstein, S. (1973): Degradation of cellular mRNA during HSV infection. *Proc. Natl. Acad. Sci. USA*, 74:2370–2374.
108. Noyes, B., and Stark, G. (1975): Nucleic acid hybridization using DNA covalently coupled to cellulose. *Cell*, 5:301–310.
109. Para, M., Goldstein, L., and Spear, P. (1982): Similarities and differences in the Fe-binding glycoprotein (gE) of herpes simplex virus types 1 and 2 and tentative mapping of the viral gene for this glycoprotein. *J. Virol.*, 41:137–144.
110. Parris, D., Dixon, R., and Schaffer, P. (1980): Physical mapping of herpes simplex virus type 1 ts mutants by marker rescue correlation of the physical and genetic maps. *Virology*, 100:275–287.
111. Paterson, B., Roberts, B., and Kuff, E. (1977): Structural gene identification and mapping by DNA:mRNA hybrid-arrested cell-free translation. *Proc. Natl. Acad. Sci. USA*, 74:4370–4374.
112. Pedersen, M., Talley-Brown, S., and Millette, R. (1981): Gene expression of herpes simplex virus. III. Effect of arabinosyladenine on viral polypeptide synthesis. *J. Virol.*, 38:712–719.
113. Pellicer, A., Robins, D., Wold, B., Sweet, R., Jackson, J., Lowy, I., Roberts, J., Sim, G., Silverstein, S., and Axel, R. (1980): Altering genotype and phenotype by DNA-mediated gene transfer. *Science*, 209:1414–1422.
114. Pereira, L., Wolff, M., Fenwick, M., and Roizman, B. (1977): Regulation of herpes macromolecular synthesis. V. Properties of α polypeptides made in HSV-1 and HSV-2 infected cells. *Virology*, 77:733–749.
115. Pizer, L., and Beard, P. (1976): The effect of herpes virus infection on mRNA in polyoma virus-transformed cells. *Virology*, 75:477–480.
116. Post, L., and Roizman, B. (1981): A generalized technique for deletion of specific genes in large genomes: α gene 22 of herpes simplex virus 1 is not essential for growth. *Cell*, 25:227–232.
117. Post, L., Mackem, S., and Roizman, B. (1981): Regulation of α genes of herpes simplex virus: Expression of chimeric genes produced by fusion of thymidine kinase with α gene promoters. *Cell*, 24:555–565.
118. Powell, K., and Purifoy, D. (1977): Nonstructural proteins of herpes simplex virus. I. Purification of the induced DNA polymerase. *J. Virol.*, 24:618–626.
119. Powell, K., Littler, E., and Purifoy, D. (1981): Nonstructural proteins of herpes simplex virus. II. Major virus-specific DNA-binding protein. *J. Virol.*, 39:894–902.
120. Powell, K., Purifoy, D., and Courtney, R. (1975): The synthesis of herpes simplex virus proteins in the absence of virus DNA synthesis. *Biochem. Biophys. Res. Commun.*, 66:262–271.
121. Preston, C. M. (1977): Cell-free synthesis of herpes simplex virus-coded pyrimidine deoxyribonucleoside kinase enzyme. *J. Virol.*, 23:455–460.
122. Preston, C. M. (1979): Control of herpes simplex virus type 1 mRNA synthesis in cells infected with wild-type virus or the temperature-sensitive mutant *ts*K. *J. Virol.*, 29:275–284.
123. Preston, C. M. (1979): Abnormal properties of an immediate-early polypeptide in cells infected with the herpes simplex virus type 1 mutant *ts*K. *J. Virol.*, 32:357–369.
124. Preston, C. (1981): Synthesis of HSV exonuclease in *Xenopus laevis* oocytes. In: *International Workshop on Herpesviruses*, edited by A. S. Kaplan, M. La Placa, F. Rapp, and B. Roizman, p. 58. Esculapio Publishing, Bologna.
125. Preston, C., and McGeoch, D. (1981): Identification and mapping of two polypeptides encoded within the herpes simplex virus type 1 thymidine kinase gene sequences. *J. Virol.*, 38:593–605.
126. Preston, V. G. (1981): Fine-structure mapping of herpes simplex virus type 1 temperature-sensitive mutations within the short repeat region of the genome. *J. Virol.*, 39:150–161.

127. Preston, V. G., Davidson, A., Marsden, H., Timbury, M., Subak-Sharpe, J., and Wilkie, N. (1978): Recombinants between herpes simplex virus types 1 and 2: Analysis of genome structures and expression of immediate-early polypeptides. *J. Virol.*, 28:499–517.
128. Proudfoot, N., and Brownlee, G. (1976): 3' non-coding region sequences in eucaryotic mRNA. *Nature*, 263:211–214.
129. Rakusanova, T., Ben-Porat, T., Himeno, M., and Kaplan, A. (1971): Early functions of the genome of herpesvirus. I. Characterization of RNA synthesized in cycloheximide-treated, infected cells. *Virology*, 46:877–889.
130. Rapp, F., and Li, J. L. (1974): Demonstration of the oncogenic potential of herpes simplex viruses and human cytomegalovirus. *Cold Spring Harbor Symp. Quant. Biol.*, 39:747–763.
131. Reyes, G., LaFemina, R., Hayward, S., and Hayward, G. (1979): Morphological transformation by DNA fragments of human herpesviruses: Evidence for two distinct transforming regions in herpes simplex virus types 1 and 2, and lack of correlation with biochemical transfer of the thymidine kinase gene. *Cold Spring Harbor Symp. Quant. Biol.*, 44:629–657.
132. Rio, D., Robbins, A., Myers, R., and Tjian, R. (1980): Regulation of SV40 early transcription *in vitro* by a purified tumor antigen. *Proc. Natl. Acad. Sci. USA*, 77:5706–5710.
133. Roizman, B. (1979): The structure and isomerization of herpes simplex virus genomes. *Cell*, 16:481–494.
134. Ruyechan, W., Morse, L., Knipe, D., and Roizman, B. (1979): Molecular genetics of herpes simplex virus. II. Mapping of the major viral glycoproteins and of the genetic loci specifying the social behavior of infected cells. *J. Virol.*, 29:677–697.
135. Sasaki, Y., Sasaki, R., Cohen, G., and Pizer, L. (1974): RNA polymerase activity and inhibition in herpesvirus-infected cells. *Intervirology*, 3:147–161.
136. Sharp, J., and Summers, W. (1981): Multiple transcription units in the *tk* region of the HSV-1 genome. In: *International Workshop on Herpesviruses*, edited by A. S. Kaplan, M. La Placa, F. Rapp, and B. Roizman, p. 59. Esculapio Publishing, Bologna.
137. Sharp, P. (1981): Speculations on RNA splicing. *Cell*, 23:643–646.
138. Sheldrick, P., Laithier, M., Lando, D., and Ryhiner, D. (1973): Infectious DNA from herpes simplex virus: Infectivity of double-stranded and single stranded molecules. *Proc. Natl. Acad. Sci. USA*, 70:3621–3625.
139. Silverstein, S., Bachenheimer, S., Frankel, N., and Roizman, B. (1973): Relationship between post-transcriptional adenylation of herpesvirus RNA and mRNA abundance. *Proc. Natl. Acad. Sci. USA*, 70:2101–2104.
140. Silverstein, S., Millette, R., Jones, P., and Roizman, B. (1976): RNA synthesis in cells infected with herpes simplex virus. XII. Sequence complexity and properties of RNA differing in extent of adenylation. *J. Virol.*, 18:977–991.
141. Skare, J., and Summers, W. (1977): Structure and function of herpesvirus genomes. I. *Eco*RI, *Xba*I, and *Hind*III endonuclease cleavage sites on herpes simplex virus type 1 DNA. *Virology*, 76:581–595.
142. Spear, P., and Roizman, B. (1980): Herpes simplex virus. In: *Molecular Biology of Tumor Viruses, Part 2: DNA Tumor Viruses*, edited by J. Tooze, pp. 615–745. Cold Spring Harbor Laboratory, Cold Spring Harbor, N.Y.
143. Stenberg, R., and Pizer, L. (1982): HSV induced changes in cellular and adenovirus RNA metabolism in an adenovirus type 5 transformed human cell line. *J. Virol.*, 42:474–487.
144. Stevens, J. G. (1975): Latent herpes simplex virus and the nervous system. *Curr. Top. Microbiol.*, 70:31–50.
145. Stevens, J. G. (1980): Herpetic latency and re-activation. In: *Oncogenic Herpesviruses, Vol. II*, edited by F. Rapp, pp. 1–17. CRC Press, Boca Raton, Fla.
146. Stevens, J., and Cook, M. (1973): Latent herpes simplex virus infection. In: *Virus Research*, edited by C. Fox and W. Robinson, pp. 437–446. Academic Press, New York.
147. Stow, N., Subak-Sharpe, J., and Wilkie, N. (1978): Physical mapping of HSV-1 mutations by marker rescue. *J. Virol.*, 28:182–192.
148. Stringer, J., Holland, L., Swanstrom, R., Pivo, K., and Wagner, E. (1977): Quantitation of herpes simplex virus type 1 RNA in infected HeLa cells. *J. Virol.*, 21:889–901.
149. Stringer, J., Holland, L., and Wagner, E. (1978): Mapping early transcripts of herpes simplex virus type 1 by electron microscopy. *J. Virol.*, 25:56–73.
150. Swanstrom, R., and Wagner, E. (1974): Regulation of synthesis of herpes simplex type 1 virus mRNA during productive infection. *Virology*, 60:522–533.

151. Swanstrom, R., Pivo, K., and Wagner, E. (1975): Restricted transcription of the herpes simplex virus genome occurring early after infection and in the presence of metabolic inhibitors. *Virology*, 66:140–150.

152. Sydiskis, R., and Roizman, B. (1967): The disaggregation of host polyribosomes in productive and abortive infection with herpes simplex virus. *Virology*, 32:678–686.

153. Thomas, P. S. (1980): Hybridization of denatured RNA and small DNA fragments transferred to nitrocellulose paper. *Proc. Natl. Acad. Sci. USA*, 77:5201–5205.

154. Van Santen, V., Cheung, A., and Kieff, E. (1981): Epstein-Barr virus RNA. VII: size and direction of transcription of virus-specified cytoplasmic RNAs in a transformed cell line. *Proc. Natl. Acad. Sci. USA*, 78:1930–1934.

155. Wadsworth, S., Jacob, R., and Roizman, B. (1975): Anatomy of herpes simplex virus DNA. II. Size, composition, and arrangement of inverted terminal repetitions. *J. Virol.*, 15:1487–1497.

156. Wagner, E. (1972): Evidence for transcriptional control of the herpes simplex virus genome in infected human cells. *Virology*, 47:502–506.

157. Wagner, E., and Roizman, B. (1969): Ribonucleic acid synthesis in cells infected with herpes simplex virus. I. Patterns of ribonucleic acid synthesis in productively infected cells. *J. Virol.*, 4:36–46.

158. Wagner, E., and Roizman, B. (1969): RNA synthesis in cells infected with herpes simplex virus. II. Evidence that a class of viral mRNA is derived from a high molecular weight precursor synthesized in the nucleus. *Proc. Natl. Acad. Sci. USA*, 64:626–633.

159. Wagner, E., Anderson, K., Costa, R., Devi, G., Gaylord, B., Holland, L. Stringer, J., and Tribble, L. (1982): Isolation and characterization of HSV-1 mRNA. In: *Herpesvirus DNA: Recent Studies on the Internal Organization and Replication of the Viral Genome*, edited by Y. Becker, pp. 45–67. Martinus Nijhoff, The Hague.

160. Wagner, E., Swanstrom, R., and Stafford, M. (1972): Transcription of the herpes simplex virus genome in human cells. *J. Virol.*, 10:675–682.

161. Wagner, M. J., Sharp, J., and Summers, W. (1981): Nucleotide sequence of the thymidine kinase gene of herpes simplex virus type 1. *Proc. Natl. Acad. Sci. USA*, 78:1441–1445.

162. Ward, R., and Stevens, J. (1975): Effect of cytosine arabinoside on viral-specific protein synthesis in cells infected with herpes simplex virus. *J. Virol.*, 15:71–80.

163. Walthen, M., Thomsen, D., and Stinski, M. (1981): Temporal regulation of human cytomegalovirus transcription at immediate-early and early times after infection. *J. Virol.*, 38:446–459.

164. Watson, R., and Clements, J. (1978): Characterization of transcription-deficient temperature-sensitive mutants of HSV-1. *Virology*, 91:364–379.

165. Watson, R., and Clements, J. (1980): A herpes simplex virus type 1 function continuously required for early and late virus RNA synthesis. *Nature*, 285:329–331.

166. Watson, R., Preston, C., and Clements, J. (1979): Separation and characterization of herpes simplex virus type 1 immediate-early mRNA's. *J. Virol.*, 31:42–52.

167. Watson, R., Sullivan, M., and Vande Woude, G. (1981): Structures of two spliced herpes simplex virus type 1 immediate-early mRNA's which map at the junctions of the unique and reiterated regions of the virus DNA S component. *J. Virol.*, 37:431–444.

168. Watson, R., Umene, K., and Enquist, L. (1981): Reiterated sequences within the intron of an immediate-early gene of herpes simplex virus type 1. *Nucleic Acids Res.*, 9:4189–4199.

169. Wigler, M., Silverstein, S., Lee, L.-S., Pellicer, A., Cheng, Y.-C., and Axel, R. (1977): Transfer of purified herpes virus thymidine kinase gene to cultured mouse cells. *Cell*, 11:223–232.

170. Wildy, P. (1973): Herpes: History and classification. In: *The Herpesviruses*, edited by A. Kaplan, pp. 1–26. Academic Press, New York.

171. Wilkie, N., and Cortini, R. (1976): Sequence arrangement in herpes simplex virus type 1 DNA: Identification of terminal fragments in restriction endonuclease digests and evidence for inversions in redundant and unique sequences. *J. Virol.*, 20:211–221.

172. Youssoufian, H., Hammer, S., Hirsch, M., and Mulder, C. (1982): Methylation of the viral genome in an *in vitro* model of herpes simplex virus latency (restriction endonucleases/5-methylcytosine/mitogens). *Proc. Natl. Acad. Sci. USA*, 79:2207–2210.

Advances in Viral Oncology, Volume 3, edited by
George Klein. Raven Press, New York © 1983.

Biochemical Aspects of Transformation By Herpes Simplex Viruses

Gary S. Hayward and Gregory R. Reyes

*Department of Pharmacology and Experimental Therapeutics, Johns Hopkins University
School of Medicine, Baltimore, Maryland 21205*

Many herpesviruses have the ability to induce tumors in experimental animals, and some occasionally exhibit this property in their natural hosts (62). In humans, herpes simplex virus type 2 (HSV-2) has for many years been suspected of being a contributing cause of squamous cell cervical carcinoma (58,89,101). However, epidemiological and serological evaluation of a possible active role for HSV-2 in this disease has been greatly complicated by (a) prior infection with the serologically cross-reactive HSV-1 virus, (b) the propensity of HSV-2 to establish long-term latent infections in ganglia innervating the genital region, followed by periodic reactivation (6,112), and (c) the lack of a suitable animal model. Even the demonstration of virus-specific DNA, RNA, or antigens in preinvasive tumor cells by *in situ* hybridization and immunomicroscopy could have the trivial explanation of preferential replication of reactivated virus in this tissue. It is not our purpose to critically evaluate the biology and etiology of the role of HSV-2 in cervical carcinoma; this has been accomplished recently for the epidemiological and serological evidence by Rawls et al. (100), for the biological aspects of transformation of cultured cells by Hampar et al. (47), and for the *in situ* hybridization results by McDougall et al. (80). We shall assume that the HSV-like subgroup of herpesviruses is indeed oncogenic and shall discuss relevant observations at the level of molecular biology and biochemical genetics and then briefly attempt to correlate them with recent findings from analysis of patient sera and tumor samples.

Examination of the mechanism of morphological transformation by HSV-2 in cultured cells shows promise of providing information about (a) whether or not one should expect to find nucleic acid sequences and antigens from a viral "oncogene" in the tumor cells, (b) a possible indirect role of the virus, such as activation of cellular "transforming" genes or RNA tumor viruses (46), and (c) the identities of any viral genes, promoters, and polypeptides that may be involved. In contrast to the situation with SV40 and adenovirus, infection of almost any mammalian cell culture with HSV leads to productive lytic infection and cell death. Perhaps the only exception to this rule is the XC line of rat cells, but these already carry the Rous sarcoma virus genome (43,77). To uncover the transforming potential of HSV in permissive cells, the lytic functions of the virus need to be inactivated. Duff and

Rapp (29,30), and subsequently many others, have clearly demonstrated that transformed cells arise at low frequencies from both primary and established rodent or
human (65) cell cultures after abortive infections with HSV under various nonpermissive protocols, including ultraviolet (UV) inactivation of the virions, the use of
temperature-sensitive (ts) mutants, and growth of the cells at high temperature
(40°C). Cell lines have been established from most of the experiments with rodent
cells (8,29,59,60), and some have been shown to produce tumors in experimental
animals (30,61,72). However, early attempts to demonstrate specific viral DNA
sequences in these cells did not give consistent or reproducible results (100), and
despite the common reports of cytoplasmic or surface viral antigens, no consensus
was achieved as to which (if any) viral polypeptides could be accurately described
as tumor or transformation antigens *(vide infra)*.

Focus formation in contact-inhibited or primary cells after transfection with isolated DNA fragments from the early region of SV40 and polyoma viruses, from
the left-hand 14% of the adenovirus type 2 genome, and from the v-*onc* genes of
avian and murine sarcoma viruses has been used successfully to define the minimal
portion of each genome that is capable of initiating transformation events (4,45).
In the DNA viruses, expression of the virus-encoded T antigen genes is necessary
in some way for both initiation and maintenance of the transformed state, although
their action may involve interactions with cellular-transformation-related polypeptides such as the 53K protein induced by SV40 infection (24,70). On the other
hand, transformation by RNA tumor viruses involves cellular "oncogenes" whose
expression is subtly altered by linkage to or nearby insertion of the strong viral
LTR promoter or enhancer sequences (7,51,92).

By analogy with the smaller DNA viruses, we might anticipate that the equivalent
sequences in herpesviruses need occupy only 1 to 3% of the genome and be expressed
at the earliest stages after infection. Despite their relatively large size and complexity
(50,118), the genomes of HSV-1 and HSV-2 have been dissected into well-defined
mapped segments with restriction enzymes (23,87,111), and there has been some
progress in describing the genome locations of individual immediate-early, delayed-
early, and late mRNAs and protein products (3,16,31,56,76,88,116). Therefore,
several groups have attempted to identify specific fragments of HSV-1 and HSV-
2 DNA that may be functionally active in intiating morphological transformation
as assayed by transfection procedures. Although no definitive answers are available
as yet, current progress based on the results of those experiments will be described
in some detail.

TRANSFECTION EXPERIMENTS WITH ISOLATED DNA FRAGMENTS

Focus Formation with Isolated HSV-1 and HSV-2 DNA Fragments

Focus formation with total sheared HSV-2 viral DNA was first briefly mentioned
by Wilkie et al. (119). Since then, three groups have published the results of focus-
formation assays with sets of isolated restriction fragments of HSV DNA extracted

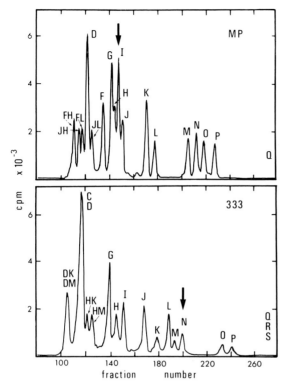

FIG. 1. Radioactivity profiles of ^{32}P-labeled HSV-1(MP) and HSV-2(333) DNA after cleavage with the *Bg*III restriction enzyme. Vertical arrows mark the positions of the minimal transforming regions defined by Reyes et al. (105), namely *Bg*III-I from HSV-1 and *Bg*III-N from HSV-2. The DNA was subjected to electrophoresis for 48 hr through 30-cm-cylinder gels of 0.6% agarose. The gels were sliced into 1-mm discs, and ^{32}P radioactivity was determined by the Cerenkov procedure. For transfection experiments, the DNA bands (not radiolabeled) were isolated from similar gels after brief staining with ethidium bromide and visualization on a long-wave UV transilluminator.

from agarose gels, and a fourth group has used isolated viral DNA fragments in a mass-culture transformation assay. Camacho and Spear (11) reported the development of foci in hamster embryo cells with one of five tested *Xba*I fragments from HSV-1(F) DNA. The 23-kb *Xba*I-F fragment consistently yielded foci of spindle-shaped cells that grew into colonies in methylcellulose. These authors also initially reported expression of an acquired viral glycoprotein in the "transformed" cells. The slightly smaller 15.8-kb *Bg*III-I fragments from the same region of the HSV-1(MP) and HSV-1(STH$_2$) genomes were also found to yield foci in a limited set of experiments described by Reyes et al. (105), using either contact-inhibited BALB/c 3T3 cells or primary hamster embryo cultures grown in low serum. Surprisingly, in the same study Reyes et al. found that totally different portions of the HSV-2(333) DNA molecule consistently gave rise to foci in both the BALB/c 3T3 cells and hamster cell systems. In a series of experiments with sets of gel-purified viral DNA fragments from digests with various different restriction enzymes, all positive fragments either consisted of, or overlapped with, a common 7.5-kb segment represented by the *Bg*III-N fragment (summarized in Fig. 2). The efficiency of transformation (approximately 6 foci per microgram of *Bg*III-N DNA) was similar to that obtained by others with isolated fragments of adenovirus DNA (115). The profiles of *Bg*III digests of ^{32}P-labeled HSV-1(MP) and HSV-2(333) DNA after electrophoretic separation through agarose gels are shown in Fig. 1, and the positions

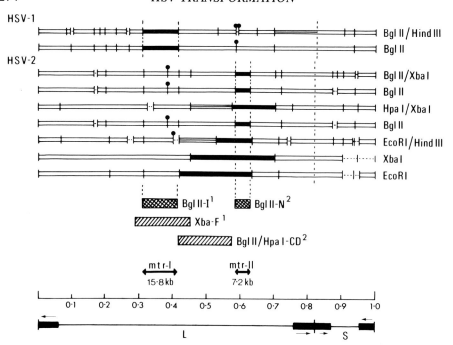

FIG. 2. Diagram showing the relative map locations of all isolated HSV DNA fragments used in our assays for the ability to initiate focus formation on monolayers of BALB/c 3T3 and hamster embryo cells. Positive fragments are given as filled bars and negative fragments as open bars. Semisolid bars indicate additional fragments that have molecular weights similar to those of the presumed positive HSV-1(STH$_2$) *Bgl*II/*Hin*dIII, HSV-2(333) *Hpa*I/*Xba*I, and HSV-2(333) *Eco*RI/*Hin*dIII species and were therefore not resolved from them during the isolation procedures. Cross-hatched areas indicate the minimal region common to all positive fragments from HSV-1 or HSV-2 DNA, and the filled circles represent cleavage sites that might possibly have inactivated focus formation with equivalent regions in the other genome. Both the HSV-1 and HSV-2 physical maps are drawn in the standard prototype orientation (56). Most of the cleavage map data come from G. Hayward, T. Buchman, and B. Roizman *(unpublished)*, as cited in Morse et al. (87). For comparison, the diagram includes the map locations of HSV-2 DNA fragments found to exhibit transforming properties in other studies (11,55).

of the *Bgl*II-I and -N fragments that gave rise to foci in our transfection experiments are arrowed.

In subsequent studies, Galloway and McDougall (39) reported that a pBR322-derived plasmid, pDG401, containing the *Bgl*II-N fragment from HSV-2(333), was also capable of giving rise to foci and forming colonies in methylcellulose assays after transfection of the *Hin*dIII-cleaved linear form into NIH/3T3 or hamster embryo cell cultures. Transformed cell lines derived from these foci yielded fibrosarcomas in nude mice. In a rather different assay, Jariwalla et al. (54) initially claimed a very high efficiency of transformation of hamster embryo fibroblast cultures with low concentrations of total HSV-2 DNA after continuous mass culture passaging and later described experiments in which the *Bgl*II-C fragment of HSV-2(S$_1$) and HSV-2(333), but not other *Bgl*II fragments, gave similar results (55). Permanent cell cultures derived from transfections with 0.1 μg of *Bgl*II[ψλεαωεδ ΔNA oρ ′″ς′″− μg of the *Bgl*II/*Hpa*I-CD fragment gave rise to tumors when injected into newborn hamsters.

Quite naturally, the apparent ability of three distinct regions of the HSV genome to initiate *in vitro* transformation has led to some confusion and skepticism. However, additional independent evidence is available in support of each finding, and potential trivial explanations involving mismapping of fragments, strain differences, and DNA translocations have been eliminated. The three morphological transforming regions, to which we shall refer as *mtr*-I (0.31–0.41), *mtr*-II (0.58–0.63), and *mtr*-III (0.42–0.57), all map adjacent to one another within the center of the unique L segment of the HSV genome (Fig. 2). Similar transfection experiments with cloned fragments of human cytomegalovirus DNA have recently led to the identification of a focus-forming region in the L segment of that genome also (90).

Biological Properties of DNA-Fragment-transformed Cell Lines

Hampar et al. (47) have recently presented a critical review of the advantages and disadvantages of primary versus established cell lines for transformation studies and have also compared the properties of BALB/c 3T3 cells transformed by UV-irradiated HSV-1 virus with those of SV40-transformed BALB/c 3T3 cells. In the experiments of Reyes et al. (105), both cell types gave foci with the *mtr*-I and *mtr*-II fragments. A primary HSV-1 *Bgl*II-I focus spreading over the BALB/c 3T3 cell monoloyer at 8 weeks after DNA transfection is shown in Fig. 3, panel (a). Both the primary and secondary foci obtained after transfection with HSV-2 *Bgl*II-N were quite distinguishable from those obtained with HSV-1 DNA; they frequently developed thick central ridges, as shown at low magnification in Fig. 3, panel (b). The "transformed" colonies of spindle-shaped hamster cells developed at 4 weeks in cultures of second-passage primary cells that were maintained after transfection in 1% fetal calf serum.

Table 1 summarizes the origins of "morphologically transformed" cell lines that were derived from transfection experiments with isolated or cloned HSV DNA fragments. In the case of the BALB/c 3T3 cells of Reyes et al. (105), all lines that were tested plated at relatively high efficiency in soft agarose and methylcellulose (see Table 2). Examples of the colonies obtained are shown in Fig. 3, panels (c) and (d). The F5A3B, F11A2B, and F11B2A lines all grew to fivefold higher saturation densities on plastic (2–3 × 10^5 cells/cm^2) than the parent BALB/c 3T3 clone A31 cells (4 × 10^4/cm^2). Similarly, the HSV-1-fragment-transformed line (although less so with the HSV-2 lines) could be readily grown and cloned in medium containing only 1% serum. The parent BALB/c 3T3 cultures did not grow in 1% serum or produce any colonies in methylcellulose or agarose. Significantly, one of the very few spontaneous BALB/c cell foci that developed in a control dish in our transfection experiments (the C2D line) grew only poorly in methylcellulose (Table 2). In assays for thymidine kinase (tk) activity in both the F5A3B and F11B2B cells, using either sensitivity to arabinosylthymine or the mobility of the

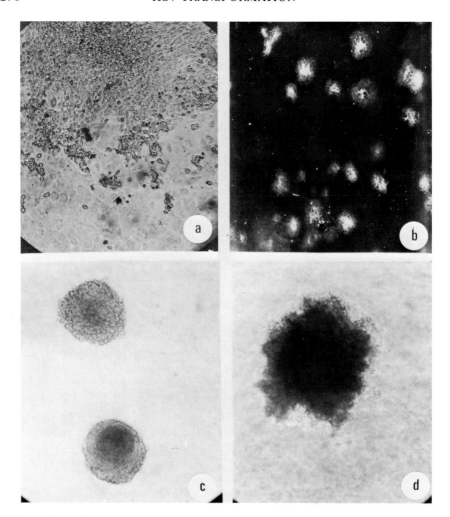

FIG. 3. Photomicrographs of foci and colonies of DNA-fragment-transformed BALB/c cells. **a:** Appearance of a primary focus on the dish from which the F5A3B cell line was derived, at 9 weeks after transfection and a subconfluent monolayer of BALB/c 3T3 clone A31 cells with the Bg/II/HindIII-IA fragment from HSV-1(STH₂) DNA. Magnification x40. **b:** Typical appearance of HSV-2 (Bg/II-N) DNA-fragment-transformed BALB/c cells as secondary foci growing on a plastic surface under dark-field illumination at low magnification (× 3). **c:** Anchorage-independent colonies of F5A3B cells growing in 0.3% soft agarose (× 40). **d:** An anchorage-independent colony of F11B2B cells growing in methylcellulose (× 40).

native enzyme from cytosol extracts in polyacrylamide gels, we found greatly increased levels of the cellular tk enzyme over that in BALB/c 3T3 cells, but no detectable virus-specific tk activity (103). At approximately the 60th to 80th passage in culture without further selection for transformed phenotype, some sublines of both our *mtr*-I- and *mtr*-II-fragment-transformed BALB/c cells reverted to a relatively normal flat epithelioid morphology.

TABLE 1. Summary and origins of HSV-DNA-fragment-transformed cell lines

Subclone designations	Input fragment	Genome map location	DNA detected (copies/cell)	Origin of cell lines
mtr-I				
Hamster embryo cells: HSV-1(F1) VI-3, VI-8, II-15, II-16	XbaI-F	0.290–0.452	No (<0.05)[a]	Camacho and Spear (11)
BALB/c 3T3 cells: HSV-1(STH₂) F5A3B, F5ABm3, F5A3Bs1	BglII/HindIII-IA	0.311–0.415	No (<0.05)[b]	Reyes et al. (105)
mtr-II				
BALB/c 3T3 cells: HSV-2(333) F11A1A, F11B2B, F11B2c1D9	BglII/XbaI-NH	0.582–0.628	Yes (0.1)[b]	Reyes et al. (105)
F12A2B	BglII-N	0.582–0.628	Yes (0.1)[b]	Reyes et al. (105)
F4A1A	HpaI/XbaI-ED	0.575–0.702	Yes (1–5)[b]	Reyes et al. (105)
F13B1A	BglII-N	0.582–0.628	No (<0.1)[b]	Reyes et al. (105)
Hamster embryo cells: HSV-2(333) HF3A1A, HF3B1Am1, HF3B2A	EcoRI/HindIII-AA, EA	0.520–0.634	No (<0.1)[b]	Reyes et al. (105)
Rat embryo cells: HSV-2(333) 401RH4	BglII-N (pDG401)	0.585–0.628	Yes (0.1)[c]	Galloway and McDougall (39)
NIH 3T3 cells: HSV-2(333) 401-NIH-1, 401-NIH-0.1	BglII-N (pDG401)	0.582–0.628		Galloway and McDougall (39)
401-I-T1, 401-0-1-T1T2	BglII-N (pDG401) tumor	0.585–0.628	Yes (0.5)[c]	Galloway and McDougall (39)
mtr-III				
Hamster embryo cells: HSV-2(S1) SDNA-CD/1	BglII/HpaI-CD	0.419–0.575	Yes (?)[d]	Jariwalla et al. (55)

[a]Less than 1×10^6 sequence complexity (67).
[b]Blot hybridization with cloned probes (103).
[c]Blot hybridization with cloned probes (39).
[d]Positive by dot blot analysis (5).

TABLE 2. *Growth of F5A3B and HF3 cells in methylcellulose*

Cell line	Passage no.	No. of colonies/No. of wells		Efficiency[a] (%)
		10^3 plated[b]	10^4 plated[b]	
F5A3B	p7	137/3	>1,200/3	4.8
F5A3B	p14	334/3	>1,200/3	11.5
F5A3B	p28	236/3	>1,200/3	8.0
F5A3B	p48	289/3	>1,200/3	9.1
F5A3Bm3	p55	164/3	>1,200/3	5.2
F5A3Bs1	p15	446/3	>1,200/3	15.0
C2D1A[c]	p7	0/3	160/3	0.5
BALB/c 3T3		0/3	0/3	<0.003
HF3A1A	p5	—	46/2[e]	0.23[e]
HF3A1A	p57	—	512/2[e]	2.6[e]
HF3B1A	p5	—	33/2[e]	0.16[e]
HF3B1Am1	p41	—	650/2[e]	3.2[e]
HF3B2A	p5	—	17/2[e]	0.08[e]
HF3B2A	p54	—	34/2	0.17
HF3B2A	p54	—	628/2[e]	3.1[e]
NBE[d]		178/2	>1,000/2	8.9
HEF (primary)	p4	—	0/8	<0.001

[a]Not corrected for plating efficiency on plastic.
[b]Number of cells plated per well.
[c]Spontaneous transformant from control dish.
[d]SV40-transformed human fibroblast line.
[e]Microcolonies (<0.1 mm diameter).

In contrast to the BALB/c mouse cell lines, the transformed cell lines derived from hamster embryo fibroblasts only gradually acquired the ability to grow in soft agarose as a function of passaging history. Again, these efficiencies are similar to those obtained initially with primary rat cell lines transformed by isolated fragments of adenovirus type 2 DNA (115). Neither the cell lines established by Camacho and Spear (11) nor those of Reyes et al. (105) were tested for tumorigenicity, but in both cases they grew in anchorage-independent methylcellulose assays, a property that usually correlates with tumorigenicity (98). The pDG401-plasmid-transformed lines derived by Galloway and McDougall (39) exhibited properties similar to those described earlier. For example, the 401-NIH lines grew at high efficiency in methyl-cellulose directly, whereas the rat embryo lines initially plated at only low efficiency in methylcellulose. The 401-NIH lines all gave tumors in 3-week-old nude mice, and tumor-derived sublines (401-1-Tu1, etc.) were in turn highly tumorigenic in newborn NIH/Swiss mice. Unlike the parent Syrian hamster embryo cells, the transformed cell lines derived by Jariwalla et al. (55), from either total *Bgl*II-cleaved DNA or the *Bgl*II/*Hpa*I-CD fragment of HSV-2 DNA, grew into colonies in low serum and in agar or agarose, but reached only slightly higher than normal saturation densities. After the 20th passage they also gradually acquired the ability to produce invasive fibrosarcomas after subcutaneous injection of 2×10^6 cells into newborn Syrian hamsters.

Secondary Transfer of the Transformed Phenotype to NIH 3T3 Cells

Minson et al. (86) first showed that the viral tk$^+$ phenotype could be transferred to new L tk$^-$ cells at a much higher efficiency with cellular DNA from biochemically transformed lines than in the original direct experiments with sheared HSV-2 DNA. They suggested that the integration events brought the tk gene into association with cellular sequences that somehow enhanced the process of biochemical transformation. Later, Copeland et al. (21) and Shih et al. (109) demonstrated transfer to NIH 3T3 cells of the morphologically transformed trait with isolated cellular DNA containing proviral forms of murine sarcoma virus, or from chemically transformed cells. We have observed similar phenomena with the F11B2B cells using the NIH 3T3 transformation assay of Andersson et al. (4). Table 3 shows the results of an experiment in which 15 to 30 μg DNA samples from several of our fragment-transformed cell lines were added to monolayer cultures of NIH 3T3 cells and assayed for focus formation. DNA from both of the *mtr*-II-transformed cell lines tested and also that from 333-8-9 cells gave foci at efficiencies similar to those reported with chemically transformed mouse cell DNA (109). Curiously, neither the *mtr*-I-transformed cell line nor a line of SV40-transformed human cells (NBE) gave positive results in this assay. Note that the transfer of the transformed phenotype occurred at a much higher efficiency (1 focus per 10^6 copies of the cell genome) than with the original viral DNA (1 focus per 2 × 10^{10} copies of the *Bgl*II-N fragment).

Activation of RNA Tumor Virus Expression

Boyd et al. (9) demonstrated by transfection procedures that isolated DNA from several herpesviruses transiently activates the expression of endogenous type C retrovirus in BALB/c 3T3 cells to levels at least 5- to 10-fold above the background

TABLE 3. *Transfection of NIH 3T3 cells with transformed cell DNA*

DNA source	Number of foci/dishes
Virus-transformed	
333-8-9 (hamster, UV, HSV-2)	9/4
72-4148 (hamster, UV, HSV-1)	14/4
NBE (human, SV40)	1/4
DNA-fragment-transformed	
F11A1A (BALB/c 3T3, HSV-2 *Bgl*II-N)	4/4
F11B2B (BALB/c 3T3, HSV-2 *Bgl*II-N)	6/4
F11B2c1D9 (BALB/c 3T3, HSV-2 *Bgl*II-N)	14/4
F5A3Bm3 (BALB/c 3T3, HSV-1 *Bgl*II-I)	0/4
Controls	
BALB/c 3T3 (mouse, contact-inhibited)	0/4
Calf thymus	0/4
No treatment	0/4

obtained with bacterial or other viral DNAs. The experiments were carried out in the presence of dexamethasone using a cocultivation infectious-center assay for xenotrophic virus in F81 feline cells and included a mitomycin C treatment step. The activity was dose-dependent up to 0.1 to 0.2 μg of HSV DNA and could be abolished by shearing the DNA below 1 to 3 × 10^6 daltons in size, by DNAse treatment, or by cross-linking. Further studies using the sets of HSV-1 lambda-phage clones constructed by Enquist et al. (32) identified three regions of HSV-1 DNA that were apparently capable of MuX virus activation in BALB/c 3T3 cells (10). The positive fragments (which each gave 10–20 foci/10^5 cells/0.25–0.5 μg of DNA) map at 0.292 to 0.316 (*Bam*HI-P), 0.455 to 0.489 (*Eco*RI-L), and 0.909 to 0.965 (*Eco*RI/*Hin*dIII-HG). The *Hin*dIII-K fragment (0.530–0.591) and the inverted repeat regions were not tested.

The significance of these observations is not yet clear. The site in *Bam*HI-P lies just inside the extreme left-hand end of *mtr*-I, and because this site is inactivated by *Eco*RI cleavage, it could be associated with the promoter for the tk gene (81,82,104). The *Eco*RI-L fragment lies within the HSV-1 equivalent of *mtr*-III and correlates closely with a site of cell–virus DNA homology *(vide infra)*.

CHARACTERIZATION OF THE MORPHOLOGICAL TRANSFORMING REGIONS OF HSV DNA

Physical and Functional Maps of the HSV-1 *Bgl*II-I Fragment

A detailed restriction map of the 15.4-kb *Bgl*II-I fragment (*mtr*-I) from HSV-1(MP) is presented in Fig. 4. This fragment lies between coordinates 0.311 and 0.415 in the prototype orientation of the viral genome. These maps were constructed from a combination of double-digestion hybridization experiments with isolated fragments and the more recent results of partial cleavage of the 5′-end-labeled plasmids containing *Bgl*II-I (pGR116 and pGR127). Figure 5 shows a diagram illustrating the relative map locations of certain viral gene products and functions that may correlate with *mtr*-I, together with a summary of our sets of pBR322-cloned subfragments covering this portion of the HSV-1 and HSV-2 genomes.

The intact promoter for the HSV-1 tk gene lies at the extreme left-hand end of the *Bgl*II-I fragment (0.312–0.313), but none of the structural tk coding sequence is retained. Two well-characterized gene products map entirely within *mtr*-I: the 115K glycoprotein gpA/B and the 128K major DNA binding protein (Fig. 5). At the right-hand end, the *Bgl*II-I fragment probably contains a portion of the viral DNA polymerase gene, which has been mapped by genetic procedures to encompass at least the sequences between 0.417 and 0.425 on an mRNA of 4.3 kb (13,116), and also a DNA replication origin (*ori*-L) between 0.405 and 0.415. This latter feature is defined by the minimum 1,500-bp sequence common to all repeat units in the class II type of tandem-repeat-defective DNA (15; G. S. Hayward, *unpublished data*). Another extraordinary feature in this section for both the HSV-1 and HSV-2 genomes is a "deletable" region surrounding the *Cla*I site at 0.402. Every

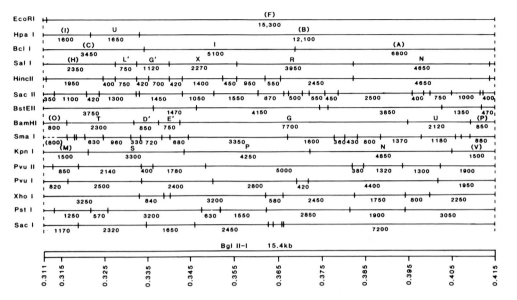

FIG. 4. Physical maps of restriction enzyme cleavage sites in the *Bgl*II-I fragment from HSV-1(MP) DNA. Most of these data were generated by partial cleavage of cloned plasmid DNA end-labeled either at the *Hind*III site on the right in pGR116 or at the *Eco*RI site just inside the left-hand boundary in pGR127. The experimental details were similar to those described in Fig. 6.

time that this site was cloned into either the pBR322 plasmid or phage lambda and grown in *Escherichia coli* (even in the recA⁻ strain HB101), a sharply defined sequence of approximately 120 bp was either rapidly deleted or methylated in such a way as to alter the apparent size of fragments containing it and to block cleavage at the *Cla*I site. Obviously, numerous other viral gene products must be encoded within the *Bgl*II-I fragment also (76,88), but it is noticeable that no mRNA or gene product that fits into the definition of the alpha or immediate-early class has yet been mapped within this region (16,116). Temperature-sensitive mutants in each of these three characterized genes have been isolated (13,20). As shown in Fig. 5, portions of the *mtr*-I region (especially within the HSV-1 *Bam*HI-G, *Bam*HI-P, and *Eco*RI-M fragments) contain the most highly conserved sequences at the DNA hybridization level among the genomes of HSV-1, HSV-2, EHV-1, PRV (pseudorabies virus), and HVT (herpesvirus tupaia from tree shrews). In contrast, the coding sequences for the tk genes, for example, are far more divergent among HSV-1, HSV-2, EHV-1, PRV, and HVT and in fact give barely detectable hybridization in some combinations (G. S. Hayward, *unpublished data*).

The question whether or not the region in HSV-2 that is equivalent to *mtr*-I can initiate transformation remains unresolved. The *Bgl*II enzyme used in most fragment-transfection experiments cleaves inside this region at coordinate 0.385, and, similarly, *Hind*III cleaves at 0.398. The two experiments reported by Reyes et al. (105) that involved *Eco*RI or *Xba*I fragments did not give sufficient numbers of

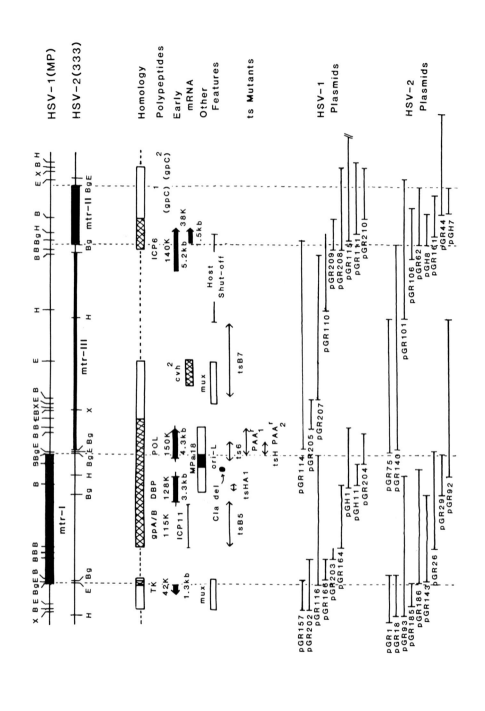

foci with the *mtr*-II region to answer this question for *mtr*-I. There is no evidence at present to suggest that the *mtr*-I-equivalent region in HSV-2 (*Bgl*II-J plus *Bgl*II-O) differs in structure or coding capacity in any significant way from that in the *Bgl*II-I fragment of HSV-1.

Physical Map and Coding Capacity of the HSV-2 *Bgl*II-N Fragment

A detailed restriction map of the 7.5-kb *Bgl*II-N fragment from HSV-2(333) DNA, constructed by partial-digestion mapping of the plasmid pGR62, is shown in Fig. 6. The location of this fragment relative to other well-characterized gene functions is illustrated in Fig. 5, together with a summary of the origins of viral DNA inserts in our sets of plasmid clones encompassing the *mtr*-II sequences. Wagner and associates (2,38) have studied the viral transcripts encoded within the *mtr*-II-equivalent region of HSV-1 (*Hin*dIII-L and *Hin*dIII-K) in some detail and have found the area to be extremely complex. It has been known for some time that the 3' end of the large 5.2-kb mRNA, which is usually regarded as an immediate-early species (IE-II) but is also greatly enhanced at delayed-early times, overlaps with *Bgl*II-N from the left-hand side (31). This mRNA species encodes the 140K ICP-6 protein, a phosphorylated, generally cytoplasmic product of the so-called alpha/beta class whose synthesis, unlike that of other delayed-early beta proteins, appears to be independent of an active 175K (ICP-4) gene product (26,84,97). The location of this gene may also correspond to the "rapid HSV-2 host shutoff" functions described by Fenwick et al. (33). A second delayed-early transcript of 1.5 kb has been shown to map within the *mtr*-II-equivalent region in HSV-1, and it apparently has a coterminal 3' end with the 5.2-kb species. Hybrid-arrest translation experiments indicate that the *Bgl*II-N fragment of HSV-2 encodes a 38K type-specific polypeptide that maps at 0.58 to 0.61 on the left-hand side of *Bgl*II-N (27), corresponding to a subregion giving rise to focus formation (D. Galloway, *personal communication*). Galloway et al. (42) also identified a 35K protein by *in vitro* translation of *Bgl*II-N-selected mRNA from HSV-2-infected cells. A number of predominantly late gene products, including gpC, have been mapped by hybridization on the right-hand side of the *mtr*-II-equivalent region in HSV-1 DNA (38,116). Similarly, two additional major late polypeptides of 61K and 56K were identified directly by *in vitro* translation from *Bgl*II-N-selected mRNA by Galloway et al.

FIG. 5. Map locations of cloned HSV DNA fragments relative to defined features of the genome within the transforming regions between 0.28 and 0.67 map units. The cross-hatched bars represent the regions of strongest homology between HSV-1 and HSV-2 DNA, and the open bars represent defined areas of low homology. Vertical dash lines depict the boundaries of the *mtr*-I *(Bgl*I-I) and *mtr*-II *(Bgl*I-N) sequences. The site of strong cell–virus homology in HSV-2 DNA *(Bam*HI-Y) is referred to as *cvh²*, and DNA fragments that activate murine xenotrophic RNA tumor virus expression are referred to as *mux* sequences. Horizontal solid arrows denote the best estimates for the positions, sizes, and orientations of several key early mRNA species. Other features are described in the text. Restriction enzyme cleavage sites are abbreviated as follows: *Bam*HI (B); *Bgl*I (Bg), *Eco*RI (E), *Hin*dIII (H), and *Xba*I (X).

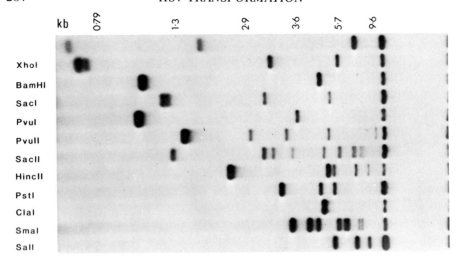

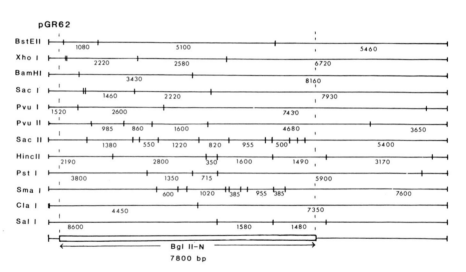

FIG. 6. Partial cleavage map of the *Bgl*II-N fragment (*mtr*-II) in pGR62 DNA. Plasmid DNA was cleaved with *Hind*III, end-labeled with ^{32}P by the polynucleotide kinase reaction, cleaved to completion with *Eco*RI, and divided into equal samples for partial digestion with the enzymes shown. The top panel shows an autoradiograph of the resulting ^{32}P-labeled fragments resolved by electrophoresis through 1.0% agarose gels. Approximate sizes of DNA fragments are given in kilobase pairs. Migration was from right to left, and the small, labeled, 23-bp *Hind*III-*Eco*RI fragment ran off the gels. The lower panel gives an interpretative physical map of the locations of cleavage sites in pGR62. The open bar represents the inserted *Bgl*II-N. fragment, which is in the parental orientation (with 0.582 on the left-hand side). Calculated distances between sites are given in base pairs. This procedure gives some distortion on the right-hand side of the map. In comparison, the pDG401 plasmid used by Galloway and McDougall (39) apparently lacks 550 bp between the *Bgl*II and *Bam*HI sites at the extreme left-hand end of *Bgl*II-N (0.585–0.588).

(42). However, there are several reasons to suspect that the structures of HSV-1 and HSV-2 DNAs may differ in this region. First, HSV-2 gpC maps farther to the right in HSV-2 than in HSV-1 (76,88). Second, an equivalent focus-forming region was not detected in HSV-1 DNA in either the work of Camacho and Spear (11) or that of Reyes et al. (105). In the former experiments the *Xba*I-E fragment (0.45–0.64) should have contained this region intact, whereas in the latter studies the *Bgl*II site at 0.585 and the *Hin*dIII site at 0.591 in HSV-1 DNA could have inactivated any potential transforming activity. Third, preliminary DNA homology studies suggest either lack of homology or the presence of extra DNA sequences within *Bgl*II-N relative to the equivalent region in HSV-1 DNA (G. S. Hayward, *unpublished data*). Fourth, although a 40K delayed-early protein has been mapped here in HSV-1 also (38), the HSV-2 35K species appears to be immunologically type-specific and may not correspond to the HSV-1 protein (42).

Coding Capacity and Cell DNA Homology in the *mtr*-III Region

A large segment of the HSV-2 genome lying between *mtr*-I and *mtr*-II, or more specifically the *Bgl*II/*Hpa*I-CD fragment (map coordinates 0.419–0.575), gave foci in the mass-culture transfection assays of Jariwalla et al. (55). However, this region, referred to here as *mtr*-III, did not give rise to foci at any time in the experiments of Reyes et al. (105), Galloway and McDougall (39), or I. Cameron and J. Macnab *(personal communication)*, except when linked to *Bgl*II-N sequences in the *Eco*RI-A fragment from 0.418 to 0.634 (E. Frost, *personal communication*) or the *Xba*I-D fragment from 0.450 to 0.702 (I. Cameron, *personal communication*). On the other hand, the cloned *Bgl*II-N (pGR60) and *Eco*RI/*Hin*dIII-AA (pGR75) fragments appear to have cell-killing effects in these mass-culture primary hamster embryo cell assays (R. Jariwalla, *personal communication*). Aurelian et al. (5) claimed that the (uncloned) cell lines established from these experiments expressed the Ag-4 antigen (= ICP-10) and retained the input viral DNA sequences. However, several cautions should be added here: (a) As shown in Fig. 7, lanes 1 to 4, the *Bam*HI-Y fragment at 0.47 to 0.49 in this region (part of pGR75) contains one of the several major sites of cell–virus DNA homology found in the HSV-2 genome (95). Repetitive sequences homologous to this site are especially prevalent in human DNA and give a pattern containing both highly dispersed elements and discrete bands after hybridization to either *Eco*RI- or *Bam*HI-cleaved genomic DNA (Fig. 7, lanes 5–12). Note that neither *mtr*-I nor *mtr*-II exhibits this kind of cell–virus homology. (b) Evidence for the presence of a viral antigen corresponding to Ag-4 in transformed cells has not yet been reproduced or confirmed by other groups, and the claim that ICP-10 is an immediate-early gene product mapping entirely within *mtr*-III is not consistent with any of the known locations of major IE mRNAs. Therefore, the possibility remains that a virus-induced cellular transformation antigen, and simple homology between *mtr*-III sequences and repetitive cellular DNA sequences, could explain some of these findings. No other well-characterized viral gene products have been clearly identified as yet from this large segment of the

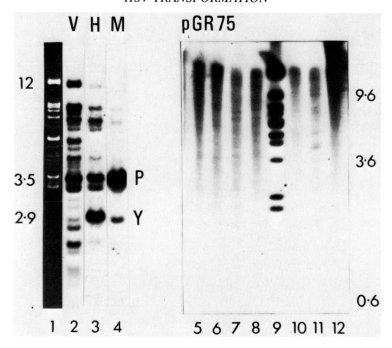

FIG. 7. Homology between HSV-2 DNA and mammalian cell genomes. Left-hand panel: Blot hybridization with cell genomic DNA probes to HSV DNA fragments on filters. Lane 1: Ethidium-bromide-stained *Bam*HI DNA fragments from HSV-2 after electrophoresis through a 1.0% aga-rose gel. Lanes 2, 3, and 4: Autoradiographs of hybrids formed between viral DNA fragments from the same gel as shown in lane 1 and ³²P-labeled probes of total viral DNA (V), human placental DNA (H), or mouse BALB/c 3T3 cell DNA (M). Right-hand panel: Blot hybridization with the pGR75 cloned viral DNA fragment probe to cleaved cell DNA on filters. The insert in this plasmid represents the *Eco*RI/*Hind*III-AA fragment from HSV-2(333) and contains the *Bam*HI-Y cell–virus homology site. Lane 5: Human placental DNA, *Eco*RI. Lane 6: Human placental DNA, *Bam*HI. Lane 7: Mouse BALB/c 3T3 cell DNA, *Eco*RI. Lane 8: Mouse BALB/c 3T3 cell DNA, *Bam*HI. Lane 9: Size standards of phage lambda DNA (mixture of *Hind*III and *Eco*RI digests). Lane 10: BSC-1 African green monkey cell DNA. Lane 11: Primary hamster kidney cell DNA. Lane 12: Chicken DNA.

HSV genome, although the genes for the 150K DNA polymerase and the cytoplasmic 140K protein (IE-II or ICP-6) partially overlap with the left- and right-hand ends of the region, respectively. The host shutoff functions, and perhaps a late polypeptide referred to as ICP-7 in the nomenclature of Morse et al. (88), may be located entirely within the *mtr*-III region. Recently, Aurelian et al. (5) have suggested that Ag-4 may indeed be equivalent to ICP-6. However, if this is the case, then only the 5′ half of the gene is being introduced into their cells by the *Bgl*II/*Hpa*I-CD fragment. Knipe et al. (63) have mapped the tsB7 mutation to this location in the HSV genome. The tsB7 virus fails to synthesize any detectable virus-specific polypeptides after infection of normally permissive cells at high temperature, and it is believed to encode a late virion polypeptide that appears to be necessary for initiation of lytic cycle functions (63).

RETENTION OF VIRAL DNA SEQUENCES IN TRANSFORMED CELLS

Early Work with UV-irradiated Virus-transformed Cell Lines

The earliest attempts using whole viral DNA probes in liquid hybridization procedures to detect HSV DNA or RNA sequences in cells transformed by UV-inactivated virus (or in tumor lines derived from them) yielded variable or inconclusive results and gave the strong impression that most of the viral sequences that might have been retained initially were gradually discarded at higher passage levels. The most commonly studied HSV-2-transformed line, 333-8-9, was developed from primary hamster cells by Duff and Rapp (29) and consists of uncloned, highly pleomorphic hyperdiploid hamster cells. Considerable amounts of viral DNA and RNA were present at early passages (19,37), but much less or none was detected after subcloning and extensive passaging (22,40,85). The subclones vary greatly in morphology (ranging from totally fibroblastic to totally epithelial), in tumorigenicity, in chromosome segregation patterns, and in viral DNA content (22). The 333-8-9 cells produce tumors in newborn hamsters and have been claimed to express virus-specific surface and cytoplasmic antigens (75). The resulting tumors, unlike those from SV40- or adenovirus-transformed cells, are highly metastatic and do not elicit tumor-specific transplantation or rejection antigens (30). In addition to the apparent expression of viral surface antigens (59,61,72), other cell lines of this type have also been shown to complement ts mutants (60,73). In the most extreme example, Park et al. (94) analyzed rescued wild-type virus from HSV-1 ts infection of HSV-2-transformed cells and found both intertypic recombinant hybrids and apparently complete recovered HSV-2 genomes. These results and others (1,18) imply that the entire HSV genome can persist in cultured cells infected under nonpermissive conditions, but the state of this DNA (integrated, episomal, or packaged) and the significance of this for transformation, tumorigenicity, and latency are unclear at present.

Interestingly, the only renaturation-kinetics study of 333-8-9 lines at relatively early passage that involved a survey with a set of isolated viral DNA fragments gave consistently positive hybridization results with probes from the region to the left of tk (0.2–0.31) and also from *mtr*-II (0.58–0.63), but only occasional or trace hybridization with probes from other regions of the HSV-2 genome (40). At late (200th) passage in uncloned 333-8-9 cells, and also in isolated subclones, we have been unable to detect viral DNA sequences by blot hybridization procedures with cloned HSV-2 DNA probes containing *mtr*-I or *mtr*-II DNA sequences (i.e., <0.1 copy/cell); however, both cloned and uncloned cultures incorporate and phosphorylate ^{125}I-iododeoxycytidine into approximately 10% of the cells, suggesting the presence of viral tk activity. (C. Flexner, G. Hayward, and P. Leitman, *unpublished data.*)

Detection of Viral RNA in Tumors by *In Situ* Hybridization

A single example of the detection of HSV-2 DNA in cervical carcinoma tissue by renaturation-kinetics analysis was reported by Frenkel et al. (36), but this result

could not be reproduced in other tumor samples (93,122) and presumably represented adventitious viral infection. Attempts to demonstrate HSV-2 RNA by *in situ*
hybridization in tumor tissue biopsy slices have apparently consistently given reproducible positive results in double-blind studies with approximately 30 to 40%
of preinvasive cervical carcinoma samples, compared with 5 to 10% scored positive
in unrelated tumors or normal tissue control samples (31a,74,79,120). The different
authors have reported varying results with tumors at later stages of development
and in nearby normal stromal tissue. These techniques are complicated by nonspecific DNA binding to certain tissues and extensive homology between many of the
same tissue samples and adenovirus type 2 DNA (74). In addition, the finding of
homology between portions of HSV-2 DNA and repetitive sequences in normal
human placental DNA suggests that great caution should be exercised in the interpretation of experiments of this kind. However, consistent detection in tumors of
RNA from specific portions of the HSV genome would go a long way toward
eliminating the concern about adventitious viral infection, as well as cross-homology
complications. Preliminary results using isolated cloned probes are now becoming
available (78,120). Both studies reported a high frequency (20–30%) of positive
in situ hybridization with sequences between 0.08 and 0.31 to the left of *mtr*-I.
McDougall et al. (78), in particular, also found sequences related to part of *mtr*-I
and to *mtr*-II (i.e., HSV-2 *Bgl*II-J and *Bgl*II-N) in 8 to 20% of the samples. Probes
from other regions in the L segment (0.38–0.58 and 0.63–0.78), as well as from
the center of the S segment, were negative. Probes from the S repeats (a major site
of cell–virus homology) gave positive *in situ* hybridization in up to 32% of tumor
samples and 8% of normal tissues. Similar studies with latently infected ganglia
(41) have also revealed a high concentration of RNA from sequences to the left of
tk (i.e., 0.08–0.31), and it should be noted here that this left portion of the L
segment gives rise to the most abundant mRNA species at late times in productive
viral infections (116).

Search for Viral DNA Sequences in Fragment-transformed Cell Lines

Hybridization with isolated viral DNA probes to transformed cell DNA after
fractionation by RPC-5 chromatography has suggested that several early passage
mtr-II lines (F11B2clD9, F4A1A1) retain viral DNA sequences, but that the F5A3B
mtr-I cell line does not (105). Further experiments (not shown) using plasmid DNA
probes containing the *Bgl*II-I or *Bgl*I-N fragments inserted into pBR322 have confirmed the apparent absence of significant stretches of viral DNA sequences in the
majority of the F5A3B cells and also in several later-passage *mtr*-II BALB/c cell
lines tested, including methylcellulose-derived subclones (at a sensitivity down to
approximately 0.1 copy/cell). Only a single BALB/c cell line tested, F4A1A1,
contained a portion of the *Bgl*II-N fragment at close to 1 copy/cell or greater (*vide
infra*). Perhaps even more surprisingly, we obtained similar negative results (less
than 0.1 copy/cell) with six separate sublines of the *mtr*-II-fragment-transformed
hamster cells (103). Leiden and Frenkel (67) also reported failure to detect viral

DNA sequences in the hamster cell lines derived from the experiments of Camacho and Spear (11), and similarly Galloway et al. (39) detected *Bgl*II-N sequences at only 0.1 copy/cell or less in their fragment-transformed hamster and NIH mouse lines. However, most interestingly, an examination of *Bgl*II-N sequences present in their NIH tumor-derived cell lines revealed portions of the right-hand side of *Bgl*II-N present at approximately 1 copy/cell (39).

These results suggest that although *Bgl*II-N and *Bgl*II-I may contain sequences necessary for initiation of focus formation, the retention of these viral sequences is unstable and may not be required for maintenance of the "morphologically transformed" phenotype in cell culture. However, perhaps some viral sequence within *Bgl*II-N is necessary for tumor formation in animals, and the passage through nude mice may clonally select for that small fraction of cells that do still retain viral sequences. The finding of different patterns of viral DNA sequences in different tumors derived from the same initial cell line (39) further supports the notion of instability and rearrangement of the integrated viral sequences. Similarly, we have observed quite different patterns of viral DNA sequences at various passage levels in the F4A1A1 cell line, even though it was originally subcloned three times (103).

Integrated Viral DNA Sequences in the F4A1A1 Cell Line

In preliminary screening of F4A1A1 DNA at the eighth passage (after four subcloning steps) using a pGR62 (*Bgl*II-N) probe, we detected a single very prominent *Bgl*II fragment of 16 kb present at approximately 1 copy/cell relative to reconstructions with authentic pGR62 or pGR101 DNA (not shown). In the same experiment, F11A1A, F12A2B, and HF3A2A DNA yielded faint hybridizing *Bgl*II bands of even higher molecular weight that we estimated to be present at 0.1 to 0.2 copy/cell. No specific bands were detectable at this sensitivity in DNAs from the F11B2c1D9, F13B3B, HF3A3A, HF3B2B, and 333-8-9 cells (at passage 200) or from the parental BALB/c 3T3 and normal hamster cell DNAs. Further analysis of the F4A1A1 cell DNA with additional restriction enzyme cleavages (e.g., *Xho*I and *Hin*dIII) revealed that higher-molecular-weight fragments (20–40 kb) transferred to the nitrocellulose at much lower efficiency than the 16-kb *Bgl*II species (Fig. 8), and therefore the results with other DNAs, especially F11A1A and F12A2B, may be greatly underestimated. The pattern of cleavages in the *Bgl*II-N complementary DNA sequences present in F4A1A1 DNA does not resemble any obvious continuous stretch of *Bgl*II-N sequences of greater than 500 bp in size. Three cloned viral DNA fragment probes representing different portions of the *Bgl*II-N sequences (pGH7, pGR106, and pGR161) (Fig. 5) all gave essentially equivalent hybridization results with F4A1A1 cell DNA (not shown), implying that the viral DNA includes sequences from the only region common to all three probes (viz., 0.607–0.610). The simplest interpretation of these and other hybridization results with F4A1A1 DNA indicates that it contains at least two and possibly four separate integration sites with very short segments of *Bgl*II-N DNA (less than 500 bp in size), with each present in multiple copies in all cells.

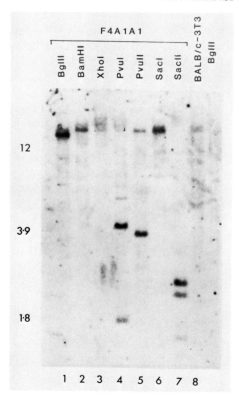

FIG. 8. Detection of HSV-2 *Bgl*II-N-related sequences by blot hybridization in an *mtr*-II-DNA-fragment-transformed cell line. Samples of F4A1A1 mouse cell DNA (15 μg per track) were cleaved with restriction enzymes, fractionated by agarose gel electrophoresis, denatured, and transferred to a nitrocellulose filter. Hybridization was carried out as described by Reyes et al. (106) with an *in vitro* nick-translated probe of pGR62 plasmid DNA. The diagram shows an autoradiograph of the resulting hybrids. Lanes 1–7: F4A1A1 genomic DNA cleaved with: 1, *Bgl*II; 2, *Bam*HI; 3, *Xho*I; 4, *Pvu*I; 5, *Pvu*II; 6, *Sac*I; 7, *Sac*II. Lane 8: Parental BALB/c 3T3 cell DNA cleaved with *Bgl*II. The positions of size standards in adjacent tracks are given in kilobase pairs.

Comparison with Biochemically Transformed Cell Lines

The idea of a direct involvement by the viral tk gene in morphological transformation has been fairly strongly refuted by several studies. First, neither the isolated *Bgl*II-I fragment nor the *Bgl*II-N fragment encodes a tk activity that can rescue Ltk⁻ cells in transfection assays involving HAT selection (105). Second, in both HSV-1 and HSV-2, fragments that do contain the tk gene map to the left of *mtr*-I and well away from *mtr*-II (105). Third, using BALB/c 3T3 clone D2 tk⁻ cells, Hampar et al. (48) showed that none of 15 HSV-1-transformed cell lines, selected as morphologically transformed foci after infection with UV-inactivated virus, simultaneously picked up the tk⁺ phenotype. Similarly, in the reverse assay, none of 47 subclones isolated from BALB/c 3T3 clone D2 tk⁻ cultures after selection for tk⁺ transformation also acquired morphologically transformed features or tumorigenicity.

There is no difficulty in detecting viral tk gene sequences in tk⁺ cell lines established by HAT selection after either infection with UV-inactivated virus (25,64,68) or transfection with isolated viral DNA fragments and recombinant cloned plasmids (96,106). However, in this case, unlike the case of morphologically transformed lines, any cells that lose the tk gene will be killed under the selective conditions employed. Some tk⁺ cell lines derived from experiments in which the entire HSV genome enters the cells also retain additional viral sequences (68,86). This was also the case in our L tk⁺ cell lines that received isolated viral DNA fragments (106). For example, the *Xba*I-F fragment from HSV-1(MP) and the *Bgl*II-G and *Hin*dIII-H fragments from HSV-2(333) each carry an intact tk gene plus large sections of adjacent viral DNA sequences covering map coordinates from 0.2 to 0.4 in the viral genome (Fig. 9) (103). Analysis of the viral DNA sequences retained in several subclones from transfections with each of these fragments has revealed at least one insertion site that carries a large proportion of the adjacent input sequences. We interpret the results of hybridization experiments of the type shown in Fig. 9 as follows: (a) Most tk⁺ cell lines contain at least one small, single-copy, integrated tk gene sequence in which the insertion event has occurred either close to the 5′ end of the tk gene or close to the 3′ end of the tk gene or both. (b) In lines in which multiple insertions have occurred, the second or third integrated

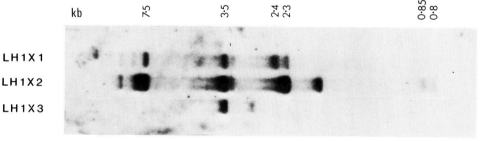

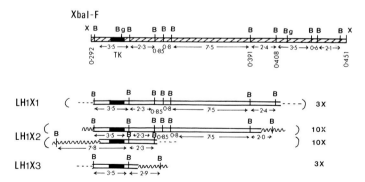

FIG. 9. Demonstration of the retention of adjacent *mtr*-I sequences in DNA-fragment-transformed L tk⁺ cell lines. Genomic DNA from three cell lines, derived from colonies appearing in HAT selection assays after transfection of L tk⁻ cells with the isolated HSV-1 *Xba*I-F fragment (0.292–0.451), was cleaved with *Bam*HI and subjected to agarose gel electrophoresis. The DNA was transferred to nitrocellulose filters and hybridized with an *in vitro* ³²P-labeled pGR116 plasmid probe (*Bgl*II-I cloned in pBR322). The top panel shows an autoradiograph of the hybrid DNA fragments formed and their approximate sizes in kilobase pairs. The lower panel presents the simplest interpretation of these results. Line LH₁X₁ carries three tandem repeat units containing all of the viral sequences between 0.296 and 0.408. Line LH₁X₂ contains two different-size inserts, each within multicopy repeat units.

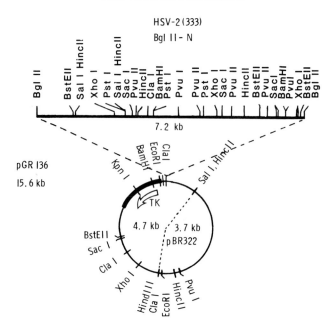

FIG. 10. Structure of the pGR136 plasmid used in tk-linked coselection experiments. The *Bg*lII-N fragment from position 0.582 to 0.628 in HSV-2(333) DNA was inserted into the *Bg*lII site 200 bp upstream from the tk promoter in the pGR18 HSV-2 tk vehicle. The pGR18 contains a 4.7-kb *Hin*dIII-*Sal*I fragment from map coordinates 0.289 to 0.320 in HSV-2 DNA. In pGR136 the *Bg*lII-N fragment occurs in an inverted orientation, with position 0.628 closest to the tk gene. An otherwise identical plasmid pGR236 carries *Bg*lII-N in the opposite or parental orientation. The several *Pst*I and *Pvu*II sites in pGR18 have been omitted from the diagram.

fragments tend to retain large stretches of adjacent sequences. (c) The secondary integrated fragments are occasionally tandemly duplicated as part of large repeat units that include stretches of cellular or carrier DNA as well as the viral sequences (106).

The hybridization experiment shown in Fig. 9 revealed that virtually the entire *mtr*-I region was retained in the LH$_1$X$_1$-fragment-transformed tk$^+$ cell line (map coordinates approximately 0.295–0.410), and slightly less was retained at one integration site in the multicopy LH$_1$X$_2$ cell line (approximately 0.295–0.385). Therefore, the *mtr*-I DNA sequence does not appear to be intrinsically unstable or deleterious in DNA-fragment-transformed cell lines. These particular L tk$^+$ cell lines could potentially be used as complementing hosts for growth and selection of "transformation-defective" virus mutants constructed by marker rescue procedures with mutagenized or biochemically deleted *mtr*-I DNA fragments. Linked coselection of *mtr*-II sequences is not possible directly with isolated viral DNA fragments because of the great distance between *Bg*lII-N and the tk gene in the HSV-2 DNA molecule. However, with the availability of cloned viral DNA fragments and tk plasmid vehicles, this obstacle can now be overcome (*vide infra*).

Coselection with the Transposition Plasmid pGR136

In an attempt to establish cell lines that stably retain either large sections or all of the *mtr*-II sequences, we constructed a transpositional plasmid (pGR136) containing the HSV-2 *Bgl*II-N fragment inserted adjacent to the HSV-2 tk gene in the pGR18 vehicle (Fig. 10). The tk⁺ cell lines established under various protocols with pGR136 (i.e., linear or circular plasmid DNA, with or without carrier L tk⁻ DNA) were then examined for retention of virus-specific DNA sequences. Cellular DNA samples from a total of 22 independent subclones were cleaved with appropriate restriction enzymes, subjected to agarose gel electrophoresis, and transferred to nitrocellulose filters for hybridization. In each case, nick-translated cloned plasmid DNAs carrying the tk gene (pGR18), the *Bgl*II-N fragment (pGR62), or the original input pGR136 plasmid were used as independent probes on three separate filters. The results were quite different from those obtained earlier with the isolated tk-containing DNA fragments. Although all lines retained intact HSV-2 tk genes, only three contained significant amounts of adjacent *Bgl*II-N sequences (2–3 kb at most), and none contained pBR322 sequences. Our interpretation of the structure of the integrated coselected sequences in several LH_2p136 cell lines is shown in Fig. 11. The three subclones that retained the most viral DNA sequences adjacent to the 5′ end of the tk gene were *cl*10, *cl*13, and *cl*18. As before, in at least two of these tk⁺ lines a second insertion was also evident in which the recombination event had occurred very close to the 5′ end of the tk gene. Because the *Bgl*II-N fragment is inserted in an inverted orientation in pGR136, each of these cell lines contains sequences from the right-hand side of *Bgl*II-N only. The dramatic contrast to findings in the LH_1X_2 and LH_2H_3 cell lines and the similarity of this result to that in the *Bgl*II-N-fragment-transformed cell lines suggest that there may be a sequence in the left-hand side of *Bgl*II-N that is deleterious to the cells or incompatible with cell survival. However, we cannot at present exclude the alternative possibility that "poison" sequences within the pBR322 DNA (71) were responsible for the lack of retention of the adjacent *Bgl*II-N sequences. A similar set of cell lines has now been established with a modified plasmid (pGR236), in which the left-hand side of the *Bgl*II-N fragment is adjacent to the tk gene, but the DNA from these lines has not yet been analyzed.

CORRELATION WITH VIRAL ANTIGENS FOUND IN TRANSFORMED CELLS AND TUMORS

Other Evidence for Involvement of *mtr*-I in Transformation: The 128K Major DNA Binding Protein

Despite the lack of focus formation in our experiments with the *mtr*-I-equivalent region from HSV-2 DNA (105) and the rather inconsistent ability to induce focus formation with *Bgl*II-I from HSV-1 (we have been unable to produce foci with the cloned pGR116 or pGR127 plasmids, which both contain an intact *Bgl*II-I fragment except for the 0.402 deletion), interest in the potential role of this region in trans-

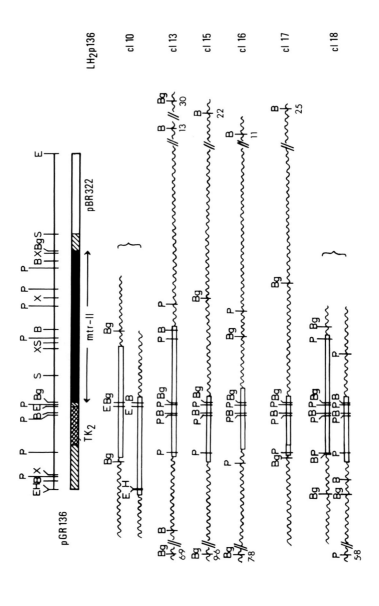

formation remains high. There are several reasons for this: First, an apparently equivalent region in equine abortion virus (EHV-1) DNA has been shown to be retained in hamster tumor cell lines derived from hamster embryo cells that were persistently infected with defective populations of EHV-1 (108). The minimal sequences of EHV-1 DNA retained in several EHV-1-transformed cell lines consistently map between 0.33 and 0.38 in the L segment of the EHV-1 genome (52,107). Second, the major viral glycoprotein gpA/B (115K, ICP-11), but not the glycoprotein gpD from the unique S segment (for example), has apparently been detected in some virus-transformed cells using monospecific antisera to the purified protein (69). Similarly, antibodies against a 118K protein that maps in this area and may correspond to gpA/B appear to occur in significantly higher levels in sera from patients with cervical carcinoma than in matched control sera (44). On the other hand, the original report of the presence of gpA/B in the hamster cells transformed with the *Xba*I-F fragment appears to have been withdrawn (P. Spear, *personal communication*).

Third, the HSV major DNA binding protein has been claimed by Dreesman et al. (28), Kaufman et al. (57), and McDougall et al. (78) to be directly detectable by immunofluorescence assays in cervical and vulva tumor samples, and also by Flannery et al. (34) in UV-inactivated HSV-transformed cells. Powell et al. (99) have extensively purified a DNA binding protein (128K, DBP) from both HSV-1- and HSV-2-infected cells and have prepared immunoprecipitating monospecific antisera against it. This protein represents a major product synthesized at delayed-early times after viral infection (99,117) and is localized exclusively in the nucleus in infected human diploid fibroblasts (Fig. 13, panels a and b). Recent evidence suggests that the viral polypeptides referred to as ICP-8, ICSP-11/12, and 143K early nonstructural (34) all represent this same major DNA binding protein. Conley et al. (20) have carried out detailed mapping studies with a mutant in this gene, concluding that the 128K protein plays a key role in "switch-on" of late viral functions, perhaps because of its functioning in viral DNA replication. The DNA sequences coding for 128K lie between 0.380 and 0.400, according to marker rescue experiments, i.e., directly adjacent to *ori*-L (Fig. 5).

FIG. 11. Maps of the integrated forms of HSV-2 DNA sequences in six LH₂p136 L tk⁺ cell lines. The top line in the diagram illustrates the structure and positions of major cleavage sites in pGR136 drawn in a linear form. The solid bar represents the *Bgl*II-N fragment sequences in the parent input pGR136 plasmid, and the hatched bar represents the HSV-2 tk gene. The simplest interpretations of viral DNA sequences detected in the genomic DNA from LH₂p136-10, -13, -15, -16, -17, and -18 are shown. Except for subline 10, the cell DNA samples were cleaved separately with *Bgl*II, *Bam*HI, and *Pvu*II. Nick-translated ³²P-plasmid DNA probes of pBR322, pGR18, and pGR136 were used in three separate blot hybridization experiments similar to that shown in Fig. 8. The open bars represent viral DNA sequences, and the wavy lines denote adjacent cell DNA sequences. The results for lines LH₂p136-10 and -18 were best interpreted as two separate integration sites. The presence of an intact 2,800-bp *Pvu*II fragment homologous to the pGR136 probe only, indicated retention of 40% of the *mtr*-II sequences adjacent to the tk gene in sublines 13 and 18. The 0.592 to 0.606 segment of *Bgl*II-N was missing from all cell lines, as demonstrated by the absence of the 1,600-bp, 980-bp, and 860-bp *Pvu*II fragments.

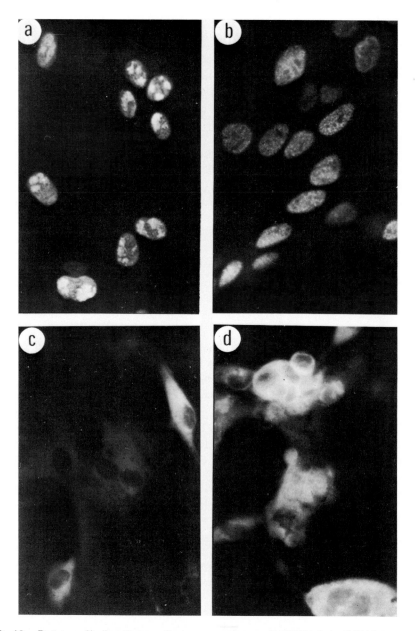

FIG. 12. Patterns of indirect immunofluorescence observed in HSV-infected HF (diploid human fibroblast) cells using mouse monoclonal hybridoma antisera (110). **a:** Anti-128K major DNA protein binding (39S) at 8 hr after infection with HSV-1 (MP). **b:** Anti-128K serum (39S) at 24 hr after HSV-1(MP) infection. **c:** Anti-140K cytoplasmic IE-II protein (2S) at 8 hr after infection with HSV-2(333). **d:** Anti-140K serum (2S) at 24 hr after HSV-2(333) infection. All infections were carried out at an m.o.i. (multiplicity of infection) of 10 pfu/ml with filtered virus stocks. FITC fluorescence from goat antimouse IgG was photographed through a ×40 oil objective under UV epifluorescence illumination. Both monoclonal ascites fluid sera were gifts from the laboratories of M. Zweig and B. Hampar (Frederick Cancer Research Center, Maryland).

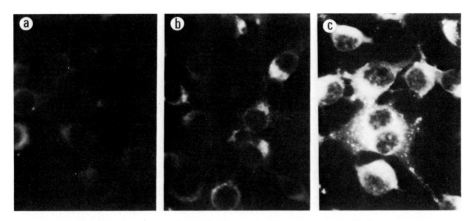

FIG. 13. Patterns of indirect immunofluorescence obtained with HSV hyperimmune sera against the LH₂p136-14 cell line. **a:** Rat preimmune serum. **b:** Rat antiserum generated against immediate-early antigens from HSV-2(HG-52)-infected primary rat embryo cells (3-hr reversal of a cycloheximide block in the presence of actinomycin D). **c:** Rat antiserum generated against early (immediate-early plus delayed-early) antigens in HG-52-infected rat embryo cells (7-hr reversal of a cycloheximide block without actinomycin D). These antisera were obtained courtesy of J. MacNab (Virology Institute, University of Glasglow, Scotland) and were diluted 1:50 before use. Absorption against methanol-fixed L tk⁻ cells quantitatively removed all of the granular perinuclear fluorescence.

Surprisingly, the monospecific antisera that were raised against the isolated 128K DBP (i.e., anti-VP143 or anti-ICSP-11/12) gave cytoplasmic fluorescence in up to 30% of the tumor tissue samples screened, in contrast to the strong nuclear fluorescence obtained in productively infected cells. A monospecific antibody against purified HSV ICSP-11/12 (99) also gives cytoplasmic fluorescence in the EHV-1-transformed cells (D. O'Callaghan, *personal communication*). The major DNA binding protein apparently represents a highly conserved group-specific antigen that cross-reacts immunologically among all viruses in the HSV-like subgroup of herpesviruses (121).

Elevated Antibody Levels to 38K in Patient Sera

Evidence of a quite different kind also implicates a 35K/38K protein in some way as a key factor in morphological transformation. Gilman et al. (44) compared the patterns of immunoprecipitated viral polypeptides in sera from patients with cervical carcinoma with those of carefully matched controls and concluded that antibodies to an HSV-2 38K type-specific protein (as well as the 118K species) occurred at statistically much higher levels and frequencies in the tumor samples, whereas those against all other viral polypeptides occurred in approximately equal amounts in both groups. These results were obtained quite independent of knowledge of the focus formation experiments of Reyes et al. (105). More recently, Suh (113) has used hyperimmune sera against HSV-2-infected cells to demonstrate that a 35K phosphorylated polypeptide is the major viral antigen immunoprecipitated from the

620-7T and 333-8-9 HSV-2-transformed cell lines and also from an *EcoRI-A-DNA*-fragment-transformed cell line (E. Frost and M. Suh, *personal communication*). This 35K protein from transformed cells gave the same *Staphylococcus aureus* V8 protease partial cleavage pattern as a viral 35K protein synthesized in HSV-2-infected cells. Both proteins were synthesized *in vitro* from poly(A)-containing RNA selected by hybridization to the *Bgl*II-N fragment. Monoclonal mouse hybridoma antibodies that immunoprecipitate an HSV-2 type-specific 38K polypeptide have been obtained by S. Bacchetti *(personal communication)* and by Goldstein (42). In our hands, the anti-38K antibody gives weak nuclear staining in HSV-2-infected cells at delayed-early times (not shown). According to Galloway et al. (42), monoclonal antibody against the 140K HSV-2 polypeptide (ICP-6) coprecipitated the HSV-2 38K protein, and vice versa, implying that these two proteins may have common or overlapping amino acid sequences.

Although we emphasize that there is no direct evidence at the present time to connect the 38K polypeptide from patient sera (44) with the 35K/38K polypeptide encoded by *Bgl*II-N from HSV-2-infected and -transformed cells (113), the exciting possibility exists that these may all be the same entity and that antibody levels to the 38K viral antigen may have prospective value in predicting the susceptibility to or progress of cervical carcinoma.

Does HSV Induce Cellular Transformation Antigens?

We do not know at present whether the correlation between the map locations of the 128K and 38K polypeptides and those for *mtr*-I and *mtr*-II is purely coincidental or is related directly or indirectly to the mechanism of transformation. Many reports of other supposedly HSV-associated tumor antigens or HSV-transformed cell antigens have appeared in the literature, e.g., TAA (17), 83K (114), and Ag-4 (5). However, most of these have not yet been shown convincingly to be viral rather than cellular proteins.

Monoclonal mouse hybridoma antibodies against several of the better characterized viral polypeptides mentioned earlier are available, although they apparently have not yet been used to examine tumor samples. Anti-128K (= major DBP or ICSP-11/12), anti-gpA/B(= 115K), anti-140K (= IE-II or ICP-6), and anti-38K were kindly provided by Berge Hampar, Tony Minson, and Silvia Bacchetti. The intracellular appearances of the DBP and 140K species in 6-hr and 24-hr HSV-1- or HSV-2-infected L tk⁻ cells, respectively, are shown in Fig. 12. However, none of these sera gave positive results by immunofluorescence in any of our fragment-transformed *mtr*-I or *mtr*-II cell lines that were tested or in the LH$_2$p127 (*Bgl*II-I) or LH$_2$136 (*Bgl*II-N) cell lines made by linked coselection with the HSV-2 tk gene. On the other hand, hyperimmune antisera prepared in either rats or mice inoculated with infected primary rat or BALB/c 3T3 cells after release from cycloheximide blockage at early stages of infection gave strong perinuclear cytoplasmic immunofluorescence against all LH$_2$p136 cell lines (Fig. 13). In neither case did the preimmune serum give any reaction, nor did these hyperimmune sera give strong reactions with nontransformed Rat-1 or BALB/c 3T3 cells. However, further investigations revealed that all transformed cells, including the parent L tk⁻ line, gave intense perinuclear granular fluorescence with these sera and that this fluorescence against LH$_2$p136 cells could be removed by absorption against L tk⁻ cells, although not by absorption against nontransformed cells. We suggest that one or both of the following situations occur: (a) Even in syngeneic animals, strong antibody reactions against cell architecture proteins such as actin cables may be mounted after injection with infected cell cultures, and these proteins register strongly as disaggregated, perinuclear granules in transformed cells (12). (b) The viral infection induces cellular proteins at early stages after infection, perhaps equivalent to the switch-on of the cellular 53K by SV40 infection (70), and these transformation-specific proteins are targets for a major antigenic response in the immunized animals. Hamster tumor antiserum that immunoprecipitated both SV40 large T antigen and the 53K protein also gave a very similar granular cytoplasmic fluorescence against L tk⁻ cells, but it gave exclusively nuclear fluorescence with the SV40-transformed human NBE cell line (not shown). Whichever of these alternatives applies, these results urge caution in the interpretation of previous claims for virus-specific cytoplasmic antigens in transformed cells based on immunofluorescence or immunoprecipitation experiments in which hyperimmune antisera against unpurified virus-infected polypeptides were used. It may not be adequate to absorb these sera only with nontransformed cells; in addition, other kinds of transformed cells or tumor samples are needed as negative controls, rather than nontransformed cells. Similarly, the positive control of absorption against HSV-infected cells does not necessarily discriminate between virus-specific antigens and induced cellular transformation-specific proteins.

CONCLUDING REMARKS

We wish to emphasize that the *mtr*-I fragment, and its apparent equivalent in equine abortion virus, is the only active transforming region identified so far among HSV-1 strains, whereas *mtr*-II and *mtr*-III have been observed only in HSV-2 DNA. We suspect that both of these functions may act in concert for full expression of the HSV-2 oncogenic phenotype, with *mtr*-II alone perhaps giving rise to only a partial transformation phenotype in much the same way as the leftmost 4.5% fragment in the adenovirus EIA region (53). Whether or not HSV-1 and HSV-2 both contain functional *mtr*-I and *mtr*-II regions remains to be determined. It may be purely coincidental, but in the experiments of Reyes et al. (105) the *Bgl*II and *Hind*III sites at 0.585 and 0.591 and HSV-2 would almost certainly have inactivated the HSV-2 equivalent of the 38K protein, and similarly the *Bgl*II and *Hind*III sites at 0.385 and 0.398 in HSV-2 DNA would probably have inactivated the HSV-2 128K major DNA binding protein. On reflection, the existence of at least two totally different mechanisms for transformation by HSV-1 and HSV-2 may not be so surprising, when one considers that current evidence favors the necessity for part of the large T antigen and perhaps also an active small T antigen for transformation by SV40 virus but clearly implicates the quite different middle T polypeptide in transformation by the structurally closely related polyoma virus (14,49,66,91). Based on previous experience with the papovaviruses and adenoviruses, it was perhaps surprising initially that the evidence favored an involvement of delayed-early genes in HSV transformation rather than the immediate-early genes that normally are required for expression of the later classes of gene products during productive infection. However, we know very little as yet about the nature of the complex HSV cascade regulation process.

In conclusion, the current biochemical evidence does not permit an unambiguous determination of the mechanism by which HSV transformation occurs, i.e., whether HSV genomes (a) carry true viral oncogenes, (b) act by a promoter insertion mechanism, or (c) invoke some other process to activate cellular transformation proteins (or all of these). Neither is there any clear, uncontested evidence that HSV does indeed play a triggering role in cervical carcinoma; the association with genital papillomavirus infections, for example, appears equally convincing to some authors (102). Nevertheless, the evidence that this subgroup of herpesviruses is oncogenic is steadily increasing, as is the likelihood that HSV-2 could play some active role in tumor formation in humans. In particular, the finding of elevated antibodies to the 38K polypeptide in cervical carcinoma sera and the detection of the 128K major DNA binding protein in tumor samples, which at least superficially correlates with the ability of the DNA fragments encoding these two proteins to initiate focus formation, provide an intriguing basis for further studies. Significant additional progress will almost certainly require the construction (or selection) of transformation-defective host-range-type mutant viruses that give aberrant focus formation phenotypes, and perhaps also the further development and utilization of well-characterized cell lines derived from human tumors (83).

ACKNOWLEDGMENTS

We thank Nancy Standish for assistance with preparation and proofreading of this manuscript and Michael McLane and Dolores Ciufo for excellent technical assistance throughout these studies. The work carried out in the authors' laboratory was supported by grants NO1 CP-71022 and RO1 CA-28473 to G.S.H. from the National Cancer Institute.

REFERENCES

1. Adler, R., Glorioso, J. C., and Levine, M. (1978): Infection by herpes simplex virus and cells of nervous system origin: Characterization of a non-permissive interaction. *J. Gen. Virol.*, 39:9–20.
2. Anderson, K. P., Frink, R. J., Devi, G. B., Gaylord, B. H., Costa, R. H., and Wagner, E. K. (1981): Detailed characterization of the mRNA mapping in the *Hin*dIII fragment K region of the herpes simplex virus type I genome. *J. Virol.*, 37:1011–1027.
3. Anderson, K. P., Stringer, J. R., Holland, L. F., and Wagner, E. K. (1979): Isolation and localization of herpes simplex virus type 1 mRNA. *J. Virol.*, 30:805–820.
4. Andersson, P., Goldfarb, M. P., and Weinberg, R. A. (1979): A defined subgenomic fragment of *in vitro* synthesized Moloney sarcoma virus DNA can induce cellular tranformation upon transfection. *Cell*, 16:63–76.

5. Aurelian, L., Manak, M. M., McKinlay, M., Smith, C. C., Klacsmann, K. T., and Gupta, P. K. (1981): "The herpesvirus hypothesis"—Are Koch's postulates satisfied? *Gynecol. Oncol.*, 12:S56–S87.

6. Baringer, J. R. (1975): Herpes simplex virus infection of nervous tissue in animals and man. *Prog. Med. Virol.*, 20:1–26.

7. Blair, D. G., McClements, W. L., Oskarsson, M. K., Fischinger, P. J., and Vande Woude, G. R. (1980): Biological activity of cloned Moloney sarcoma virus DNA: Terminally redundant sequences may enhance transformation efficiency. *Proc. Natl. Acad. Sci. USA*, 77:3504–3508.

8. Boyd, A. L. (1975): Characterization of single-cell clonal lines derived from HSV-2-transformed mouse cells. *Intervirology*, 6:156–167.

9. Boyd, A. L., Derge, J. G., and Hampar, B. (1978): Activation of endogenous type C virus in BALB/c mouse cells by herpesvirus DNA. *Proc. Natl. Acad. Sci. USA*, 75:4558–4562.

10. Boyd, A. L., Enquist, L., Vande Woude, G. F., and Hampar, B. (1980): Activation of mouse retrovirus by herpes simplex virus type 1 cloned DNA fragments. *Virology* 103:228–231.

11. Camacho, A., and Spear, P. G. (1978): Transformation of hamster embryo fibroblasts by a specific fragment of the herpes simplex virus genome. *Cell*, 15:993–1002.

12. Carley, W. W., Barak, L. S., and Webb, W. W. (1981): F-actin aggregates in transformed cells. *J. Cell Biol.*, 90:797–802.

13. Chartrand, P., Stow, N. D., Timbury, M. C., and Wilkie, N. M. (1979): Physical mapping of *paa*ʳ mutations of herpes simplex virus type 1 and type 2 by intertypic marker rescue. *J. Virol.*, 31:265–276.

14. Chowdhury, K., Light, S. E., Garon, C. F., Ho, Y., and Israel, M. A. (1980): A cloned polyoma DNA fragment representing the 5' half of the early gene region is oncogenic. *J. Virol.*, 36:566–574.

15. Ciufo, D. M., and Hayward, G. S. (1981): Tandem repeat defective DNA from the L-segment of herpes simplex virus genomes. In: *Herpesvirus DNA: Developments in Molecular Virology, Vol. 1*, edited by Y. Becker, pp. 107–128. Martinus-Nijhoff, Boston.

16. Clements, J. B., Watson, R. J., and Wilkie, N. M. (1977): Temporal regulation of herpes simplex virus type 1 transcription: Location of transcripts on the viral genome. *Cell*, 12:275–285.

17. Cocchiara, R., Tarro, G., Flaminio, G., Di Gioia, M., Smeraglia, R., and Geraci, D. (1980): Purification of herpes simplex virus tumor associated antigen from human kidney carcinoma. *Cancer*, 46:1594–1601.

18. Colberg-Poley, A. M., Isom, H. C., and Rapp, F. (1979): Reactivation of herpes simplex virus type 2 from a quiescent state by human cytomegalovirus. *Proc. Natl. Acad. Sci. USA*, 76:5948–5951.

19. Collard, W., Thornton, H., and Green, M. (1973): Cells transformed by human herpesvirus 2 transcribe virus-specific RNA sequences shared by herpesvirus type 1 and 2. *Nature [New Biol.]*, 243:264–266.

20. Conley, A. J., Knipe, D. M., Jones, P. C., and Roizman, B. (1981): Molecular genetics of herpes simplex virus. VII. Characterization of a temperature sensitive mutant produced by *in vitro* mutagenesis and defective in DNA synthesis and accumulation of gamma polypeptides. *J. Virol.*, 37:191–206.

21. Copeland, N. G., Zelenetz, A. D., and Cooper, G. M. (1979): Transformation of NIH/3T3 mouse cells by DNA of rous sarcoma virus. *Cell*, 17:993–1002.

22. Copple, C. D., and McDougall, J. K. (1976): Clonal derivatives of a herpes type 2 transformed hampster cell line (333-8-9): Cytogenetic analysis, tumorigenicity and virus sequence detection. *Int. J. Cancer*, 17:501–510.

23. Cortini, R., and Wilkie, N. M. (1978): Physical maps for HSV type 2 DNA with five restriction endonucleases. *J. Gen. Virol.*, 39:259–280.

24. Crawford, L. V., Pim, D. C., Gurney, E. G., Goodfellow, P., and Taylor-Papadimitriou, J. (1981): Detection of a common feature in several human tumor cell lines—a 53,000-dalton protein. *Proc. Natl. Acad. Sci. USA*, 78:41–45.

25. Davis, D. B., and Kingsbury, D. T. (1976): Quantitation of the viral DNA present in cells transformed by UV-irradiated herpes simplex virus. *J. Virol.*, 17:788–793.

26. Dixon, R. A. F., and Schaffer, P. A. (1980): Fine-structure mapping and functional analysis of temperature-sensitive mutants in the gene encoding the herpes simplex virus type 1 immediate-early protein VP175. *J. Virol.*, 36:189–203.

27. Docherty, J. J., Subak-Sharpe, J. H., and Preston, C. M. (1981): Identification of a virus-specific

polypeptide associated with a transforming fragment (*Bgl*II-N) of herpes simplex virus type 2 DNA. *J. Virol.*, 40:126–132.

28. Dreesman, G. R., Burek, J., Adam, E., Kaufman, R. H., and Melnick, J. L. (1980): Expression of herpesvirus-induced antigens in human cervical cancer. *Nature*, 283:591–593.

29. Duff, R., and Rapp, F. (1971): Properties of hamster embryo fibroblasts transformed *in vitro* after exposure to ultraviolet-irradiated herpes simplex virus type 2. *J. Virol.*, 8:469–477.

30. Duff, R., and Rapp, F. (1973): Oncogenic transformation of hamster embryo cells after exposure to inactivated herpes simplex virus type 1. *J. Virol.*, 12:209–217.

31. Easton, A. J., and Clements, B. J. (1980): Temporal regulation of herpes simplex virus type 2 transcription and characterization of virus immediate-early in mRNAs. *Nucleic Acids Res.*, 8:627–645.

31a. Elgin, R. P., Sharp, F., MacLean, A. B., Macnab, J. C. M., Clements, J. B., and Wilkie, N. M. (1981): Detection of RNA complementary to herpes simplex virus DNA in human cervical squamous cell neoplasms. *Cancer Res.*, 41:3597–3603.

32. Enquist, L. W., Madden, M. J., Schiop-Stansly, P., and Vande Woude, G. F. (1979): Cloning of herpes simplex type 1 DNA fragments in a bacteriophage lambda vector. *Science*, 203:541–544.

33. Fenwick, M., Morse, L. S., and Roizman, B. (1979): Anatomy of herpes simplex virus DNA. XI. Apparent clustering of functions affecting rapid inhibition of host DNA and protein synthesis. *J. Virol.*, 29:825–827.

34. Flannery, V. L., Courtney, R. J., and Schaffer, P. A. (1977): Expression of an early non-structural antigen of herpes simplex virus in cells transformed *in vitro* by herpes simplex virus. *J. Virol.*, 21:284–291.

35. Omitted in proof.

36. Frenkel, N., Roizman, B., Cassai, E., and Nahmias, A. (1972): A DNA fragment of herpes simplex 2 and its transcription in human cervical cancer tissues. *Proc. Natl. Acad. Sci. USA*, 69:3784–3789.

37. Frenkel, N., Locker, H., Cox, B., Roizman, B., and Rapp, F. (1976): Herpes simplex virus DNA in transformed cells: Sequence complexity in five hamster cell lines and one derived hamster tumor. *J. Virol.*, 18:885–893.

38. Frink, R. J., Anderson, K. and Wagner, E. K. (1981): Herpes simplex type 1 *Hin*dIII fragment L encodes spliced and complementary mRNA species. *J. Virol.*, 39:539–572.

39. Galloway, D. A., and McDougall, J. K. (1981): Transformation of rodent cells by a cloned DNA fragment of herpes simplex virus type 2. *J. Virol.*, 38:749–760.

40. Galloway, D. A., Copple, C. D., and McDougall, J. K. (1980): Analysis of viral DNA sequences in hamster cells transformed by herpes simplex virus type 2. *Proc. Natl. Acad. Sci. USA*, 77:880–884.

41. Galloway, D. A., Fenoglio, C. M., and McDougall, J. K. (1981): Limited transcription of the herpes simplex virus genome when latent in human sensory ganglia. *J. Virol.*, 41:686–691.

42. Galloway, D. A., Goldstein, L. C., and Lewis, J. B. (1982): Identification of proteins encoded by a fragment of herpes simplex virus type 2 DNA that has transforming activity. *J. Virol.*, 42:530–537.

43. Garfinkle, B., and McAuslan, B. R. (1974): Transformation of cultured mammalian cells by viable herpes simplex virus subtypes 1 and 2. *Proc. Natl. Acad. Sci. USA*, 71:220–224.

44. Gilman, S. C., Docherty, J. J., Clarke, A., and Rawls, W. E. (1980): The reaction patterns of herpes simplex virus type 1 and type 2 proteins with the sera of patients with uterine cervical carcinoma and matched controls. *Cancer Res.*, 40:4640–4647.

45. Graham, F. L., Abrahams, P. J., Mulder, C., Heijneker, H. L., Warnaar, S. O., De Vries, F. A. J., Fiers, W., and Van der Eb., A. J. (1974): Studies on *in vitro* transformation by DNA and DNA fragments of human adenoviruses and simian virus 40. *Cold Spring Harbor Symp. Quant. Biol.*, 39:637–650.

46. Hampar, B., and Boyd, A. L. (1978): Interaction of oncornaviruses and herpesviruses: A hypothesis proposing a co-carcinogenic role for herpesviruses in transformation. In: *Oncogenesis and Herpesvirus III Part 2*, edited by G. de The, W. Henle, and F. Rapp, pp. 583–589. IARC Scientific Publications, Lyon.

47. Hampar, B., Boyd, A. L., Derge, J. G., Zwieg, M., Eader, L., and Showalter, S. D. (1980): Comparison of properties of mouse cells transformed spontaneously or by ultraviolet light-irradiated herpes simplex virus or by simian virus 40. *Cancer Res.*, 40:2213–2222.

48. Hampar, B., Derge, J. G., Boyd, A. L., Tainsky, M. A., and Showalter, S. D. (1981): Herpes simplex virus (type 1) thymidine kinase gene does not transform cells morphologically. *Proc. Natl. Acad. Sci. USA*, 78:2616–2619.
49. Hassell, J. A., Topp, W. C., Rifkin, D. B., and Moreau, P. (1980): Transformation of rat embryo fibroblasts by cloned polyoma virus DNA fragments containing only part of the early region. *Proc. Natl. Acad. Sci. USA*, 77:3978–3982.
50. Hayward, G. S., Jacob, R. J., Wadsworth, S. C., and Roizman, B. (1975): Anatomy of herpes simplex virus DNA. IV. Evidence for four populations of molecules that differ in the relative orientations of their long and short components. *Proc. Natl. Acad. Sci. USA*, 74:4243–4247.
51. Hayward, W. S., Neel, B. G., and Astrin, S. M. (1981): Activation of a cellular *onc* gene by promotor insertion in ALV-induced lymphoid leukosis. *Nature*, 290:475–480.
52. Henry, B. E., Robinson, R. A., Dauenhauer, S. A., Atherton, S. S., Hayward, G. S., and O'Callaghan, D. J. (1981): Structure of the genome of equine herpesvirus type 1. *Virology*, 115:97–114.
53. Houweling, A., Van den Elsen, P. J., and Van der Eb, A. J. (1980): Partial transformation of primary rat cells by the leftmost 4.5% fragment. *Virology*, 105:537–550.
54. Jariwalla, R. J., Aurelian, L. and Ts'o, P. O. P. (1979): Neoplastic transformation of cultured Syrian hamster embryo cells by DNA of herpes simplex virus type 2. *J. Virol.*, 30:404–409.
55. Jariwalla, R. J., Aurelian, L., and Ts'o, P. O. P. (1980): Tumorigenic transformation induced by a specific fragment of DNA from herpes simplex virus type 2. *Proc. Natl. Acad. Sci. USA*, 77:2279–2283.
56. Jones, P. C., Hayward, G. S., and Roizman, B. (1977): Anatomy of herpes simplex virus DNA: VII. RNA is homologous to noncontiguous sites in both the *L* and *S* components of viral DNA. *J. Virol.*, 21:268–276.
57. Kaufman, R. H., Dreesman, G. R., Burek, J., Kornhonen, M. O., Matson, D. O., Melnick, J. L., Powell, K. L., Purifoy, D. J. M., Courtney, R. J., and Adam, E. (1981): Herpesvirus-induced antigens in squamous-cell carcinoma in situ of the vulva. *N. Engl. J. Med.*, 305:483–488.
58. Kessler, I. I. (1976): Human cervical cancer as a venereal disease. *Cancer*, 36:783–791.
59. Kessous, A., Bibor-Hardy, V., Suh, M., and Simard, R. (1979): Analysis of chromosomes, nucleic acids, and polypeptides in hamster cells transformed by herpes simplex virus type 2. *Cancer Res.*, 39:3225–3234.
60. Kimura, S., Esparza, J., Benyesh-Melmick, M., and Schaffer, P. A. (1974): Enhanced replication of temperature-sensitive mutants of herpes simplex virus type 2 (HSV-2) at the non-permissive temperature in cells transformed by HSV-2. *Intervirology*, 3:162–169.
61. Kimura, S., Flannery, V. L., Levy, B., and Schaffer, P. A. (1975): Oncogenic transformation of primary hamster cells by herpes simplex virus type 2 (HSV-2) and an HSV-2 temperature-sensitive mutant. *Int. J. Cancer*, 15:786–798.
62. Klein, G. (1972): Herpesvirus and oncogenesis. *Proc. Natl. Acad. Sci. USA*, 69:1056–1064.
63. Knipe, D. M., Batterson, W., Nosal, C., Roizman, B., and Buchan, A. (1981): Molecular genetics of herpes simplex virus. VI. Characterization of a temperature-sensitive mutant defective in the expression of all early viral gene products. *J. Virol.*, 38:539–547.
64. Kraiselburd, E., Gage, L. P., and Weissbach, A. (1975): Presence of a herpes simplex virus DNA fragment in an L-cell clone obtained after infection with irradiated herpes simplex type 1. *J. Mol. Biol.*, 97:533–542.
65. Kucera, L. S., and Gusdon, J. P. (1976): Transformation of human embryonic fibroblasts by photodynamically inactivated herpes simplex virus, type 2 at supra-optimal temperature. *J. Gen. Virol.*, 30:257–261.
66. Lania, L., Gandini-Attardi, D., Griffiths, M., Cooke, B., de Cicco, D., and Fried, M. (1980): The polyoma virus 100K large T antigen is not required for the maintenance of transformation. *Virology*, 101:217–232.
67. Leiden, J. M., and Frenkel, N. (1981): HSV DNA fragments in herpesvirus transformed cells. In: *Herpesvirus DNA: Developments in Molecular Virology, Vol. 1*, edited by Y. Becker, pp. 197–212. Martinus-Nijhoff, Boston.
68. Leiden, J. M., Frenkel, N., and Rapp, R. (1980): Identification of the herpes simplex virus DNA sequences present in six herpes simplex virus thymidine kinase-transformed mouse cell lines. *J. Virol.*, 33:272–285.
69. Lewis, J. C., Kucera, L. S., Eberle, R., and Courtney, R. J. (1982): Detection of herpes simplex virus type 2 glycoproteins expressed in virus-transformed rat cells. *J. Virol.*, 42:275–282.

70. Linzer, D. I. H., and Levine, A. J. (1979): Characterization of a 54K dalton cellular SV40 tumor antigen present in SV40-transformed cells and uninfected embryonal carcinoma cells. *Cell*, 17:43–52.

71. Lusky, M., and Botchan, M. (1981): Inhibition of SV40 replication in simian cells by specific pBR322 DNA sequences. *Nature*, 293:79–81.

72. Macnab, J. C. M. (1979): Tumour production by HSV-2 transformed lines in rats and the varying response to immunosuppression. *J. Gen. Virol.*, 43:39–56.

73. Macnab, J. C. M., and Timbury, M. C. (1976): Complementation of ts mutants by a herpes simplex virus ts-transformed cell line. *Nature*, 261:233–235.

74. Maitland, N. J., Kinross, J. H., Busuttil, A., Ludgate, S. M., Smart, G. E., and Jones, K. W. (1981): The detection of DNA tumour virus-specific RNA sequences in abnormal human cervical biopsies by *in situ* hybridization. *J. Gen. Virol.*, 55:123–137.

75. Marquez, E., and Rapp, F. (1975): Presence of herpesvirus-associated antigens on the surfaces transformed tumor and metastatic cells and enhanced antigenicity of transformed cell using 5-iodo 2' deoxy-uridine. *Intervirology*, 6:64–71.

76. Marsden, H. S., Stow, N. D., Preston, V. G., Timbury, M. C., and Wilkie, N. M. (1978): Physical mapping of herpes simplex virus-induced polypeptides. *J. Virol.*, 28:624–642.

77. McAuslan, B. R., Garfinkle, B., Adler, R., Devinney, D., Florkiewicz, R., and Shaw, J. E. (1974): Transformation of cells by herpes simplex virus-fact or fantasy. *Cold Spring Harbor Symp. Quant. Biol.*, 39:765–772.

78. McDougall, J. K., Crum, C. P., Fenoglio, C. M., Goldstein, L. C., and Galloway, D. A. (1982): Herpesvirus-specific RNA and protein in carcinoma of the uterine cervix. *Proc. Natl. Acad. Sci. USA*, 79:3853–3857.

79. McDougall, J. K., Galloway, D. A., and Fenoglio, C. (1980): Cervical carcinoma: detection of herpes simplex virus RNA in cells undergoing neoplastic change. *Int. J. Cancer*, 25:1–8.

80. McDougall, J. K., Galloway, D. A., Crum, C., Levine, R., Richart, R., and Fenoglio, C. M. (1981): Detection of nucleic acid sequences in cervical tumors. *Gynecol. Oncol.*, 12:S42–S55.

81. McKnight, S. L. (1980): The nucleotide sequence and transcript map of the herpes simplex virus thymidine kinase gene. *Nucleic Acids Res.*, 8:5949–5964.

82. McKnight, S. L., Gavis, E. R., Kingsbury, R., and Axel, R. (1981): Analysis of transcriptional regulatory signals of the HSV thymidine kinase gene: Identification of an upstream control region. *Cell*, 25:385–398.

83. Melnick, J. L., Adam, E., Lewis, R., and Kaufman, R. H. (1979): Cervical cancer cell lines containing herpesvirus markers. *Intervirology*, 12:111–114.

84. Middleton, M., Reyes, G. R., Macnab, J., Buchan, A., and Hayward, G. S. (1982): Expression of cloned herpes virus genes: I. Detection of antigens from HSV-2 immediate-early regions in transfected cells. *J. Virol.*, 43:1091–1101.

85. Minson, A. C., Thouless, M. E., Eglin, R. P., and Darby, G. (1976): The detection of virus DNA sequences in herpes type 2 transformed hampster cell line (333-8-9). *Int. J. Cancer*, 17:493–500.

86. Minson, A. C., Wildy, P., Buchan, A., and Darby, G. (1978): Introduction of the herpes simplex virus thymidine kinase gene into mouse cells using virus DNA or transformed cell DNA. *Cell*, 13:581–587.

87. Morse, L. S., Buchman, T. G., Roizman, B., and Schaffer, P. A. (1977): Anatomy of herpes simplex virus DNA. IX. Apparent exclusion of some parental DNA arrangements in the generation of intertypic (HSV-1 × HSV-2) recombinants. *J. Virol.*, 24:231–248.

88. Morse, L. S., Pereira, L., Roizman, B., and Schaffer, P. A. (1978): Anatomy of HSV DNA. XI. Mapping of viral genes by analysis of polypeptides and functions specified by HSV-1 × HSV-2 recombinants. *J. Virol.*, 26:389–410.

89. Nahmias, A. J., Josey, W. E., Naib, Z. M., Luce, C. F., and Duffey, A. (1971): Antibodies to herpes simplex types 1 and 2 in humans. 2. Women with cervical cancer. *Am. J. Epidemiol.*, 91:529–537.

90. Nelson, J. A., Fleckenstein, B., Galloway, D. A., and McDougall, J. K. (1982): Transformation of NIH 3T3 cells with cloned fragments of human cytomegalovirus strain AD169. *J. Virol.*, 43:83–91.

91. Novak, Y., Dilworth, S. M., and Griffin, B. E. (1980): Coding capacity of a 35% fragment of the polyoma virus genome is sufficient to initiate and maintain cellular transformation. *Proc. Natl. Acad. Sci. USA*, 77:3278–3282.

92. Oskarrson, M., McClements, W. L., Blair, D. G., Maizel, J. V., and Vande Woude, G. F. (1980):

Properties of a normal mouse cell DNA sequence (sarc) homologous to a src sequence of Moloney sarcoma virus. *Science*, 207:1222–1224.

93. Pagano, J. S. (1975): Diseases and mechanisms of persistent DNA virus infection: Latency and cellular transformation. *J. Infect. Dis.*, 132:209–223.

94. Park, M., Lonsdale, D. M., Timbury, M. C., Subak-Sharpe, J. H., and Macnab, J. C. M. (1980): Genetic retrieval of viral genome sequences from herpes simplex virus transformed cells. *Nature*, 285:412–415.

95. Peden, K., Mounts, P., and Hayward, G. S. (1982): Homology between mammalian cell DNA sequences and human herpesvirus genomes detected by a high complexity probe hybridization procedure. *Cell*, 31:71–80.

96. Pellicer, A., Wigler, M., Axel, R., and Silverstein, S. (1978): The transfer and stable integration of the HSV thymidine kinase gene into mouse cells. *Cell*, 14:133–141.

97. Pereira, L., Wolff, M. H., Fenwick, M., and Roizman, B. (1977): Regulation of herpesvirus macromolecular synthesis. V. Properties of alpha-polypeptides made in HSV-1 and HSV-2 infected cells. *Virology*, 77:733–749.

98. Pollack, R., Risser, R., Conton, S., Freedman, V., Shin, S.-I., and Rifkin, D. B. (1975): Production of plasminogen activator and colonial growth in semi-solid medium are *in vitro* correlates of tumorigenicity in the immune deficient nude mouse. In: *Proteases and Biological Control*, edited by E. Reich, D. B. Rifkin, and E. Shaw, pp. 885–889. Cold Spring Harbor Laboratory, Cold Spring Harbor, N.Y.

99. Powell, K. L., Littler, E., and Purifoy, D. J. M. (1981): Nonstructural proteins of herpes simplex virus. II. Major virus-specific DNA-binding protein. *J. Virol.*, 39:894–902.

100. Rawls, W. E., Bacchetti, S., and Graham, F. L. (1977): Relation of herpes simplex viruses to human malignancies. *Curr. Top. Microbiol. Immunol.*, 77:72–98.

101. Rawls, W. E., Tompkins, W. A. F., Figueroa, M. E., and Melnick, J. L. (1968): Herpes virus type 2: Association with carcinoma of the cervix. *Science*, 161:1255–1257.

102. Reid, R., Stanhope, C. R., Herschman, B. R., Booth, E., Phibbs, G. D., and Smith, J. P. (1982): Genital warts and cervical cancer. Evidence of an association between sub-clinical papillomavirus infection and cervical malignancy. *Cancer*, 50(2):377–387.

103. Reyes, G. R. (1982): Morphological and biochemical transformation with the DNA of herpes simplex virus. Ph.D. thesis, Johns Hopkins School of Medicine.

104. Reyes, G. R., Jeang, K.-T., and Hayward, G. S. (1982): Transfection with the isolated herpes simplex virus thymidine kinase genes: I. Minimal size of the active fragments from HSV-1 and HSV-2. *J. Gen. Virol.*, 62:191–206.

105. Reyes, G. R., LaFemina, R., Hayward, S. D., and Hayward, G. S. (1979): Morphological transformation by DNA fragments of human herpesviruses: Evidence for two distinct transforming regions in herpes simplex virus types 1 and 2 and lack of correlation with biochemical transfer of the thymidine kinase gene. *Cold Spring Harbor Symp. Quant. Biol.*, 44:629–641.

106. Reyes, G. R., McLane, M. W., and Hayward, G. S. (1982): Transfection with the isolated herpes simplex virus thymidine kinase genes: II. Evidence for amplification of viral and adjacent cellular DNA sequences. *J. Gen. Virol.*, 60:209–224.

107. Robinson, R. A., Tucker, P. W., Dauenhauer, S. A., and O'Callaghan, D. J. (1981): Molecular cloning of equine herpesvirus type 1 DNA: Analysis of standard and defective viral genomes and viral sequences in oncogenically transformed cells. *Proc. Natl. Acad. Sci. USA*, 78:6684–6688.

108. Robinson, R. A., Vance, R. B., and O'Callaghan, D. J. (1980): Oncogenic transformation by equine herpesvirus. II. Coestablishment of persistent infection and oncogenic transformation of hamster embryo cells by equine herpesvirus type 1 preparation enriched for defective interfering particles. *J. Virol.*, 36:204–219.

109. Shih, C., Shilo, B. Z., Goldfarb, M. P., Dannenberg, A., and Weinberg, R. A. (1979): Passage of phenotypes of chemically transformed cells via transfection of DNA and chromatin. *Proc. Natl. Acad. Sci. USA*, 76:5714–5718.

110. Showalter, S. D., Zweig, M., and Hampar, B. (1981): Monoclonal antibodies to herpes simplex virus type 1 proteins, including the immediate-early protein ICP-4. *Infect. Immun.*, 34:684–692.

111. Skare, J., and Summers, W. C. (1977): Structure and function of herpesvirus genomes II. *Eco*RI, *Xba*I and *Hind*III endonuclease cleavage sites on herpes simplex virus type 1 DNA. *Virology*, 76:581–596.

112. Stevens, J. G. (1975): Latent herpes simplex virus and the nervous system. *Curr. Top. Microbiol. Immunol.*, 70:31–50.

113. Suh, M. (1982): Characterization of a polypeptide present in herpes simplex virus type 2-transformed and -infected hamster embryo cells. *J. Virol.*, 41:1095–1098.
114. Suh, M., Kessous, A., Poirier, N., and Simard, R. (1980): Immunoprecipitation of polypeptides from hamster embryo cells transformed by herpes simplex virus type 2. *Virology*, 104:303–311.
115. Van der Eb, A. J., Mulder, C., Graham, F. L., and Houweling, A. (1977): Transformation with specific fragments of adenovirus DNAs. I. Isolation of specific fragments with transforming activity from adenovirus 2 and 5 DNAs. *Gene*, 2:115–132.
116. Wagner, E. K. (1983): *This volume.*
117. Wilcox, K. W., Kohn, A., Sklyanskaya, E., and Roizman, B. (1980): Herpes simplex virus phosphoproteins. I. Phosphate cycles on and off some viral polypeptides and can alter their affinity for DNA. *J. Virol.*, 33:167–182.
118. Wilkie, N. M. (1976): Physical maps for HSV type 1 DNA for restriction endonucleases *Hind*III, *Hpa*I and *Xba*I. *J. Virol.*, 20:222–233.
119. Wilkie, N. M., Clements, J. B., Macnab, J. C. M., and Subak-Sharpe, J. H. (1974): The structure and biological properties of herpes simplex virus DNA. *Cold Spring Harbor Symp. Quant. Biol.*, 39:657–666.
120. Wilkie, N. M., Elgin, R. P., Sanders, P. G., and Clements, J. B. (1981): In: *Interactions between Virus and Host Molecules.* Academic Press, New York.
121. Yeo, J., Killington, R. A., Watson, D. H., and Powell, K. L. (1981): Studies on cross-reactive antigens in the herpesviruses. *Virology*, 108:256–266.
122. zur Hausen, H., Schulte-Holthausen, H., Wolf, H., Dorries, K., and Egger, H. (1974): Attempts to detect virus-specific DNA in human tumors. II. Nuclei acid hybridization with complementary RNA of human herpes group viruses. *Int. J. Cancer*, 13:657–664.

Note added in proof

Recently Dutia (*J. Gen. Virol.*, 64:513–521, 1983) found that the HSV-1 tsG and HSV-2 ts8 mutations, which give rise to novel temperature-sensitive ribonucleotide reductase activity in infected cells, map within HSV-1 *Bam*HI-O at genome coordinates 0.578–0.603. This result raises the possibility that the 140K and 38K polypeptides may represent coprecipitating A and B subunits of a putative virus encoded ribonucleotide reductase enzyme. In support of this notion Huszar and Bacchetti (*Nature*, 302:76–79, 1983) report co-precipitation of both polypeptides with antiserum prepared against a partially purified ribonucleotide reductase enzyme induced in HSV-2 infected cells and also with monoclonal antibodies that neutralize or immunoprecipitate the induced reductase activity.

Advances in Viral Oncology, Volume 3, edited by
George Klein. Raven Press, New York © 1983.

Oncogenic Transformation by
Herpesvirus saimiri

*Ronald C. Desrosiers and **Bernhard Fleckenstein

*New England Regional Primate Research Center, Harvard Medical School,
Southborough, Massachusetts 01772; and **Institute for Clinical Virology, University of
Erlanger-Nürnberg, D8520 Erlangen, West Germany

Studies of growth transformation and tumor induction by retroviruses, papovaviruses, and adenoviruses have implicated a few basic strategies by which a virus can change the normal pattern of cell division into an abnormal one. Many tumor viruses appear to carry their own transforming genes. Retroviruses that have their own transforming genes (oncogenes) appear to have acquired this DNA sequence from the host cell, but there is no evidence for cellular sequences homologous to the transforming DNA regions of papovaviruses and adenoviruses. Some other retroviruses do not carry a gene coding for a transformation-specific protein and do not transform cells in culture, yet still can produce slowly developing tumors in animals. In this latter case, retrovirus DNA integrates near a cellular oncogene, activating its expression. In contrast to the situation with these model tumor virus systems, little is known at a molecular level about any herpesvirus-induced oncogenic transformation. Which, if any, of these schemes is important for herpesvirus-induced oncogenic transformation remains to be elucidated. The dearth of specific information on herpesvirus-induced transformation is probably due, at least in part, to the much greater genetic complexity of herpesviruses and their more complicated life cycle. The herpesviruses are also a very diverse group; mechanisms of oncogenic transformation determined for one member probably will not be applicable to an unrelated member. The greater genetic complexity of herpesviruses as compared with the other model tumor viruses mentioned earlier could perhaps result in more complex mechanisms for oncogenic transformation, conceivably requiring more than one region of the genome.

Herpesvirus saimiri offers several advantages for study of oncogenic transformation in a herpesvirus system. First of all, there can be no doubt that *H. saimiri* is a tumor virus; tumors are induced rapidly and reproducibly in various species of New World primates. In fact, the reproducible response is a tremendous aid to many types of studies. The ability to grow *H. saimiri* lytically in cultured New World primate monolayer cells furnishes a distinct advantage over Epstein-Barr virus (EBV), for which no truly permissive system is known. The only sources of EBV are some transformed lymphoid cell lines that produce virus at relatively low levels. Such a permissive system facilitates production of purified virions and virion DNA and also facilitates study of the synthesis of viral RNA and proteins and their control. In addition to the considerable information already available on the biology of the *H. saimiri* system, modern gene technology has engendered increasing information on the structure and characteristics of viral DNA from lytic infection and as it exists in tumor cells. Numerous lymphoid tumor cell lines are available, and these may be used to study the persistence of viral DNA and the factors responsible for growth transformation. Finally, two nononcogenic variants have arisen independently following tissue culture manipulation, and these promise to be valuable aids in the quest to understand the tumorigenicity of this virus.

The biological aspects of this virus have been thoroughly summarized in previous reviews (10,16,17,25,29,30) and thus will be dealt with only brieflyhere.

BACKGROUND

Natural History

H. saimiri was first isolated at the New England Regional Primate Research Center from kidney cells of a squirrel monkey *(Saimiri sciureus)* explanted into culture (51). Numerous subsequent investigations have shown that squirrel monkeys are natural hosts for this virus. More than 90% of squirrel monkeys, whether wild-caught or colony-born, have been infected with this virus (20,22). Infection by *H. saimiri* has been shown in two ways: demonstration of seroconversion to positive antibody status (usually within the first 2 years of life) and isolation of virus present latently in peripheral lymphocytes. Natural or experimental infection of squirrel monkeys produces no obvious clinical symptoms. Serological surveys of other primates have shown that most other species are not naturally infected with *H. saimiri* (21). Spider monkeys *(Ateles geoffroyi)* sometimes appear positive in serological assays because they harbor a related virus, *Herpesvirus ateles*, which has demonstrated DNA base sequence homology with *H. saimiri* (27) and can cross-react immunologically (21). The presence of *H. saimiri-* and *H. ateles* reactive antibodies in 4 of 4 woolly monkeys *(Lagothrix lagothricha)* may mean that this species is another natural host for one of these viruses or that this species harbors a related, cross-reacting virus (21).

H. saimiri is present latently in peripheral lymphocytes of most squirrel monkeys, and this conveniently permits isolation of virus without major surgical invasion or killing of the animal. A small sample of whole blood or separated lymphocytes can simply be cocultivated with permissive cells in culture until outgrowth of virus, usually 5 to 10 days later. About 10^5 to 10^6 lymphocytes from a healthy squirrel monkey are required to recover virus. Studies using fractionated lymphocytes have shown that *H. saimiri* is harbored in T cells (17,75). Cell-free *H. saimiri* has also been recovered from oral secretions of squirrel monkeys (20), and it seems likely that the virus is transmitted horizontally by exposure to saliva or virus-containing aerosols.

Laboratory Propagation

H. saimiri has demonstrated permissive growth in several types of cultured New World primate cells (49). Owl monkey kidney (OMK) cell lines growing in monolayers appear to be the best choice for lytic growth of *H. saimiri*. Cells other than those of nonhuman primate origin support the growth of *H. saimiri* either not at all or very inefficiently. Optimal yields of virus following low-multiplicity infection are only about 20 infectious particles per cell; based on yields of DNA from purified virions, the number of DNA-containing particles produced per cell is around 100 times this amount. The time course of the infectious cycle is protracted longer than 36 hr, even at multiplicities of infection greater than 1 (56). At low multiplicities of infection (0.01–0.1), maximum virus yields and complete cytopathic effect (CPE) are not reached until 4 to 7 days after infection. Infection of cultured OMK cells appears to be somewhat asynchronous. Foci of CPE appear and develop at different rates in an infected cell monolayer, and *H. saimiri* always produces heterogeneously sized plaques under agar whether or not the virus has just been plaque-purified.

Tumor Induction

Table 1 summarizes the susceptibility of commonly used New World primate species and rabbits to tumor induction by *H. saimiri*. Although there has been one positive report (55), Old World primates generally are not susceptible (43,53,61). The response of tamarin marmosets (*Saguinus* species) is the most rapid and reproducible among all animals tested. All infected tamarin marmosets have suc-

TABLE 1. *Induction of tumors by* H. saimiri *in selected species*

| Species | Tumor incidence (%) | | References |
	H. saimiri strain S295C	H. saimiri strain 11	
Saguinus oedipus[a]	100	100	43,54,73
Saguinus fuscicollis-nigricollis[b]	100	100	43,73
Callithrix jacchus[c]	0–10	100[h]	4,43–45,77
Aotus trivirgatus[d]	50–100	100	1,7,36,50,52,54
Oryctolagus cuniculus[e]	20–80	0[h]	8
Oryctolagus cuniculus[f]	10–50	NT[i]	63
Oryctolagus cuniculus[g]	100[h]	NT	3

[a]Cotton-top marmoset.
[b]White-lip marmoset.
[c]Common marmoset.
[d]Owl monkey.
[e]New Zealand white rabbit.
[f]ACCRB inbred strain of New Zealand white rabbit.
[g]IIIJ inbred strain of New Zealand white rabbit.
[h]Less than 10 animals tested.
[i]NT = not tested.

cumbed to a rapidly progressing malignant T cell lymphoma. For cotton-top marmosets *(Saguinus oedipus)*, the time course to death has depended on the size of the inoculum; 10^5 infectious particles result in death, usually 21 to 28 days post inoculation. Because the cotton-top marmoset is an endangered species, their use for terminal experiments is not practical in most cases. However, other readily available New World primate species may be conveniently used. The responses of these other species vary with respect to percentage of animals that succumb, time course to death, and pathology. These features have been extensively summarized in previous reviews (10,16,25,29,30). The choice of virus strain used is clearly a factor in the responses in some species. For example, strains 11 and OMI appear to induce tumors quite consistently in common marmosets *(Callithrix jacchus)* and owl monkeys *(Aotus trivirgatus)*, but strain S295C, at least at its current state of cell culture passage, frequently results in a lower percentage of tumor incidence and/or a longer time course to death. Even with a given strain of *H. saimiri*, different studies have reported different percentages of tumor incidence and survival time. Evaluation of these differences and conclusions about species susceptibility are difficult because of the large number of variables that could possibly affect the outcome of such studies. These variables include the size of the inoculum, the passage history of the virus, and the age and genetic history of the animals. The susceptibility of certain species of rabbits, first observed by Daniel et al. (8), has also been noted by other investigators (3,63).

The pathological findings also vary with the animal species and the *H. saimiri* strain. Varied pathological features include malignant lymphoma of the reticulum cell, immature poorly differentiated or well-differentiated lymphocytic types, and various forms of leukemia. The marked leukemic responses in some species with some strains of *H. saimiri* are valuable to molecular biologists. For example, *H. saimiri* strain S295C infection of white-lip marmosets *(Saguinus fuscicollis–Saguinus nigricollis)* results in marked leukemia, with white cell counts greater than 10^8 cells/ml. Lymphocyte preparations from such leukemic animals provide a rich and convenient source of essentially pure tumor cells for studies of the state of *H. saimiri* DNA and its expression (12).

In Vitro Transformation

Attempts to transform lymphocytes *in vitro* by *H. saimiri* have been surprisingly unsuccessful. Several groups have experienced difficulties in trying to achieve immortalization of peripheral leukocytes by *H. saimiri* in cell culture. In one of numerous experiments we obtained a cotton-top marmoset cell line from infecting blood lymphocytes with *H. saimiri* strain OMI, employing squirrel monkey fibroblasts as a feeder layer. The cell line, designated H1591, has grown continuously now for more than 3 years. The sharp contrast between high oncogenicity in animals and poor transforming potential *in vitro* is remarkable. On the other hand, it should also be considered that the oncogenicity in tamarins and other monkeys may be more a reflection of a state of paralysis in the cellular immune system of the tumor-developing host than a reflection of the transforming power of the virus. It may be that the primary target for transformation is a more immature stem cell, rather than a well-differentiated peripheral lymphocyte, or it may be that some unknown factors that contribute to transformation *in vivo* are lacking in the *in vitro* transformation. L. A. Falk *(personal communication)* has obtained several continuously growing T lymphocyte cell lines; T lymphocytes from cotton-top marmosets were stimulated with concanavalin A, grown in culture medium containing T cell growth factor (Interleukin 2), and then infected with *H. saimiri*.

In contrast to *H. saimiri*, *H. ateles* has reproducibly transformed monkey lymphocytes *in vitro*. Peripheral or splenic lymphocytes of tamarin marmosets *(S. oedipus, S. fuscicollis, S. labiatus)* and common marmosets *(C. jacchus)* can be immortalized by cocultivation with lethally X-irradiated *H. ateles*-producing cell lines (24) or by cell-free virus particles (19). Attempts to transform lymphoid or epithelial cells by intact or fragmented DNA of *H. saimiri* or *H. ateles* have been unsuccessful, at least so far.

STRUCTURE OF VIRION DNA

Wild-Type Viruses

H. saimiri has a genome structure that is different from the DNA organization of all herpesviruses characterized previously. Most strikingly, the genomes of *H. saimiri* contain manyfold repetitive DNA that amounts to over 25% of virion DNA, and the high $G+C$ content of repetitive DNA results in an extreme intramolecular heterogeneity in base composition. Two types of DNA molecules are found in *H. saimiri* particles: (a) M genomes (M-DNA) represent the majority of virion DNA. M-DNA contains the entire genetic information of the virus, because transfection into permissive cell cultures or whole animals results in propagation of the virus (26,28). (b) H genomes are defective, because they consist of repetitive DNA only and possess very little genetic information.

M genomes are linear double-stranded DNA molecules ranging from 145 to 165 kilobase pairs (kb) (32), with an average $G+C$ content of 45.4% (26). The M-DNA molecule is composed of an internal segment of unique-sequence L-DNA (36% $G + C$, 110 kb) that is framed by two terminal stretches of repetitive H-DNA (71% $G + C$) (5) (Fig. 1). Each repeat unit of H-DNA has 1.4 kb, the repeats are strictly arranged in tandem, and the two terminal stretches of H-DNA in M genomes are directed in the same orientation. The lengths of individual H-DNA ends vary from 21 μm to less than 1 μm, and the H-DNA segments of M-DNA molecules seem to differ in length by integer numbers of repeat units. The number of repeat units at each end can vary from about 1 to 40, and M-DNA in all contains a variable number of H-DNA repeat units ranging from about 25 to 40.

H genomes are long chains of repetitive DNA in strict head-to-tail arrangements, with a length about the same as that found in M genomes. Reassociation kinetics

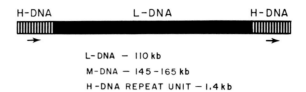

L-DNA — 110 kb

M-DNA — 145 - 165 kb

H-DNA REPEAT UNIT — 1.4 kb

FIG. 1.   Structure of virion M-DNA molecule. The L-DNA region is indicated by the black area, and each H-DNA repeat unit is indicated by vertical lines. The number of repeat units at either end can vary from 1 to 40, and the total number of repeat units in most M-DNA molecules ranges from 25 to 40.

and cleavage comparisons with restriction endonucleases indicate complete homology between H-DNA sequences from H genomes and M genomes. *H. saimiri* particles originating from transfection with M-DNA contain the same relative amounts of H genomes as regular stocks, indicating that H genomes are made from H sequences of M-DNA in each cycle of replication (26). The H-DNA repeat unit has recently been completely sequenced (W. Bear, E. Knust, B. Fleckenstein, and B. Barrell, *unpublished data*).

Cleavage comparisons of DNAs from more than 20 independent *H. saimiri* isolates with numerous restriction endonucleases have yielded distinct but related patterns, indicating that the basic genome structure is the same for all strains (13). Physical maps were constructed for several virus isolates, such as prime strain S295C, strain 11, SMHI, and OMI, with endonucleases *Aos*I, *Bam*HI, *Cla*I, *Eca*I, *Eco*RI, *Kpn*I, *Sac*II, *Sal*I, *Sma*I, and *Xho*I (30). The cleavage maps have indicated colinear arrangement of DNA sequences within the L-DNA segments of all strains. The colinearity of gene maps among *H. saimiri* strains has also been demonstrated by construction of recombinants; the *H. saimiri* recombinants were generated by cotransfection of OMK cells with long overlapping restriction fragments of virion DNA from different strains (41). Cross-hybridization experiments using CoT analysis have not detected significant base pair divergence among strains. A more quantitative determination of the degree of base pair homology was obtained by measuring melting-temperature (T_m) depression of heteroduplex molecules. In these experiments, less than 3°C were found for ΔT_m between L-DNA homoduplex and heteroduplex molecules, indicating at most a 2% base pair divergence for DNA sequences covering most of the length of L-DNA (41).

However, marked variability has been detected in the homology of the leftmost segments of L-DNA. Ten strains of *H. saimiri* fell into two groups (A and B) based on homology of restriction fragments from within this region. The sizes of these segments in five group A viruses varied between 7 and 10 kb. Fragments from within this region of any group A virus hybridized with corresponding fragments of other group A viruses, but little or no hybridization was detected to DNA of group B viruses. Similar results were obtained in the reverse experiment using a labeled group B virus fragment as hybridization probe. *H. saimiri* strains 11 and OMI were classified as group A, and prime strain S295C and strain SMHI were assigned to group B (C. Mulder, E. Szomolanyi, P. Medvecsky, R. Desrosiers, J. Koomey, L. Falk, and B. Fleckenstein, *unpublished data*).

Nononcogenic Variants

Attenuation of *H. saimiri* has been achieved in two laboratories, resulting in normally growing virus strains that have lost their oncogenic potential. Cell culture manipulation and plaque purification of strain 11 resulted in a nononcogenic variant termed 11att (66). This nononcogenic variant did not produce lymphoma in cotton-top or common marmosets. Infection with 11att could not protect cotton-top marmosets from developing malignant lymphomas after challenge inoculation with wild-type virus, but it did cause a significant delay in the time course of tumor development. However, it was found that tumors could be prevented in common marmosets by vaccination with *H. saimiri* strain 11att (76). Cleavage comparisons of M-DNAs from *H. saimiri* strains 11 and 11att have revealed that an L-DNA segment of approximately 1.7 kb has been deleted from the leftmost part of the L-DNA region of strain 11 during the process of attenuation. No other difference could be detected between DNAs of strain 11att and the wild-type strain 11 (C. Mulder, J. Koomey, L. Falk, and R. Desrosiers, *unpublished data*). The 1.7-kb deletion was found to be a stable property of the attenuated virus, whether examined after continuous passage in cell culture or after isolation from persistently infected marmosets (18).

Strain SMHI was attenuated by long-term persistent infection of semipermissive Vero cells (9). The attenuated strain, designated strain SMHIatt replicates normally in OMK cell cultures, induces an antibody response in cotton-top marmosets and owl monkeys, and conveys partial protection of these animals against challenge with wild-type virus. Virion DNA from *H. saimiri* SMHIatt exhibits several structural alterations in comparison with the parental wild-type virus. A deletion of 5.7 kb was found in the left end of the L-DNA, probably encompassing the left L-H-DNA junction or immediately adjacent to it. This deletion is larger than, but seems analogous to, the deletion in 11att. In addition, the M-DNA of SMHIatt has acquired a fragment of L-DNA that is inserted into its H-DNA sequences. This segment (11 kb) represents an inverted repetition of a 5.5-kb region of the right end of L-DNA. DNA preparations from SMHIatt also have yielded variable amounts of defective DNA molecules, consisting of a tandemly repeated portion of 12.4-kb L-DNA plus 1.2-kb H-DNA. This type of defective genome has totally replaced the H-genome-type defectives that are normally found in wild-type strains. These alterations have resulted in a significantly lower proportion of repetitive H-DNA sequences in SMHIatt. Analytical density centrifugation has shown that SMHIatt contains 17% H-DNA only, contrasting with 29% H-DNA in wild-type SMHI.

It is not clear at the present time by what mechanisms the attenuated *H. saimiri* strains 11att and SMHIatt have lost their oncogenic properties. The attenuated strains may have lost their ability to transform or immortalize lymphoid T cells because of a change in a putative transforming protein. Alternatively, the attenuated viruses may express a virion antigen or nonstructural protein differently, resulting in different presentation of transformed cell surfaces to immune cells and elimination through normal functions of the immune system. It may also be possible that a viral protein that suppresses normal T cell functions in wild-type infection is not formed by the attenuated strains. It is striking that both attenuated *H. saimiri* strains have developed a deletion in the same region of the genome, but there is no proof as yet that this deletion by itself is responsible for the attenuation. Further experiments, including animal inoculations with recombinants between attenuated and wild-type viruses, will be necessary to define the role of the left-terminal L-DNA in transformation, tumor induction, and attenuation.

VIRAL DNA IN TUMORS AND TRANSFORMED CELL LINES

Genome Copy Number

Abundant amounts of *H. saimiri* DNA have been found by hybridization techniques in lymphomatous tissues, tumor cell lines, and *in vitro* immortalized lymphoid cells. Both types of viral sequences, L- and H-DNA, have been detected by measurement of reassociation kinetics using ^{3}H-labeled viral DNA as probes. In four separate spleen and lymph node biopsies from tumor-bearing cotton-top marmosets, 0.0115% to 0.108% of total cell DNA hybridized with H-DNA, and 0.014% to 0.075% of total cell DNA hybridized with L-DNA (31). These values for L-DNA would represent 7 to 38 complete M genome equivalents per cell. The biopsy and autopsy material used for DNA extraction, of course, contained a mixture of virus-transformed malignant cells, uninfected normal tissue constituents, and, perhaps, lytically and abortively infected cells. Thus, it is not possible to estimate accurately the number of viral genome equivalents per neoplastic cell. The presence of multiple viral genomes in tumors appears analogous to the detection of EBV DNA in Burkitt's lymphoma and nasopharyngeal carcinoma (58,78) and Marek's disease virus DNA in chicken lymphomas (57).

Permanently growing T cell lines have been cultured from lymph nodes, spleen, thymus, and peripheral leukocytes of tumor-bearing tamarin marmosets *(S. oedipus, S. fuscicollis, S. nigricollis)* (23,31,62). *H. saimiri*-transformed lymphoid tumor lines grow mainly as suspension cultures, forming small clumps and larger cell aggregates of 100 cells or more. Tumor cells continue to preserve T-cell-specific markers, such as rosette formation with sheep red blood cells (17,69). In general, certain percentages of the cells (about 1–10%) in recently established tumor lines produce infectious virus particles. After several months of growth *in vitro*, virus production decreases to much lower or undetectable levels. Some cell lines lose the ability to produce virus entirely within the first year of cultivation, whereas others maintain a low level of virus production over several years. CoT analysis with H- and L-DNA of *H. saimiri* has indicated that most lymphoid tumor cell lines contain multiple viral genome copies. Various tumor cell lines contain about 80 to 280 genome equivalents per diploid cell, and there seems to be no correlation with the amount of viral DNA in the cells and the ability of cells to produce virus. A lower proportion of *H. saimiri* DNA was found in the cell line H1591, which was established by *in vitro* immortalization of marmoset lymphocytes with strain OMI (29,31,37,40).

Sequence Arrangement

The similarities between *H. saimiri* and EBV prompted a search for nonintegrated circular viral DNA in *H. saimiri*-transformed cells. Persistence of nonintegrated circles of EBV DNA in transformed cells is well documented (46). All *H. saimiri*-transformed cell lines investigated so far have been found to contain circular viral DNA. Werner et al. (70) found large covalently closed circles in the nonproducer cell line 1670 by electron microscopy of superhelical DNA fractions, and, similarly, circular *H. saimiri* DNA was demonstrated in the tumor cell lines 70N2 and L77/ 5, in lymphoid cells transformed *in vitro*, and in tumor biopsies (40).

Partial denaturation mapping and length measurements in the electron microscope have revealed unusual features of circular viral DNA from transformed cells. Circles isolated from the nonproducer cell line 1670 have 200 kb; thus, they are considerably larger than M-DNA of virus particles. Examination of many circular molecules from 1670 cells with partially denatured L sequences has shown that two L-DNA regions (L1 = 89 kb, L2 = 52 kb) are separated by two regions of repetitive H-DNA (H1 = 35 kb, H2 = 26 kb). Computer alignment of denaturation histograms has indicated that L2 sequences are a subset of L1 sequences, and the common sequences are oriented in the same direction (70,71). These results indicate that a segment of 20 kb is absent from the circles of 1670 cells. When DNA from 1670 cells was digested with restriction endonucleases, electrophoresed through agarose gels, transferred to nitrocellulose filters, and hybridized to ^{32}P-labeled virion L-DNA, the deletion was placed between 55 and 75 kb from the left end of virion L-DNA (11). Thus, despite a size that exceeds that of virion DNA by 30%, circular DNA molecules of 1670 cells are a form of defective genome. When cloned virion DNA fragments from within this 55- to 75-kb region of L-DNA were used as hybridization probes to blots of 1670 DNA, these sequences were not detected at a sensitivity level where 0.1 genome equivalent per cell could have been found (S. Schirm, C. Kaschka-Dierich, and B. Fleckenstein, *unpublished data*).

Circular viral DNA from the nonproducer cell line 70N2 has been found to have a structure similar to that of nonintegrated genomes of 1670 cells. Long (L1 = 86 kb) and short (L2 = 28 kb) L-DNA sequences, both in the same orientation, are intespersed between a long stretch (H1 = 38 kb) and a short stretch (H2 = 28 kb) of repetitive H-DNA. Thus, both cell lines have higher relative proportions of repetitive H-DNA than virion M-DNA. The L1 and H1 regions of 1670 cells and 70N2 cells are about the same length; however, the H2 region of 70N2 cells is slightly shorter, and the L2 region is markedly shorter than the corresponding parts of 1670 circles. Thus, the viral genetic complexities of cell line 70N2 and 1670 are very nearly the same (11,40).

H. saimiri circular DNA molecules of the *in vitro*-immortalized H1591 cell line consist of a single L-DNA segment and a single H-DNA segment. The L-DNA region has been found to have 65 kb; this is much shorter than virion L-DNA. Denaturation patterns indicate that the missing sequences correspond mostly to the right half of L-DNA of virus particles. On the other hand, the length of H-DNA (78 kb) far exceeds the total amount of repetitive DNA in virion M genomes (40).

The stability of circular *H. saimiri* DNA in established lymphoid tumor cell lines after multiple culture passage is remarkable. The high amount of repetitive DNA in tandem orientation could easily be available for recombination events that would result in altered sizes of H-DNA segments. This may suggest that there are mechanisms to avoid recombination processes in persisting viral circles in lymphoid cells. On the other hand, our laboratories have found evidence for a pronounced heterogeneity of viral DNA in the early passages of cell line H1591. Possibly, structural variability is characteristic of early cell lines, and long-term selection by continuous passage may result in lines with stable persisting circular DNA of apparent uniform composition.

The conversion of *H. saimiri*-producing lymphoid cell lines to nonproducer status seems to parallel deletions within DNA. This is reminiscent of EBV-transformed cells; the nonproducing Raji cell line also has deletions of unique EBV DNA sequences (6). However, the regions missing in *H. saimiri*- transformed cells are far longer than the deletions observed in persisting EBV genomes.

So far, it has not been possible to determine to what extent, if at all, *H. saimiri* DNA is integrated into the genome in transformed cells. Difficulties arise from the size of viral genomes, the relatively high amount of circular viral DNA present in transformed cells, and the similar densities of viral DNA and cellular DNA. Entanglement of circular molecules or density changes due to modified bases could pretend an association with the cellular genome on separation steps. When freshly prepared DNA from *H. saimiri*-transformed cells has been analyzed by isopyknic centrifugation in dye-salt gradients, a minor proportion of viral sequences has been found at a lower density than superhelical DNA. Because relaxation of large superhelical herpesvirus circles can occur because of trace amounts of intracellular nucleases and other causes, this approach will probably be inappropriate to answer the question whether or not integrated *H. saimiri* DNA exists. Sensitive hybridizations using cloned L-DNA fragments have not resulted in detection of any fragments other than those present in the circular molecules of known structure (S. Schirm, C. Kaschka-Dierich, and B. Fleckenstein, *unpublished data*).

DNA Methylation

5-Methylcytosine (m^5C) is the only modified base that has been detected in mammalian cell DNA. Methyl groups are added to particular cytosines postreplicatively by DNA methylase using *S*-adenosylmethionine as the methyl donor. Some 3 to 5% of the cytosines in mammalian cell DNA are methylated in this manner; m^5C occurs by far most frequently in the dinucleotide 5'CG3', but m^5C does appear rarely outside this dinucleotide (68). In double-stranded DNA, CG is a palindromic sequence, and the C in both strands is found methylated. If a region of double-stranded DNA containing CG dinucleotides methylated on both strands is replicated, a resultant double-stranded DNA molecule will initially contain hemimethylated DNA (i.e., parental strand methylated and daughter strand unmethylated). Because partially purified mammalian cell DNA methylases seem most active with hemimethylated DNA (33,38), methylated sites may tend to be inherited (64,65).

Some 50 to 90% of CG dinucleotides in various mammalian cell DNAs are methylated (34). Germ cell DNA appears to be completely or nearly completely methylated. During the course of differentiation, methyl groups are lost from specific CG sites in a tissue-specific manner (47,48). Demethylases have not been found in mammalian cells, but completely unmethylated CG dinucleotide base pairs could arise from failure to methylate through two rounds of DNA replication. Specific programs in the course of differentiation must result in the tissue-specific demethylation patterns (15,35). In this sense, methylated CG sites are not strictly inherited. Similarly, the results of studies of foreign DNA introduced into cells by transfection and of X-chromosome DNA are not entirely consistent with strict inheritance of methylated CG sites. Many of the CG methylations are inherited through many generations, but a significant portion are not inherited (60,67,72,74). Unmethylated sites appear to be more strictly inherited (59,60,67,72,74). Further work will be needed to understand the forces operating when the presence or absence of methylation at specific sites is not inherited.

Three lines of evidence indicate that *H. saimiri* virion DNA produced from lytic infection of OMK cells is unmethylated, or nearly so: (a) Nucleoside composition analysis of highly purified virion DNA by high-performance liquid chromatography has shown that the level of m^5C is at least 30 times less than the level in host cell DNA. This is less than 10 methyl groups per L-DNA region. (b) von Acken et al. (4) have analyzed radiolabeled virion DNA using thin-layer chromatography, and their reported limits of detection indicate less than one methyl group per virion M-DNA molecule. (c) No detectable differences in cleavage patterns of virion DNA have been observed between *Hpa*II and *Msp*I (CCGG) (14). The specificities of these isoschizomers are shown in Table 2. These results indicate less than one methylated CCGG, on average, per virion L-DNA molecule.

In contrast to the situation with virion DNA, extensive methylation has been detected in viral DNA of tumor cells. Several restriction endonucleases have been used in addition to *Hpa*II and *Msp*I to analyze viral DNA methylation in tumor cells (12,14). No evidence was found for methylation of the 5'C in the dinucleotide CC using restriction endonucleases *Hae*III (GGCC) and *Msp*I (CCGG); however, methylation of CG was detected. *Hpa*II (CCGG) and *Sma*I (CCCGGG) primarily were used to detect H-DNA CG methylation. In the original study, three virus-producing cell lines (77/5, 1926, and H1591) and two nonproducing cell lines (1670 and 70N2) were examined for H-DNA methylation. The level of H-DNA methylation in producing cell lines was less than 10% of CG sites, whereas in the nonproducing cell lines it was greater than 50% of CG sites. We suggested at that time

TABLE 2. *Sequence specificities
of restriction endonucleases
Hpall and MspI*[a]

Sequence	Hpall	MspI
CCGG	+	+
CMGG[b]	−	+
MCGG	+	−
MMGG	−	−

[a]The ability or inability to cleave the indicated sequence is noted by a plus or minus, respectively.
[b]M = 5-methylcytosine.

that perhaps viral DNA methylation plays some role in the control of viral expression in tumor cells. We have since found that producing cell lines also have less L-DNA methylation than nonproducing cell lines, but significant levels of L-DNA methylation (15–80% of CG sites) were detected in the virus-producing cell lines (12). However, only a small fraction of cells (less than 0.1%) are able to produce virus, and it seems likely that completely unmethylated viral genomes are present together with intracellular viral DNA containing unmethylated H-DNA regions and variably methylated L-DNA regions in the producing cell cultures. H-DNA is also not significantly methylated in tumor cells taken directly from tumor-bearing animals.

*Hpa*II and *Fnu*DII (CGCG) have been used for analysis of L-DNA CG methylation in tumor cells taken directly from tumor-bearing animals (12). Most *Hpa*II and *Fnu*DII sites in viral L-DNA in these tumor cells were not cleaved, apparently because of methylation. From band intensities of Southern blot autoradiograms it was estimated that 28 of 32 sites were methylated in more than 90% of the molecules, but four sites were unmethylated in more than 95% of the molecules in tumor cells taken directly from tumor-bearing animals. The map locations of the four unmethylated CG sites in L-DNA of tumors are shown in Fig. 2. Two of the *Hpa*II sites and two of the *Fnu*DII sites were specifically unmethylated. We find it remarkable that the numbers and locations of the unmethylated sites appeared identical in four different tumor samples (one owl monkey and three white-lip marmosets). The nonproducer cell line 1670, in continuous culture for over 7 years, contained specifically unmethylated *Hpa*II and *Fnu*DII sites similar to those found in fresh tumor cells (12).

The density of DNA in cesium chloride gradients is lowered by methylation of the cytosine ring in the 5-position (42). The density of viral DNA from 1670 and 70N2 cells in cesium chloride gradients is lower than would be expected for unmodified DNA and perhaps reflects the degree of CG methylation. Treatment of nonproducer cells with the potent inducer of herpesvirus expression TPA (12-*O*-tetradecanoylphorbol-13-acetate) resulted in a density of viral DNA closer to that

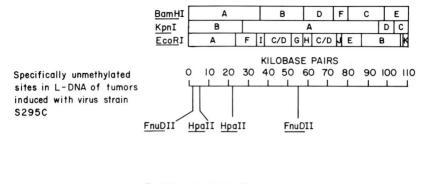

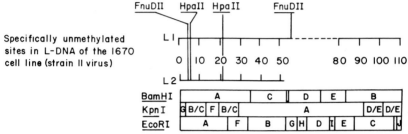

FIG. 2. Locations of specifically unmethylated sites in L-DNA. The terminal cleavage site in each map is the first *Sma* I site in H-DNA. Virion L-DNA cleavage maps were adapted from Fleckenstein and Mulder (30).

expected for unmodified DNA (39). Further work, including restriction endonuclease digestion and Southern blotting, will be needed to demonstrate an effect of TPA on the level of DNA methylation.

As mentioned earlier, unmethylated DNA introduced into cultured cells via transfection usually remains stably unmethylated for many generations. The situation with *H. saimiri* contrasts with this; the viral DNA invariably is extensively methylated following stable association with the growth-transformed cell. If a cellular methylase is methylating *H. saimiri* DNA, it remains to be explained how this particular methylation pattern arises. The unmethylated CG sites may be naturally refractory to methylation. Alternatively, the observed methylated and unmethylated sites could arise by chance in the millions of infected lymphocytes in the animal; if this results in expression of transformation-specific products and outgrowth of transformed cells, this particular methylation pattern could be selected for and passed on to daughter cells.

Unfortunately, nothing is known about the origins of viral RNA in tumor cells. The large numbers of correlations of hypomethylated regions of DNA with gene expression naturally prompt us to speculate if viral RNA in tumor cells might be derived from regions containing unmethylated CG sites. In contrast to the large amounts of viral DNA, the level of *H. saimiri* RNA in marmoset tumor cells is low, at least as low as EBV RNA in human transformed cells.

CONCLUDING REMARKS

Several approaches have been used in the attempt to gain an understanding of the mechanisms responsible for oncogenic transformation by *H. saimiri*. These approaches, not significantly different from those used previously to study other model tumor virus systems, have included studies of (a) structure, sequence arrangement, and characteristics of viral DNA in tumor cells, (b) expression of viral DNA in tumor cells, and (c) mutants defective in oncogenic transformation.

Viral DNA in tumor cells has been shown to be present largely as covalently closed circular DNA. If there is any viral DNA integrated with host cell sequences in the tumor cells thus far examined, it is a small percentage of the total. Now that it is known that many viruses carry their own oncogenes, it does not seem necessary to invoke an integration event for oncogenic transformation. For viruses that carry their own transforming genes, it seems necessary only that the genetic information become stably associated with the cells and that appropriate sequences be expressed. This could conceivably be accomplished for the large-genome herpesviruses by the formation of the circular DNA structure.

Further analyses have revealed large deletions of viral DNA information in several nonproducer cell lines. These deletions include the 55- to 75-kb L-DNA region in tumor cell lines 1670 and 70N2 and an even larger deletion in the *in vitro*-immortalized cell line H1591. Because the 55- to 75-kb L-DNA region is present at less than 0.1 genome copy per cell, its continued presence is apparently not necessary to maintain the immortalized growth phenotype.

Analysis of methylated and unmethylated CG sites in viral DNA has revealed a pattern common to the four tumor samples thus far examined. The methylation patterns appear identical in tumors from different animal species (owl monkey and white-lip marmosets), and the pattern is even similar in the continuously passaged 1670 cell line. This raises the possibility that the observed methylation pattern or some aspects of it could be important for maintenance of the growth-transformed phenotype. It seems reasonable to speculate whether or not viral RNA in tumor cells might be derived from the few regions containing unmethylated sites. If the *H. saimiri* protein product or products are responsible for oncogenic transformation, identification of the structure and origin of viral RNA in tumor cells will be an important step toward determining if these viral RNAs must be expressed to achieve oncogenic transformation. The demonstration of specific methylated and unmethylated sites has provided potential insight into how expression of these regions may be controlled.

Further study of the two nononcogenic variants should reveal whether or not the deletions at the left junction of unique and repetitive DNA are responsible for the loss of oncogenicity and also should reveal the nature of the lesion. In perhaps the least interesting scenario, an altered viral protein or antigen that allows an infected animal to overcome tumor cell growth with the aid of its immune system could trivially explain the lack of oncogenicity. A suitable *in vitro* transformation or immortalization assay must be developed to test the nononcogenic variants as well as other variants and laboratory constructs. A genetic system of complementation groups has not been developed for *H. saimiri* but eventually may be needed to determine loci required for oncogenic transformation. Nevertheless, several pieces of evidence have intimated a possible role for the leftmost L-DNA region in oncogenic transformation: (a) This region of DNA continues to be present in nonproducer lines that contain large deletions in other L-DNA regions. (b) This left L-DNA region is sometimes present in tumor cell lines with a molarity double that of other regions. (c) Two of four specifically unmethylated sites are located in this region. (d) The two nononcogenic variants have independently acquired deletions in this region.

ACKNOWLEDGMENTS

Work described in this chapter was supported by grants RR00168 to the New England Regional Primate Research Center from the Division of Research Resources (NIH), 1 RO1 CA 31363-01 from the National Institutes of Health, and 1511-C-1 from the American Cancer Society, Massachusetts Division, and by grants from Wilhelm-Sander-Stiftung and Deutsche Forschungsgemeinschaft (SFB 118).

REFERENCES

1. Ablashi, D. V., Loeb, W. F., Valerio, M. G., Adamson, R. H., Armstrong, G. R., Bennett, D. G., and Heine, U. (1971): Malignant lymphoma with lymphatic leukemia in owl monkeys induced by *Herpesvirus saimiri. J. Natl. Cancer Inst.*, 47:837–855.
2. Ablashi, D. V., Pearson, G., Rabin, H., Armstrong, G., Easton, J., Valerio, M., and Cicmanec, J. (1978): Experimental infection of *Callithrix jacchus* marmosets with *Herpesvirus ateles, Herpesvirus saimiri* and Epstein-Barr virus. *Biomedicine*, 29:7–10.
3. Ablashi, D. V., Sundar, K. S., Armstrong, G., Golway, P., Valerio, M., Bengali, Z., Lemp, J., and Fox, R. R. (1980): *Herpesvirus saimiri*-induced malignant lymphoma in inbred strain III/J rabbits *(Oryctolagus cuniculus). J. Cancer Res. Clin. Oncol.*, 98:165–172.
4. von Acken, U., Simon, D., Grunert, F., Doring, H.-P., and Kröger, H. (1979): Methylation of viral DNA *in vivo* and *in vitro. Virology*, 99:152–157.
5. Bornkamm, G. W., Delius, H., Fleckenstein, B., Werner, F.-J., and Mulder, C. (1976): Structure of *Herpesvirus saimiri* genomes: Arrangement of heavy and light sequences in the M-genome. *J. Virol.*, 25:154–161.
6. Bornkamm, G. W., Delius, H., Zimber, V., Hudewentz, J., and Epstein, M. A. (1980): Comparison of Epstein-Barr virus strains of different origin by analysis of the viral DNAs. *J. Virol.*, 35:603–618.
7. Cicmanec, J. L., Loeb, W. F., and Valerio, M. G. (1974): Lymphoma in owl monkeys *(Aotus trivirgatus)* inoculated with *Herpesvirus saimiri*: Clinical, hematological, and pathological findings. *J. Med. Primatol.*, 3:8–17.
8. Daniel, M. D., Melendez, L. V., Hunt, R. D., King, N. W., Anver, M., Fraser, C. E. O., Barahona, H., and Baggs, R. B. (1974): *Herpesvirus saimiri*: VII. Induction of malignant lymphoma in New Zealand white rabbits. *J. Natl. Cancer Inst.*, 53:1803–1807.
9. Daniel, M. D., Silva, D., Koomey, J. M., Mulder, C., Fleckenstein, B., King, N. W., Hunt, R. D., Seghal, P., and Falk, L. A. (1979): *Herpesvirus saimiri*: Strain SMHI modification of oncogenicity. In: *Advances in Comparative Leukemia Research*, edited by D. S. Yohn, B. A. Lapin, and J. R. Blakeslee, pp. 395–396. Elsevier/North Holland, Amsterdam.
10. Deinhardt, F. (1973): *Herpesvirus saimiri*. In: *The Herpesviruses*, edited by A. Kaplan, pp. 595–625. Academic Press, New York.
11. Desrosiers, R. C. (1981): *Herpesvirus saimiri* DNA in tumor cells—deleted sequences and sequence rearrangements. *J. Virol.*, 39:497–509.

12. Desrosiers, R. C. (1982): Specifically unmethylated CG sites in *Herpesvirus saimiri* DNA in tumor cells. *J. Virol.*, 43:427–435.
13. Desrosiers, R. C., and Falk, L. A. (1982): *Herpesvirus saimiri* strain variability. *J. Virol.*, 43:352–356.
14. Desrosiers, R., Mulder, C., and Fleckenstein, B. (1979): Methylation of *Herpesvirus saimiri* DNA in lymphoid tumor cell lines. *Proc. Natl. Acad. Sci. USA*, 76:3839–3843.
15. Ehrlich, M., and Wang, R. (1981): 5-Methylcytosine in eucaryotic DNA. *Science*, 212:1350–1357.
16. Falk, L. A. (1980): Simian herpesviruses and their oncogenic properties. In: *Oncogenic Herpesviruses, Vol. I*, edited by F. Rapp, pp. 145–173. CRC Press, Boca Raton, Fl.
17. Falk, L. A. (1980): Biology of *Herpesvirus saimiri* and *Herpesvirus ateles*. In: *Viral Oncology*, edited by G. Klein, pp. 813–832. Raven Press, New York.
18. Falk, L. A., Desrosiers, R., and Hunt, R. D. (1980): *Herpesvirus saimiri* infection in squirrel and marmoset monkeys. In: *Viruses in Naturally Occurring Cancer*, edited by M. Essex, G. Todaro, and H. zur Hausen, pp. 137–143. Cold Spring Harbor Laboratory, Cold Spring Harbor, N.Y.
19. Falk, L. A., Johnson, D., and Deinhardt, F. (1978): Transformation of marmoset lymphocytes *in vitro* with *Herpesvirus ateles*. *Int. J. Cancer*, 21:652–657.
20. Falk, L. A., Nigida, S. M., Deinhardt, F. W., Cooper, R. W., and Hernandez-Camacho, J. I. (1973): Oral excretion of *Herpesvirus saimiri* in captive squirrel monkeys and incidence of infection in feral squirrel monkeys. *J. Natl. Cancer Inst.*, 51:1987–1989.
21. Falk, L. A., Nigida, S. M., Deinhardt, F., Wolfe, L. G., Cooper, R. W., and Hernandez-Camacho, J. I. (1974): *Herpesvirus ateles*: Properties of an oncogenic herpesvirus isolated from circulating lymphocytes of spider monkeys (*Ateles* sp.). *Int. J. Cancer*, 14:473–482.
22. Falk, L. A., Wolfe, L. G., and Deinhardt, F. (1972): Epidemiology of *Herpesvirus saimiri* infection in squirrel monkeys. *J. Med. Primatol.*, 111:151–158.
23. Falk, L. A., Wolfe, L. G., Hoekstra, J., and Deinhardt, F. (1972): Demonstration of *Herpesvirus saimiri* associated antigens in peripheral lymphocytes from infected marmosets during *in vitro* cultivation. *J. Natl. Cancer Inst.*, 48:523–530.
24. Falk, L. A., Wright, J., Wolfe, L., and Deinhardt, F. (1974): *Herpesvirus ateles*: Transformation *in vitro* of marmoset splenic lymphocytes. *Int. J. Cancer*, 14:244–251.
25. Fleckenstein, B. (1979): Oncogenic herpesviruses of nonhuman primates. *Biochim. Biophys. Acta*, 560:301–342.
26. Fleckenstein, B., Bornkamm, G., and Ludwig, H. (1975): Repetitive sequences in complete and defective genomes of *Herpesvirus saimiri*. *J. Virol.* 15:398–406.
27. Fleckenstein, B., Bornkamm, G., Mulder, C. Werner, F. J., Daniel, M. D., Falk, L. A., and Delius, H. (1978): *Herpesvirus ateles* DNA and its homology with *Herpesvirus saimiri* nucleic acid. *J. Virol.*, 21:361–373.
28. Fleckenstein, B., Daniel, M. D., Hunt, R. D., Werner, F.-J., Falk, L. A., and Mulder, C. (1978): Tumor induction with DNA of oncogenic primate herpesviruses. *Nature*, 274:57–59.
29. Fleckenstein, B., and Desrosiers, R. (1982): *Herpesvirus saimiri* and *Herpesvirus ateles*. In: *The Herpesviruses*, Vol. 1, edited by B. Roizman, pp. 253–332. Plenum Press, New York.
30. Fleckenstein, B., and Mulder, C. (1980): Molecular biological aspects of *Herpesvirus saimiri* and *Herpesvirus ateles*. In: *Viral Oncology*, edited by G. Klein, pp. 799–812. Raven Press, New York.
31. Fleckenstein, B., Müller, I., and Werner, F.-J. (1977): The presence of *Herpesvirus saimiri* genomes in virus transformed cells. *Int. J. Cancer*, 19:546–554.
32. Fleckenstein, B., and Wolf, H. (1974): Purification and properties of *Herpesvirus saimiri* DNA. *Virology*, 58:55–64.
33. Gruenbaum, Y., Cedar, H., and Razin, A. (1982): Substrate and sequence specificity of a eucaryotic DNA methylase. *Nature*, 295:620–622.
34. Gruenbaum, Y., Stein, R., Cedar, H., and Razin, A. (1981): Methylation of CpG sequences in eucaryotic DNA. *F.E.B.S. Lett.*, 124:67–71.
35. Holliday, R., and Pugh, J. E. (1975): DNA modification mechanisms and gene activity during development. *Science*, 187:226–232.
36. Hunt, R. D., Melendez, L. V., King, N. W., Gilmore, C. E., Daniel, M. D., Williamson, M. E., and Jones, T. C. (1970): Morphology of a disease with features of malignant lymphoma in marmosets and owl monkeys inoculated with *Herpesvirus saimiri*. *J. Natl. Cancer Inst.*, 44:447–465.

37. Johnson, D. R., Ohno, S., Kaschka-Dierich, C., Fleckenstein, B., and Klein, G. (1981): Relationship between *Herpesvirus ateles* associated nuclear antigens (HATNA) and the number of viral genome equivalents in HVA carrying lymphoid lines. *J. Gen. Virol.*, 52:221–226.
38. Jones, P. A., and Taylor, S. M. (1981): Hemimethylated duplex DNAs prepared from 5-azacytidine treated cells. *Nucleic Acids Res.*, 9:2933–2947.
39. Kaschka-Dierich, C., Bauer, I., Fleckenstein, B., and Desrosiers, R. C. (1981): Episomal and nonepisomal herpesvirus DNA in lymphoid tumor cell lines. In: *Haematology and Blood Transfusion, Vol. 26,* edited by R. Neth, R. Gallo, T. Graf, M. Mannweiler, and H. Winkler, pp. 197–203. Springer-Verlag, Berlin.
40. Kaschka-Dierich, C., Bauer, I., Schirm, S., and Fleckenstein, B. (1982): Structure of nonintegrated, covalently closed circular viral DNA in *Herpesvirus saimiri* and *Herpesvirus ateles* transformed cells. *J. Virol.*, 44:295–310.
41. Keil, G., Muller, I., Fleckenstein, B., Koomey, J. M., and Mulder, C. (1980): Generation of recombinants between different strains of *Herpesvirus saimiri*. In: *Viruses in Naturally Occurring Cancer,* edited by M. Essex, G. Todaro, and H. zur Hausen, pp. 145–161. Cold Spring Harbor Laboratory, Cold Spring Harbor, N.Y.
42. Kirk, J. T. O. (1967): Effect of methylation of cytosine residues on the buoyant density of DNA in cesium chloride solution. *J. Mol. Biol.*, 28:171–172.
43. Laufs, R., and Fleckenstein, B. (1972): Susceptibility to *Herpesvirus saimiri* and antibody development in Old and New World monkeys. *Med. Microbiol. Immunol.*, 158:227–236.
44. Laufs, R., and Melendez, L. V. (1973): Latent infection of monkeys with oncogenic herpesvirus. *Med. Microbiol. Immunol.*, 158:299–308.
45. Laufs, R., Steinke, H., Steinke, G., and Petzold, D. (1974): Latent infection and malignant lymphoma in marmosets *(Callithrix jacchus)* after infection with two oncogenic herpesviruses from primates. *J. Natl. Cancer Inst.*, 53:195–199.
46. Lindahl, T., Adams, A., Bjursell, G., Bornkamm, G. W., Kaschka-Dierich, C., and Jehn, V. (1976): Covalently closed circular duplex DNA of Epstein-Barr virus in a human lymphoid cell line. *J. Mol. Biol.*, 102:511–530.
47. Mandel, J., and Chambon, P. (1979): DNA methylation: Organ specific variations in the methylation pattern within and around ovalbumin and other chicken genes. *Nucleic Acids Res.*, 1:2081–2103.
48. McGhee, J. D., and Ginder, G. (1979): Specific DNA methylation sites in the vicinity of the chicken β-globin genes. *Nature*, 280:419–420.
49. Melendez, L. V., Daniel, M. D., Garcia, F. G., Fraser, C. E. O., Hunt, R. D., and King, N. W. (1969): *Herpesvirus saimiri*. I. Further characterization studies of a new virus from the squirrel monkey. *Lab. Animal Care*, 19:372–377.
50. Melendez, L. V., Daniel, M. D., Hunt, R. D., Fraser, C. E. O., Garcia, F. G., King, N. W., and Williamson, M. E. (1970): *Herpesvirus saimiri*. V. Further evidence to consider this virus as the etiological agent of a lethal disease in primates which resembles a malignant lymphoma. *J. Natl. Cancer Inst.*, 44:1175–1181.
51. Melendez, L. V., Daniel, M. D., Hunt, R. D., and Garcia, F. G. (1968): An apparently new herpesvirus from primary kidney cultures of the squirrel monkey *(Saimiri sciureus)*. *Lab. Animal Care*, 18:374–381.
52. Melendez, L. V., Hunt, R. D., Daniel, M. D., Blake, B. J., and Garcia, F. G. (1971): Acute lymphocytic leukemia in owl monkeys inoculated with *Herpes-saimiri*. *Science*, 171:1161–1163.
53. Melendez, L. V., Hunt, R. D., Daniel, M. D., Fraser, C. E. O., Barahona, H. H., Garcia, F. G., and King, N. W. (1972): *Herpesvirus saimiri* and *Herpesvirus ateles*, the first oncogenic herpesvirus of primates—a review. In: *Oncogenesis and Herpesviruses,* edited by P. M. Biggs, G. de Thé, and L. N. Payne, pp. 451–461. IARC Press, Lyon.
54. Melendez, L. V., Hunt, R. D., Daniel, M. D., Garcia, F. G., and Fraser, C. E. O. (1969): *Herpesvirus saimiri*. II. Experimentally induced malignant lymphoma in primates. *Lab. Animal Care*, 19:378–386.
55. Melendez, L. V., Hunt, R. D., Daniel, M. D., and Trum, B. F. (1970): New World monkeys, herpesvirus and cancer. In: *Infections and Immunosuppression in Sub-human Primates,* edited by H. Balner and W. J. B. Beveridge, pp. 111–117. Munksgaard, Copenhagen.
56. Morgan, D. G., and Epstein, M. A. (1977): Sequential immunofluorescence and infectivity studies on the replication of *Herpesvirus saimiri* on owl monkey kidney cells. *J. Gen. Virol.*, 34:61–72.

57. Nazerian, K., Lindahl, T., Klein, G., and Lee, L. F. (1973): DNA of Marek's disease virus in virus-induced tumors. *J. Virol.*, 12:841–846.
58. Nonoyama, M., and Pagano, J. S. (1973): Homology between Epstein-Barr virus DNA and viral DNA from Burkitt's lymphoma and nasopharyngeal carcinoma determined by DNA-DNA reassociation kinetics. *Nature*, 242:44–47.
59. Pellicer, A., Robbins, D., Wold, B., Sweet, R., Jackson, J., Lowy, I., Roberts, J., Sim, G. K., Silverstein, S., and Axel, R. (1980): Altering genotype and phenotype by DNA-mediated gene transfer. *Science*, 209:1414–1422.
60. Pollack, Y., Stein, R., Razin, A., and Cedar, H. (1980): Methylation of foreign DNA sequences in eucaryotic cells. *Proc. Natl. Acad. Sci. USA*, 77:6463–6467.
61. Rabin, H. (1971): Assay and pathogenesis of oncogenic viruses in nonhuman primates. *Lab. Anim. Sci.*, 21:1032–1049.
62. Rabson, A. S., O'Connor, G. T., Lorenz, D. E., Kirchstein, R. L., Legallais, F. Y., and Tralka, T. S. (1971): Lymphoid cell culture line derived from lymph node of marmoset infected with *Herpesvirus saimiri*. *J. Natl. Cancer Inst.*, 46:1099–1109.
63. Rangan, S. R. S., Martin, L. N., Enright, F. M., and Allen, W. P. (1976): *Herpesvirus saimiri* induced malignant lymphoma in rabbits. *J. Natl. Cancer Inst.*, 57:151–156.
64. Razin, A., and Riggs, A. (1980): DNA methylation and gene function. *Science*, 210:604–610.
65. Riggs, A. D. (1975): X inactivation, differentiation and DNA methylation. *Cytogenet. Cell Genet.*, 14:9–25.
66. Schaffer, P., Falk, L. A., and Deinhardt, F. (1975): Attenuation of *Herpesvirus saimiri* for marmosets after successive passage in cell culture at 39°C. *J. Natl. Cancer Inst.*, 55:1243–1246.
67. Stein, R., Gruenbaum, Y., Pollack, Y., Razin, A., and Cedar, H. (1982): Clonal inheritance of the pattern of DNA methylation in mouse cells. *Proc. Natl. Acad. Sci. USA*, 79:61–75.
68. Van der Ploeg, L. H. T., Groffey, J., and Flavell, R. A. (1980): A novel type of secondary modification of two CCGG residues in the human globin gene locus. *Nucleic Acids Res.*, 8:4563–4574.
69. Wallen, W. C., Neubauer, R. H., Rabin, H., and Cicmanec, J. L. (1973): Nonimmune rosette formation by lymphoma and leukemia cells from *Herpesvirus saimiri* infected owl monkeys. *J. Natl. Cancer Inst.*, 51:967–975.
70. Werner, F.-J., Bornkamm, G. W., and Fleckenstein, B. (1977): Episomal viral DNA in a *Herpesvirus saimiri* transformed lymphoid cell line. *J. Virol.*, 22:794–803.
71. Werner, F.-J., Desrosiers, R. C., Mulder, C., Bornkamm, G. W., and Fleckenstein, B. (1978): Physical mapping of viral episomes in *Herpesvirus saimiri* transformed lymphoid cells. In: *Persistent Viruses*, edited by J. Stevens, G. Todaro, and G. F. Fox, pp. 189–200. Academic Press, New York.
72. Wigler, M., Levy, D., and Perucho, M. (1981): The somatic replication of DNA methylation. *Cell*, 24:33–40.
73. Wolfe, L. G., Falk, L. A., and Deinhardt, F. (1971): Oncogenicity of *Herpesvirus saimiri* in marmoset monkeys. *J. Natl. Cancer Inst.*, 47:1145–1162.
74. Wolfe, S., and Migeon, B. (1982): Studies of x chromosome DNA methylation in normal human cells. *Nature*, 295:667–671.
75. Wright, J., Falk, L. A., Collins, D., and Deinhardt, F. (1976): Mononuclear cell fraction carrying *Herpesvirus saimiri* in persistently-infected squirrel monkeys. *J. Natl. Cancer Inst.*, 57:959–962.
76. Wright, J., Falk, L. A., Wolfe, L. G., and Deinhardt, F. (1980): *Herpesvirus saimiri*: Protective effect of attenuated strain against lymphoma induction. *Int. J. Cancer*, 26:477–482.
77. Wright, J., Falk, L. A., Wolfe, L. G., Ogden, J., and Deinhardt, F. (1977): Susceptibility of common marmosets *(Callithrix jacchus)* to oncogenic and attenuated strains of *Herpesvirus saimiri*. *J. Natl. Cancer Inst.*, 59:1475–1478.
78. zur Hausen, H., Schulte-Holthausen, H., Klein, G., Henle, W., Henle, G., Clifford, P., and Santesson, L. (1970): EBV DNA in biopsies of Burkitt tumors and anaplastic carcinomas of the nasopharynx. *Nature*, 228:1056–1058.

Advances in Viral Oncology, Volume 3, edited by
George Klein. Raven Press, New York © 1983.

Hepatitis B Virus and Primary Hepatocellular Carcinoma

W. Thomas London

Institute for Cancer Research, Philadelphia, Pennsylvania 19111

Nearly all of the research on the etiology and pathogenesis of primary hepato-cellular carcinoma (PHC) in experimental animals has been concerned with chemical carcinogens. Ironically, it now appears that in humans, a virus, the hepatitis B virus (HBV), is implicated in the etiology of nearly all cases of PHC. In these cases, persistent infection with HBV is a necessary, and possibly sufficient, cause of the cancer. That is, prevention of infection with HBV probably will prevent most cases of PHC. Other factors in the environment, such as aflatoxins, cycads, nitrosamines, and alcohol, may also damage the liver and may influence the rate at which PHCs develop in individuals infected with HBV, but there is no direct evidence that these factors are required for the development of liver cancer in humans. An effective vaccine against HBV is now being produced in the United States, France, and The Netherlands. It is likely that the vaccine will be widely administered to populations living in areas endemic for HBV infection. Within 5 to 10 years it should be possible to learn whether or not the vaccine prevents chronic liver disease. If it does, it will be reasonable to conclude, without waiting 30 years for definitive proof, that it will also prevent PHC.

PREVALENCE AND DISTRIBUTION OF PHC

Despite its relative rarity in the United States and Europe, PHC may be the most common cancer in humans worldwide. In Taiwan, not only is it the most common malignant neoplasm, accounting for 20% of all cancers, but also it is the second leading cause of death (3). Beasley suggested that even this high incidence may be a significant underestimate of the true frequency of PHC. Many deaths in Taiwan that are attributed to cirrhosis on death certificates probably are due to PHC (2).

In mainland China, Li and Shiang (21) reported that there are 100,000 deaths per year from PHC in a population of 850 million, or 11.7 per 100,000. This, again, is a minimum estimate. The actual mortality from PHC may be two or three times that. Similarly high death rates from PHC have also been observed among the black populations of Africa. About half of the world's population lives in areas of high incidence for PHC, and in these areas this tumor may account for 1 million deaths per year (22).

CLINICAL AND PATHOLOGICAL FEATURES OF PHC

PHC in adults arises in 70 to 90% of cases involving a liver with cirrhosis, less commonly in association with chronic active hepatitis, and in less than 10% of cases involving a histologically normal liver (13). In children, hepatocellular cancers usually are found in otherwise normal livers. Such tumors are rare, even in areas of the world with high incidences of PHC among adults. The relation of childhood tumors to HBV has not been investigated adequately.

Histologically, most PHCs consist of neoplastic hepatocytes arranged in trabecular patterns, often with acinuslike structures. Some tumors are highly anaplastic and lack trabecular organization. Trabeculae are two to eight cells thick and usually are separated by vascular spaces lined by endothelial cells. Kupffer cells are rarely found within tumor foci. The tumors tend to invade and grow in intravascular spaces, particularly portal veins, and they may cause portal hypertension. Neoplastic hepatocytes resemble normal hepatocytes morphologically and frequently maintain many normal functions, e.g., glycogen and albumin synthesis. A distinguishing characteristic of malignant hepatocytes in all species studied is lack of stainable iron (58). This probably reflects a change in isoferritin content from the normal liver isoferritin (which binds large amounts of iron) to an isoferritin with a more acidic isoelectric point (which retains less iron) (11).

CHARACTERISTICS OF HBV

Before discussing the epidemiologic studies relating HBV to PHC, it is necessary to briefly review the characteristics of human HBV and HBV-like viruses in other species. The virion of HBV is a 42-nm particle containing an outer coat and an inner core. Table 1 lists the antigenic components of the virion and the antibodies they elicit. When an individual is infected with HBV, the viral surface antigen is made in excess and circulates in the blood as 22-nm spherical particles and as elongated particles of variable lengths and 22 nm in width. These noninfectious particles can be separated from other components in serum, and they are the materials used to make the currently available vaccines against hepatitis B (6).

The core of the virus contains the following constituents: (a) the DNA genome, (b) a DNA polymerase, (c) a protein kinase, and (d) a 19,000-dalton protein that carries the HBcAg determinant. A 15,000-dalton subunit of the core protein carries the HB_eAg determinant (30). As originally demonstrated by Summers et al. (51),

TABLE 1. *Nomenclature of antigens and antibodies associated with HBV*

Antigen	Antibody
HB_sAg: hepatitis B surface antigen	Anti-HB_s: antibody to HB_sAg
HB_cAg: hepatitis B core antigen	Anti-HB_c: antibody to HB_cAg
HB_eAg: hepatitis B e antigen	Anti-HB_e: antibody to HB_eAg

the genome of the virus is a double-strand circular DNA molecule with a single-strand region of variable length (Fig. 1). The DNA polymerase is capable of incorporating nucleotides *in vitro* into the incomplete strand to form a complete, double-strand DNA molecule of about 3,200 base pairs (bp). On the basis of studies with the duck hepatitis B virus (DHBV), a virus similar in morphology, genome size and structure, and tissue tropism to human HBV, Summers and Mason (49,50) have proposed a scheme for the replication of viruses of the HBV class (Fig. 1). It involves transcription of a genome-length RNA strand from the complete (minus) DNA strand. This is followed by copying of the RNA molecule into a new single-strand (minus-strand) DNA. The RNA strand is degraded as the new DNA strand is formed. Finally, the plus-strand DNA is copied off the minus strand; the minus strand is not degraded, and the plus strand frequently is not completed before the virus is assembled and discharged from the infected cell. The evidence for this model of replication is provided by Mason et al. (28,50). It is not known whether the polymerase found in the virus is coded for by the host or by the virus. It also is not known whether one enzyme can carry out the three different polymerase steps (DNA → RNA, RNA → DNA, DNA → DNA) required for this model of repli-

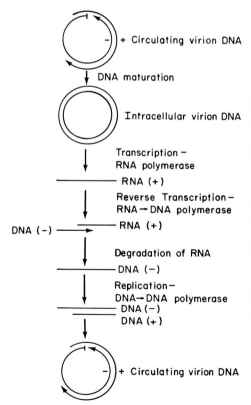

FIG. 1. Proposed pathway for replication of genome for HBV-like viruses. Formation of closed-circular, covalently linked, double-strand DNA occurs after the virus penetrates the cell. A full genome-length RNA intermediate is transcribed from the DNA minus strand. The RNA intermediate is reverse-transcribed to minus-strand DNA, and the RNA strand is degraded. Plus-strand DNA is synthesized by the DNA polymerase incorporated into the core of the virion. Virions are assembled and discharged from the cell before formation of the DNA plus strand has been completed. The various single-strand intermediates of genomic replication are found within protein cores that may form the core of the virion. Observations supporting this model are given elsewhere (28,50) (Adapted from Summers and Mason, ref. 50.)

cation or whether two or three different enzymes are needed. Integration of the viral genome is not required in this model, but it is possible that RNA is transcribed from an integrated rather than a free viral genome.

The RNA transcripts and succeeding steps of replication appear to occur within protein cores. Also, whether or not these structures are composed of the same viral proteins as the cores of mature virions is not known.

Albin and Robinson have identified a protein kinase activity in hepatitis B virions (1). The enzyme is located in the core of the virion and phosphorylates *in vitro* serine residues in the core antigen. The functional significance of these properties in virus replication or hepatocarcinogenesis is not clear. One possibility is that the phosphate serves as a linkage site for glycosylation of core polypeptides.

The host responses to HBV may be broadly separated into those associated with transient infections and those associated with persistent infections (Fig. 2). Transient infection, with development of anti-HB$_s$, leads to protection against subsequent infection with HBV and reduced risk of chronic liver disease. Until recently it had been thought that the disappearance of HB$_s$Ag from the peripheral blood and the appearance of anti-HB$_s$ meant that virus had also been cleared from the liver. This

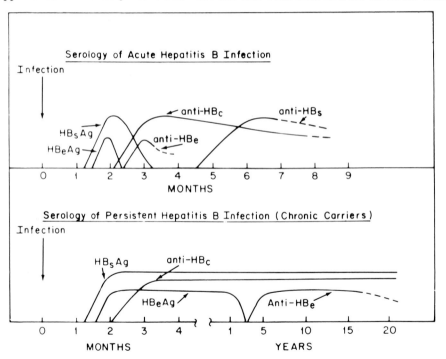

FIG. 2. Responses to HBV infection. The upper panel shows the serological responses of individuals who have transient infections with HBV. The lower panel shows the responses of individuals who have persistent infections. Individuals with HB$_s$Ag in their sera have circulating complete virions and free viral DNA in their livers. Persistent infections are associated with integrated viral DNA in hepatocytes (9).

may be the general case, but in some instances whole virus or viral DNA may be retained in the liver (9). The circumstances leading to this outcome need to be elucidated.

Persistent infections are characterized by persistance of HB_sAg in the peripheral blood and of HBV DNA in the liver of the host for many years, perhaps for the lifetime of the individual. Persons are classified as chronic carriers of HBV on the basis of persistence of HB_sAg in their sera for more than 6 months (25). Persistent infections are associated with an increased risk of developing chronic active hepatitis, cirrhosis, and PHC. HBV infections in adults are transient in 90 to 95% of cases, whereas infections of infants less than 6 months old are persistent in 90% of cases.

It is believed that most of the infections in infancy are transmitted by exposure to the blood of carrier mothers during birth (20,36,48). Mother-to-child transmission accounts for about 40% of the carriers in endemic areas and probably a greater proportion of the infections that eventually lead to PHC. This point will be elaborated further in the discussion of the epidemiology of PHC. Prevention of mother-to-child transmission can be effected by administering hepatitis B hyperimmune globulin (HBIG) to babies born to carrier mothers shortly (a few hours) after birth. A subsequent dose of HBIG probably should be given 1 to 2 months after birth, and that should be followed by immunization with the hepatitis B vaccine. A clinical trial in Japan of a program of this type has prevented all persistent infections and more than 90% of transient infections in infants (K. Nishioka, *personal communication*).

EPIDEMIOLOGIC EVIDENCE RELATING HBV TO PHC

As studies of the HBV-PHC relationship have accumulated over the past 15 years, the evidence favoring an etiologic role for the virus has become progressively stronger. International differences in incidences and mortality rates for PHC have been recognized for many years. The international distribution of HBV carriers appeared to correlate roughly with PHC incidence and mortality (5).

Studies of HBV infection in patients with PHC and controls were begun in the late 1960s. The initial investigations, using insensitive methods to detect HB_sAg, showed weak association or no association (44). As radioimmunoassay and other sensitive methods were introduced, large differences between patients and controls were detected. Fifty to 80% of PHC patients in endemic areas were found to be $HB_sAG(+)$, as compared with 5 to 15% of controls. When anti-HB_c was included in the testing profile, 80 to 90% of patients were positive, compared with 15 to 35% of controls (22). The incidence of anti-HB_s was generally lower among patients than among controls. From these kinds of studies, the relative risk for PHC among HBV carriers in endemic areas was estimated to be 15 to 30 times that for noncarriers (18). Prince (40) estimated that the relative risks for HBV carriers in western Europe and the United States were similar to those for carriers in Africa and Asia. From this he concluded that environmental carcinogens, such as aflatoxins and nitrosamines, which are unequally distributed in areas of high and low incidences of PHC, do not contribute significantly to the development of PHC in HBV carriers.

Because PHC usually arises in a liver affected by cirrhosis or chronic hepatitis, it was considered important to investigate the role of HBV in these diseases in areas with high incidences of PHC. Case–control studies in such areas again showed very high frequencies of HBV infection among patients as compared with controls. For example, Hann et al. (17) found that in Korea more than 90% of the patients with cirrhosis attending the Liver Clinic at Seoul National University Hospital were $HB_sAg(+)$, as were 75% of the patients with chronic active hepatitis, compared with 6 to 14% antigen positivity in matched controls.

Another retrospective epidemiologic approach was taken by Larouzé et al. (19) based on earlier observations of family clustering of HBV carriers and PHC (35). They hypothesized that because many chronic carriers of HBV develop as a result of infections acquired from carrier mothers at birth or during early infancy and because individuals infected early in life are chronic carriers longer than are carriers of similar age infected later in life, a higher incidence of carriers should be found among mothers of PHC patients than among mothers of appropriate controls if the duration of persistent HBV infection is related to the risk of hepatocarcinogenesis. They found that 71% of 28 mothers of PHC patients in Senegal were $HB_sAg(+)$, as compared with 13% of controls matched for age, sex, and neighborhood. Similar observations have been made in Korea (17) and Taiwan (2). These observations suggest that prevention of mother-to-child transmission will have a major impact on the prevention of PHC in endemic areas.

Markers of HBV infection can be searched for in the tumor and nontumor portions of the livers of patients with PHC and compared with the incidence of markers in controls. HB_sAg can be identified in tissues either by histochemical techniques (orcein stain) or, more specifically, by immunohistological methods (immunoperoxidase). Using these methods, many investigators have found that HB_sAg is commonly found in the nonneoplastic hepatocytes of livers containing PHC. In a particularly well controlled study of tissues obtained at autopsy, Nayak et al. (31) found that more than 90% of livers of patients with PHC in India contained HB_sAg, compared with 3% of livers from individuals without PHC (Table 2).

The case–control approach can also be applied to the identification, localization, and characterization of HBV DNA in hepatic tumor and nontumor tissues. This

TABLE 2. *Frequencies of HB_sAg and HB_cAg in livers of patients with PHC or cirrhosis and controls*

HBV component	PHC	Cirrhosis	Controls
HB_sAg	47/50 (94%)	41/58 (71%)	1/54
HB_cAg	9/41 (22%)	12/39 (31%)	0/25

Data from Nayak et al. (31).

will be discussed in greater detail later in this review. For the moment it is sufficient to state that HBV DNA is integrated into the genome of PHC cells and that both free (virion) DNA and integrated HBV DNA are found in nontumor tissues. Patients without PHC and without liver disease generally lack viral DNA (10,43).

Epidemiologically, the most convincing and most powerful studies are prospective. In the case of HBV and PHC, an extraordinary study is being carried out in Taiwan by Beasley and his colleagues (2,3). They are following 22,707 individuals for the development of PHC. The subjects of the study are Chinese men living in Taiwan and employed in the civil service. They belong to an insurance program that provides an annual physical examination and records all deaths and causes of death. The men were recruited into the study between December 1975 and June 1978. They were tested for HBV markers at the time of recruitment and were classified as $HB_sAg(+)$ or $HB_sAg(-)$. As of September 1, 1981, 70 cases of PHC had occurred among the 3,454 $HB_sAg(+)$ individuals, and only 1 case among the 19,253 negative individuals. Thus, the relative risk of developing PHC among carriers is 390 times that for noncarriers. More than 98% of the cases of PHC (the attributable risk) have occurred in carriers. In the one instance where PHC developed in an $HB_sAg(-)$ individual, that person lacked anti-HB_s but had circulating anti-HB_c antibody. The likelihood is that he had been a carrier prior to recruitment for this study.

Thus, HBV infection precedes the development of PHC. On the basis of studies of families of patients, it appears likely that a majority of individuals who ultimately develop PHC acquire their infections at birth or during the first year of life from a carrier mother or older sibling. This would suggest an interval of 40 years or more from the onset of infection to the development of clinically detectable cancer.

MOLECULAR BIOLOGY OF HBV IN PHC

Cloned HBV DNA has been used by several groups as a specific probe to detect HBV DNA sequences in liver and serum. Whether the viral DNA is free or integrated into the host cell genome has been determined by digesting the DNA extracted from liver tissues with restriction enzymes, separating the DNA fragments by electrophoresis on agarose gels, transferring the separated DNA to nitrocellulose filters by the method of Southern (47), and hybridizing with ^{32}P-labeled HBV DNA. Bands that hybridize with the labeled probe are visualized by autoradiography. Virion DNA is about 3.2 kilobase pairs (kb) in length; fragments larger than 3.2 kb indicate the presence of integrated sequences.

Using these techniques, several groups have identified integrated HBV DNA in PHC tissues (10,16,42). The most extensive experience has been reported from the laboratories of Shafritz in New York (43) and Tiollais in Paris (9). Shafritz and associates studied 20 patients with PHC from South Africa. They extracted DNA from 10- to 20-mg samples of liver tissue obtained by needle biopsy. Considering the sensitivity of the transfer-hybridization procedure and the fact that not all cells in the biopsy specimens were tumor cells or hepatocytes, they probably were able to detect one HBV DNA sequence per cell if almost all liver or tumor cells contained such a sequence. Nevertheless, they found HBV DNA integrated into the host cell DNA in 15 of 20 cases, 12 of 12 being $HB_sAg(+)$ and 3 of 8 being $HB_sAg(-)$ but anti-$HB_s(+)$.

Tiollais's group extracted DNA from 30-mg samples of tissue from patients with PHC from different geographic locations. Among 15 patients who were $HB_sAg(+)$ and/or anti-$HB_c(+)$, all demonstrated integrated HBV DNA sequences in tumor tissue. Following this experience, these investigators studied 32 European patients who had PHC but were $HB_sAg(-)$. All had integrated HBV DNA in their tumors. Twenty of these patients were alcoholics who were thought to have had PHC on the basis of alcohol-induced cirrhosis. Seven of the alcoholics had no serological markers of HBV infection. If the work by Tiollais's group is supported by the findings of other investigators, this would indicate that virtually all human PHCs are caused by HBV (9).

Both Shafritz's and Tiollais' groups have observed HBV DNA banding patterns on Southern blots that are identical in samples of tissue from different portions of a single tumor, suggesting that the tumors are clonal. That is, the first neoplastic cell contained HBV DNA integrated at a particular site or sites, and all the descendants of that cell contain the same integrated sequences at the same sites. The banding patterns differ from tumor to tumor, both in the number of bands and in the positions of the bands visualized, implying that a unique integration site may not be involved. To test this hypothesis, however, the cellular sequences flanking the integrated viral sequences must be cloned and compared with each other. Such experiments are just beginning to be done.

Both the French and American investigators have demonstrated integrated HBV DNA in nontumor tissues of livers containing PHCs and in the livers of patients chronically infected with HBV but without PHC. For example, 6 of 51 French alcoholics without PHC had integrated HBV DNA in their livers (9). Banding patterns rather than smears were observed, implying that a particular virus can integrate at only a limited number of sites in a given host or that cells with HBV DNA integrated at certain sites are protected from the cytotoxic factors killing other hepatocytes and that the death of other hepatocytes promotes the proliferation of the cells with viral sequences integrated at certain sites. These hypotheses are not mutually exclusive, and both could be correct.

In some patients with PHC the banding patterns of integrated HBV DNA were indentical in tumor and nontumor tissues. This observation requires confirmation, but if it is correct it suggests that although integration may be a necessary step in the development of a tumor, neither the integration event nor the site of integration is critical for the development of a tumor.

Brechot et al. (9) have observed integrated HBV DNA sequences in children as early as 8 months after the onset of chronic HBV infection. They have also seen integrated viral DNA in patients with chronic active hepatitis, with or without cirrhosis, who have no serological markers of HBV infection. On the other hand, they have also shown that patients who have completely recovered from acute HBV infection (histologically normal liver, anti-HB$_s$ in the serum) do not have free or integrated HBV DNA in their livers. Thus, integration of HBV DNA is a common event in the course of HBV infection. It is not known whether it is a necessary part of the life cycle of the virus or a frequent, but random, event. It is not clear if a particular site on the virus is involved in integration. Understanding the role of HBV DNA integration in the virus cycle and the effects of integration on the host cell should lead to a greater understanding of the role of the virus in hepato-carcinogenesis.

HBV-LIKE VIRUSES IN ANIMALS AND THEIR RELATIONSHIPS TO PHC IN THEIR HOSTS

By 1971 it was apparent that HBV had characteristics that distinguished it from other viruses known at that time. On the basis of these features, Blumberg et al. (7) postulated that HBV was the first example a new class of viruses, which they called "Icrons," a combination of an acronym for the Institute for Cancer Research in Philadelphia, where HBV was discovered, and a neuter Greek ending. The purpose in assigning a name was to stimulate the search for viruses like HBV.

In the early 1970s we (Blumberg and London) were told by Robert Snyder, director of the Penrose Research Laboratory of the Philadelphia Zoological Garden, that a colony of woodchucks *(Marmota monax)* he had been observing at the zoo had a high incidence of chronic hepatitis and hepatocellular carcinoma. We obtained serum specimens from these animals and tested them for HB$_s$Ag and anti-HB$_s$ by the precipitin methods in use in our laboratory at that time. We did not detect either antigen or antibody, but we retained the sera in our bank of biological specimens.

Summers became interested in the molecular biology of HBV in 1975 and soon thereafter began looking for HBV-like viruses in animals other than humans. He tested the woodchuck serum samples in our collection for a DNA polymerase activity like that seen in HBV. That is, he assayed the sera for incorporation of labeled nucleotides into a double-strand DNA product of about 3,000 bp. He found that 15% of the sera contained such an activity. Fractions containing the polymerase activity were isolated on cesium chloride gradients and examined in the electron microscope. Particles 42 nm in diameter virtually identical to human HBV virions (Dane particles) and smaller 22-nm spherical and rod-shaped forms similar to HB$_s$Ag particles were seen (52).

Antigenic cross-reactivities of the core and surface antigens of the woodchuck virus with the comparable antigens in HBV were identified (57). At the DNA level, Galibert et al. (15) found greater than 70% homology between the nucelotide sequences of the genomes of the two viruses. Summers demonstrated that the virus was localized in the liver, and therefore he named it the woodchuck hepatitis virus (WHV) (52,53).

Biologically, WHV behaves similarly to HBV. Woodchucks persistently infected with WHV develop chronic hepatitis and eventually PHC. In an ongoing study of 27 animals chronically infected with WHV, 5 animals have died of pneumonia or other intercurrent infections, but 20 of 22 remaining animals have developed PHC. No liver cancers have occurred in animals not persistently infected with WHV (J. Summers, *personal communication*). In our colony, 7 of 7 persistently infected woodchucks have developed PHC in less than 2 years, and no tumors have developed in more than 50 uninfected or transiently infected woodchucks *(unpublished data)*.

In the wild, woodchucks die at younger ages than in captivity. Snyder (45), using release and capture experiments, estimated the mean age at death for wild animals as 14.9 months and the median as 8 months. In the protected environment of the zoo, the mean and median age at death was about 55 months. In the zoo, about 25% of the colony died of PHC, at ages ranging from 2 to 8 years. Among 1,007 animals shot in the wild and autopsied, only 4 cases of PHC were identified. Thus, in the wild, the selective effect of PHC is small, because most animals die before they can develop PHC (46). Chronically infected animals do reproduce, however, and maternal transmission is probably a major factor in maintenance of WHV in free-living woodchuck populations. Whether or not WHV affects fertility or fecundity is unknown.

The frequency of WHV infection in woodchucks varies greatly in different locations. Tyler (55) found that 24% of 166 animals trapped within 220 km of Philadelphia were $WH_sAg(+)$, and 42% had anti-WH_s (the nomenclature for WHV antigens and antibodies follows the same pattern used for HBV). In other areas of the United States, no infected animals have been found. This is again similar to the variation in the incidence of HBV infection observed in human populations.

Also, as in humans, WHV DNA is integrated into the tumor cell genome of PHCs in woodchucks, and the tumors are clonal with respect to the integrated viral DNA (34,53). In some animals, more than one tumor is seen. In these animals, each tumor demonstrates a different banding pattern. This indicates that WHV can integrate at several sites and that either (a) the site of integration is not critical for tumor formation or (b) there are many targets in the cellular genome that are susceptible to malignant transformation.

One difference in behavior between the viruses in woodchucks and humans is that in nontumor liver tissues of animals with PHC or in livers of animals with chronic hepatitis without PHC, banding patterns of WHV DNA are not detected. Rather, smears of radioactivity appear on Southern blots. By digesting cellular DNA with restriction enzymes that do not cut WHV DNA and inserting the resulting fragments into plasmid vectors, Summers's group (34) showed that WHV is integrated into nontumor tissue. The smears on the Southern blots indicate that integration occurs at many different sites in different hepatocytes.

Ogston et al. (33) studied the sequence and structure of WHV DNA in woodchuck tumors. They cloned single integrations from two tumors in two different animals and determined their structures by restriction mapping and heteroduplex electron microscopy. They found that the viral sequences in both integrations were extensively rearranged and that there were deletions of the viral genome in both tumors. Cellular DNA sequences also appeared to be rearranged in the region of the integrations. Hairpin structures in the integrated sequences were seen in the electron microscope. This behavior of WHV DNA *in vivo* is similar to that of other DNA viruses (SV40) in tissue culture (8). How these structures relate to tumor formation is uncertain.

Other HBV-like viruses have now been identified in Pekin ducks, as noted earlier (29), and in ground squirrels (27). The virus in ground squirrels (ground squirrel hepatitis B virus, GSHV) is very similar morphologically, antigenically, and in genome size and structure to HBV and WHV. Biologically, however, it behaves differently. The virus does not appear to produce acute or chronic hepatitis or liver cancer, even though it does cause chronic infections (41). Understanding the basis for this difference in biological behavior may provide an important insight into how HBV and WHV "cause" cancer.

The duck hepatitis B virus (DHBV) was detected originally by Summers et al. *(unpublished data)* in sera from domestic ducks collected in the People's Republic of China. In some regions of China where PHC is common in humans it is also common in domestic ducks. Investigators in China suggested that the tumors in humans and ducks were caused by a chemical carcinogen in human food and in table scraps fed to domestic ducks. Blumberg, during a trip to China in 1977, suggested that the ducks were infected with an Icron (4). In collaboration with T.-T. Sun, sera were collected from 33 domestic ducks purchased in Chi-tung County, north of Shanghai. Viruslike particles were seen in 11 of these sera, and the same sera contained an HBV-like endogenous DNA polymerase activity and DNA molecules that were similar in size and structure to HBV and WHV. Subsequently, Mason, Seal, and Summers (29) discovered that about 14% of Pekin ducks *(Anas domesticus)* in the United States (the major commercially bred duck in the United States) were infected with the same or a very similar virus.

Studies from Mason's laboratory have revealed the following: (a) The virion of DHBV is morphologically similar to the virions of HBV, WHV, and GSHV. (b) The surface antigen particles are larger and more heterogeneous than the analogous particles in humans, woodchucks, and ground squirrels. (c) There is no antigenic cross-reactivity between DHBV and the other HBV-like viruses. (d) The virus replicates in the liver and to a lesser extent in the pancreas. (e) As noted earlier, the replicative cycle of HBV-like viruses has been delineated by the study of the duck virus (28,50).

The question whether or not DHBV induces liver disease and liver cancer is not resolved. In the United States, studies of young (less than 1 year old) persistently infected ducks have not demonstrated inflammatory or neoplastic liver disease. However, M. Omata and associates *(unpublished data)* have studied the sera and tissues of Pekin ducks collected in China and Japan. In their studies there was an association between the presence of DHBV in serum and chronic hepatitis, cirrhosis, and, in one case, liver cancer.

Transovarian transmission is the major and perhaps only means of transmission of DHBV in nature. O'Connell, Urban, and London *(unpublished data)* have found DHBV in the sera of duck embryos as early as 5 days after incubation and evidence of viral replication at 12 days of incubation. Persistent infections appear to be the rule, although how long after hatching virus replication continues has not been determined.

It is likely that HBV-like viruses are widespread in nature. How they are related to each other, from which species they originated, and which features are related to disease induction are areas for future research.

ROLE OF HBV IN THE PATHOGENESIS OF PHC

On the basis of the epidemiological and molecular biological evidence, it appears certain that HBV and WHV play an essential role in the pathogenesis of PHC in humans and woodchucks. The mechanisms involved, however, are uncertain. Most of the virological research on hepatocarcinogenesis has concentrated on identifying a single event by which a "normal" hepatocyte is transformed into a malignant cell. For example, Ogston et al. (33) discussed the following three models: (a) The virus contains a transforming gene. Expression of this gene in the infected cell induces the transformed phenotype. Integration is not necessary for expression of the trans-forming gene, but it is a method for stabilizing the inheritance of the gene. If this hypothesis is correct, each tumor cell must contain one complete, active, integrated copy of the transforming gene (54). (b) The integrated viral sequence contains a promoter that inappropriately activates the transcription and translation of a cellular oncogene (promotor-insertion hypothesis) (32). It is the product of the oncogene that produces the transformed phenotype. This hypothesis requires the presence, in every malignant cell, of an integrated viral DNA sequence with promoter activity upstream from a cellular oncogene. (c) Virus-induced rearrangements of cellular DNA decrease the expression of a (hypothetical) cellular gene whose product inhibits cell division (37). Descendants of such a cell would produce a clone of proliferating cells. If this model is correct, cellular DNA rearrangements should occur at the same locus in all PHC cells.

Thus far, no convincing evidence has been produced to support or reject any of these models. Study of WHV and cellular DNA sequences in woodchuck tumors may ultimately determine if any of these models is correct.

In the past, several investigators have considered developmental models of car-cinogenesis based on the notion that cancer results from a combination of cellular proliferation and a block in differentiation (26,37–39). An event at the DNA level is probably responsible for such a process, but it is not necessary to postulate the specific molecular event in order to consider a biological model of this kind.

Blumberg and I (23,24) have proposed a model in which HBV selectively kills the most mature hepatocytes and stimulates the proliferation of immature liver cells. HBV DNA integrated at certain sites in the cellular genome inhibits differentiation without affecting cell division. By this process, a clone of proliferating hepatocytes may arise that is characterized by the presence of integrated HBV DNA and im-maturity. This simple model is compatible with the clinical, pathological, bio-chemical, and molecular information that is currently available.

In devising our model, Blumberg and I considered the following phenomena concerning HBV infection and PHC: (a) PHC is associated with persistent but not with transient HBV infections. (b) There is a long "incubation" period (20–40 years) between the onset of HBV infection and the development of PHC. (c) HB$_s$Ag is commonly found in nonneoplastic hepatocytes but rarely in the tumor cells of a liver containing PHC. (d) Integrated viral DNA is found in both tumor and nontumor cells of a liver containing PHC. (e) PHCs in humans (and lower animals) frequently produce proteins (e.g., alpha-fetoprotein) that usually are synthesized by immature or fetal hepatocytes.

Our model postulates that the liver contains two (or more) populations of hepatocytes: (a) cells that are susceptible to productive infection with HBV, hereafter called S cells; (b) cells that are resistant (or relatively resistant) to productive infection, hereafter called R cells. According to the model, R cells are less mature hepatocytes, and S cells are fully differentiated hepatocytes. An R cell can divide and differentiate into one R cell and one S cell (normal replacement) or two S cells (which would not leave a cell for subsequent divisions) or two R cells (which would result in the accumulation of immature cells). An S cell either cannot divide at all or can divide only one or two more times and then give rise to only other S cells. Integration of HBV genomes can occur in either R or S cells.

In the liver, the stimulus for cell division is the death or removal of hepatocytes. Persistent infection with HBV leads to continuous cell death and, hence, to continuous regeneration. Because S cells are the cells that become productively infected, they are at greatest risk of dying. R cells do not replicate virus and have a greater reproductive capacity than S cells. Therefore, R cells are likely to increase and S cells to decrease in number if infection continues. That is, HBV infection selects against mature, differentiated cells and promotes the growth of immature, less differentiated cells.

Integration of HBV DNA in S cells may occur (possibly as part of the normal virus cycle), but this will not have tumorigenic potential, both because of the limited capacity of differentiated hepatocytes for cell division and because of the susceptibility of S cells to productive infection with HBV. Integration of HBV DNA into R cells may have tumorigenic significance. R cells are already being stimulated to proliferate by the death of S cells. Integration, by causing rearrangements of host cell DNA (33), may interfere with differentiation, thereby increasing the probability that division of an R cell will yield only other R cells. Thus, a proliferating clone of immature cells can arise. As this clone expands, it may, by the process of clonal evolution (14), develop the phenotypic characteristics of a malignant neoplasm. A clinically evident tumor will not result, however, unless the stimulus to cell division is maintained by the death of S cells. In those instances in which PHC develops in the absence of persistent HBV infection of nonneoplastic hepatocytes, the model assumes that other hepatotoxic agents (e.g., alcohol, aflatoxin) are continuing the selective pressure on S cells. There must, of course, be some stage at which the R cell clone acquires sufficient autonomy that it does not require external stimuli for continued growth, but we assume that this is late in the process.

Productive infection with HBV probably does not directly lyse S cells, but their survival may be shortened by one or a combination of several mechanisms. Virus replication may compromise host cell metabolism sufficiently to eventually kill the cell. Second, infected S cells may be subject to cellular immune responses to viral–cellular antigen complexes on their surfaces (12). Third, infected S cells may be more vulnerable to the effects of toxic oxygen radicals than uninfected hepatocytes. Vierucci et al. (56) have shown that HBV proteins cause the release, without being phagocytized, of superoxide anions from polymorphonuclear leukocytes.

The model helps to explain why HBV produces primarily persistent infections early in life and mainly transient infections after infancy. According to the model, the liver of the fetus will be composed mostly of R cells and will not be able to support replication of HBV. Lee et al. (20) have shown that HBV is present in amniotic fluid and in the gastrointestinal tract of babies born to HBV-infected mothers. Nevertheless, such babies do not produce virus detectable in their blood until 6 weeks of age.

After birth, further division and differentiation occur, giving rise to S cells that permit viral replication. Infection with HBV at this time leads to a persistent infection, because as S cells become infected and die, new S cells are continuously becoming available, by the normal processes of growth and development, to maintain the infection. Later in life the reverse is true; most cells in the liver are mature hepatocytes, and few are immature R cells. Infection may result in the death of large numbers of S cells (acute hepatitis), and too few S cells are differentiated from R cells to maintain the infection.

The integrated viral DNA seen in nontumor cells (9,43) is, according to the model, present in S cells. Such cells can be quite stable. HBV DNA can be integrated into precisely the same cellular site in an S cell and an R cell, but only the R cell can become a tumor.

Recently, Urban, O'Connell, and I (*unpublished data*) have observed incomplete replication of DHBV in duck embryos after 10 days of incubation and complete replication after 12 days of incubation. This observation supports the notion that enzymes or other substances produced by more mature hepatocytes are required for the complete cycle of virus replication. Further studies of the duck embryo system may provide information as to whether or not integration is part of the virus replication cycle and, if so, when in the replicative sequence it occurs. Studies of persistent WHV infection in woodchucks and the effects of these infections on hepatocyte populations in the woodchuck liver may permit direct evaluation of the model in a system in which PHCs occur naturally.

SUMMARY

HBV infection can now be considered the "cause" of most cases of PHC in humans. By judicious use of hepatitis B hyperimmune globulin and the hepatitis B vaccine, most infections with HBV can be prevented. Primary prevention strategies are now being developed and instituted in many countries, including Taiwan, the People's Republic of China, Japan, and the United States. It is very probable that as a result of these public health programs the incidence of this common and lethal tumor will begin to fall within the next 20 years.

ACKNOWLEDGMENTS

This work was supported by USPHS grants CA-06551, RR-05539, CA-06927, and CA-22780 from the National Institutes of Health and by an appropriation from the Commonwealth of Pennsylvania.

REFERENCES

1. Albin, C., and Robinson, W. S. (1980): Protein kinase activity in hepatitis B virus. *J. Virol.*, 34:297–302.
2. Beasley, R. P. (1982): Hepatitis B virus as the etiologic agent in hepatocellular carcinoma — epidemiologic consideration. *Hepatology*, 2:21S–26S.
3. Beasley, R. P., Lin, C.-C., Hwang, L.-Y., and Chien, C.-S. (1981): Hepatocellular carcinoma and hepatitis B virus. A prospective study of 22,707 men in Taiwan. *Lancet*, 2:1129–1132.
4. Blumberg, B. S. (1981): Viruses similar to hepatitis B virus. *Hum. Pathol.*, 12:1107–1113.
5. Blumberg, B. S., Larouzé, B., London, W. T., Werner, B., Hesser, J. E., Millman, I., Saimot, G., and Payet, M. (1975): The relation of infection with the hepatitis B agent to primary hepatic carcinoma. *Am. J. Pathol.*, 81:669–682.
6. Blumberg, B. S., and Millman, I. (1972): Vaccine against viral hepatitis and process. Serial No. 864,788 filed 10/8/69; patent 36 36 191 issued 1/18/72, U.S. Patent Office, 1972.
7. Blumberg, B. S., Millman, I., Sutnick, A. I., and London, W. T. (1971): The nature of Australia antigen and its relation to antigen-antibody complex formation. *J. Exp. Med.*, 134:320–329.
8. Botchan, M., Stringer, J., Mitchison, T., and Sambrook, J. (1980): Integration and excision of SV40 DNA from the chromosome of a transformed cell. *Cell*, 20:143–152.
9. Brechot, C., Pourcel, C., Hadchouel, M., Dejean, A., Louise, A., Scotto, J., and Tiollais, P. (1982): State of hepatitis B virus DNA in liver diseases. *Hepatology*, 2:27S–34S.
10. Brechot, C., Pourcel, C., Louise, A., Rain, B., and Tiollais, P. (1980): Presence of integrated hepatitis B virus DNA sequences in cellular DNA of human hepatocellular carcinoma. *Nature*, 286:533–535.
11. Drysdale, J. W. (1977): Ferritin phenotypes: Structure and metabolism. In: *Iron Metabolism*, pp. 41–67. Ciba Foundation Symposium 51. Elsevier/North Holland, Amsterdam.
12. Eddleston, A. L. W. F., Mondelli, M., Mieli-Vergani, G., and Williams, R. (1982): Lymphocyte cytotoxicity to autologous hepatocytes in chronic hepatitis B virus infection. *Hepatology*, 2:122S–127S.
13. Edmondson, H. A., and Peters, R. L. (1977): Liver. In: *Pathology*, ed. 7, edited by W. A. D. Anderson and J. M. Kissane, pp. 1321–1438. C. V. Mosby, St. Louis.
14. Foulds, L. (1969): *Neoplastic Development, Vol. 1.* Academic Press, London.
15. Galibert, F., Chen, T. N., and Mandart, E. (1982): Nucleotide sequence of a cloned woodchuck hepatitis virus genome: Comparison with the hepatitis B virus sequence. *J. Virol.*, 41:51–65.
16. Gerin, J. L., Shih, J. W.-K., and Huyer, B. H. (1982): Biology and characterization of hepatitis B virus. In: *Viral Hepatitis, 1981*, edited by W. Szmuness, H. J. Alter, and J. E. Maynard, pp. 49–56. Franklin Institute Press, Philadelphia.
17. Hann, H.-W., Kim, C. Y., London, W. T., Whitford, P., and Blumberg, B. S. (1982): Hepatitis B virus and primary hepatocellular carcinoma: Family studies in Korea. *Int. J. Cancer*, 30:47–51.
18. Larouzé, B., Blumberg, B. S., London, W. T., Lustbader, E. D., Sankale, M., and Payet, M. (1977): Forecasting the development of primary hepatocellular carcinoma by the use of risk factors: Studies in West Africa. *J. Natl. Cancer Inst.*, 58:1557–1561.
19. Larouzé, B., London, W. T., Saimot, G., Werner, B. G., Lustbader, E. D., Payet, M., and Blumberg, B. S. (1976): Host responses to hepatitis B infection in patients with primary hepatic carcinoma and their families. A case/control study in Senegal, West Africa. *Lancet*, 2:534–538.
20. Lee, A. K., Ip, H. M., and Wong, V. C. (1978): Mechanisms of maternal-fetal transmission of hepatitis B virus. *J. Infect. Dis.*, 138:668–671.
21. Li, F. P., and Shiang, E. L. (1980): Cancer mortality in China. *J. Natl. Cancer Inst.*, 65:217–221.
22. London, W. T. (1981): Primary hepatocellular carcinoma. *Hum. Pathol.*, 12:1085–1097.
23. London, W. T., and Blumberg, B. S. (1981): Hepatitis B virus and primary hepatocellular car-

cinoma. In: *Cancer: Achievements, Challenges and Prospects for the 1980's Vol. 1*, edited by
J. H. Burchenal and H. F. Oettgen, pp. 161–183. Grune & Stratton, New York.

24. London, W. T., and Blumberg, B. S. (1982): A cellular model of the role of hepatitis B virus in
    the pathogenesis of hepatocellular carcinoma. *Hepatology*, 2:10S–14S.

25. London, W. T., Drew, J. S., Lustbader, E. D., Werner, B. G., and Blumberg, B. S. (1977): Host
    responses to hepatitis B infection in patients in a chronic hemodialysis unit. *Kidney Int.*, 12:51–
    58.

26. Lotem, J., and Sachs, L. (1974): Different blocks in the differentiation of myeloid leukemic cells.
    Proc. Natl. Acad. Sci. USA, 71:3507–3511.

27. Marion, P. L., Oshiro, L. S., Regnery, D. C., Scullard, G. H., and Robinson, W. S. (1980): A
    virus in Beechey ground squirrels that is related to hepatitis B virus in humans. *Proc. Natl. Acad.
    Sci. USA*, 77:2941–2945.

28. Mason, W. S., Aldrich, C., Summers, J., and Taylor, J. M. (1982): Asymmetric replication of
    duck hepatitis B virus DNA in liver cells. Free minus-stranded DNA. *Proc. Natl. Acad. Sci. USA*,
    79:3997–4001.

29. Mason, W. S., Seal, G., and Summers, J. (1980): A virus of Pekin ducks with structural and
    biological relatedness to human hepatitis B virus. *J. Virol.*, 36:829–836.

30. Miyakawa, Y., and Mayumi, M. (1982): HB$_e$Ag-anti-HB$_e$ system in hepatitis B virus infection.
    In: *Viral Hepatitis, 1981*, edited by W. Szmuness, H. J. Alter, and J. E. Maynard, pp. 183–194.
    Franklin Institute Press, Philadelphia.

31. Nayak, N. C., Dhar, A., Sachdeva, R., Mittal, A., Seth, H. N., Sudarsanam, D., Reddy, B.,
    Waghaolikar, U. L., and Reddy, C. R. R. M. (1977): Association of human hepatocellular car-
    cinoma and cirrhosis with hepatitis virus surface and core antigens in the liver. *Int. J. Cancer*,
    20:643–654.

32. Neel, B. G., Hayward, W. S., Robinson, H. L., Fang, J., and Astrin, S. M. (1981): Avian leukosis
    virus-induced tumors have common proviral integration sites and synthesize discrete new RNA's:
    Oncogenesis by promoter insertion. *Cell*, 23:323–334.

33. Ogston, C. W., Jonak, G. J., Rogler, C. E., Astrin, S. M., and Summers, J. (1982): Cloning and
    structural analysis of integrated woodchuck hepatitis virus sequences from hepatocellular carci-
    nomas of woodchucks. *Cell*, 29:385–394.

34. Ogston, C. W., Jonak, G. J., Rogler, C. E., Tyler, G. V., Snyder, R. L., Astrin, S. M., and
    Summers, J. W. (1982): Integrated woodchuck hepatitis virus DNA in hepatocellular carcinomas
    from woodchucks. In: *Viral Hepatitis, 1981*, edited by W. Szmuness, H. J. Alter, and J. E.
    Maynard, pp. 809–810. Franklin Institute Press, Philadelphia.

35. Ohbayashi, A., Okochi, K., and Mayumi, M. (1972): Familial clustering of Australia antigen and
    patients with chronic liver disease or primary liver cancer. *Gastroenterology*, 62:618–625.

36. Okada, K., Kamiyama, I., Inomata, M., Imai, M., Miyakawa, Y., and Mayumi, M. (1976): e
    Antigen and anti-e in the serum of asymptomatic carrier mothers as indicative of positive and
    negative transmission of hepatitis B virus to their infants. *N. Engl. J. Med.*, 294:746–749.

37. Osgood, E. E. (1957): A unifying concept of the etiology of the leukemias, lymphomas and
    cancers. *J. Natl. Cancer Inst.*, 18:155–166.

38. Pierce, G. B., Nakane, P. K., and Mazurkiewicz, J. E. (1974): Natural history of malignant stem
    cells. In: *Differentiation and Control of Malignancy of Tumor Cells*, edited by W. Nakahara, T.
    Ono, T. Sugimura, and H. Sugano, p. 453. Universtiy of Tokyo Press, Tokyo.

39. Potter, V. R. (1978): Phenotypic diversity in experimental hepatomas: The concept of partially
    blocked ontogeny. *Br. J. Cancer*, 38:1–23.

40. Prince, A. M. (1980): Evidence suggesting that hepatitis B virus is a tumor-inducing virus in man.
    An estimate of the risk of development of hepatocellular cancer in chronic HB$_s$Ag carriers and
    controls. In: *The Role of Viruses in Human Cancer, Vol. 1*, edited by G. Giraldo and E. Beth,
    pp. 141–155. Elsevier/North Holland, Amsterdam.

41. Robinson, W. S., Marion, P., Feitelson, M., and Siddiqui, A. (1982): The Hepadna virus group:
    Hepatitis B and related viruses. In: *Viral Hepatitis, 1981* edited by W. Szmuness, H. J. Alter,
    and J. E. Maynard, pp. 57–68. Franklin Institute Press, Philadelphia.

42. Shafritz, D. A., and Kew, M. C. (1981): Identification of integrated hepatitis B virus DNA
    sequences in human hepatocellular carcinomas. *Hepatology*, 1:1–8.

43. Shafritz, D., Shouval, D., Sherman, H. I., Hadziyannis, S. J., and Kew, M. C. (1981): Integration
    of hepatitis B virus DNA into the genome of liver cells in chronic liver disease and hepatocellular
    carcinoma. *N. Engl. J. Med.*, 305:1067–1073.

44. Smith, J. B., and Blumberg, B. S. (1969): Viral hepatitis, postnecrotic cirrhosis and hepatocellular carcinoma. *Lancet*, 2:953.
45. Snyder, R. L. (1977): Longevity and disease patterns in captive and wild woodchucks, *Proc. Am. Assoc. Zool. Parks and Aquariums*, pp. 535–552.
46. Snyder, R. L., and Summers, J. (1980): Woodchuck hepatitis virus and hepatocellular carcinoma. In: *Viruses in Naturally Occurring Cancers*, edited by M. Essex, G. Todaro, and H. zur Hausen, pp. 447–457. Cold Spring Harbor Laboratory, Cold Spring Harbor, N.Y.
47. Southern, E. M. (1975): Detection of specific sequences among DNA fragments separated by gel electrophoresis. *J. Mol. Biol.*, 98:503–517.
48. Stevens, C. E., Beasley, R. P., Tsui, J., and Lee, W. (1975): Vertical transmission of hepatitis B antigen in Taiwan. *N. Engl. J. Med.*, 292:771–774.
49. Summers, J., and Mason, W. S. (1982): Properties of the hepatitis B-like viruses related to their taxonomic classification. *Hepatology*, 2:61S–66S.
50. Summers, J., and Mason, W. S. (1982): Replication of the genome of a hepatitis B-like virus by reverse transcription of an RNA intermediate. *Cell*, 29:403–415.
51. Summers, J., O'Connell, A., and Millman, I. (1975): Genome of hepatitis B virus: Restriction enzyme cleavage and structure of DNA extracted from Dane particles. *Proc. Natl. Acad. Sci. USA*, 72:4597–4601.
52. Summers, J., Smolec, J. M., and Snyder, R. (1978): A virus similar to human hepatitis B virus associated with hepatitis and hepatoma in woodchucks. *Proc. Natl. Acad. Sci. USA*, 75:4533–4537.
53. Summers, J., Smolec, J. M., Werner, B. G., Kelly, T. J., Tyler, G. V., and Snyder, R. L. (1980): Hepatitis B virus and woodchuck hepatitis virus are members of a novel class of DNA viruses. In: *Viruses in Naturally Occurring Tumors*, edited by M. Essex, G., Todaro, and H. zur Hausen, pp. 459–470. Cold Spring Harbor Laboratory, Cold Spring Harbor, N.Y.
54. Topp, W. C., Lane, D., and Pollack, R. (1980): Transformation by SV40 and polyoma virus. In: *DNA Tumor Viruses*, edited by J. Tooze, pp. 205–296. Cold Spring Harbor Laboratory, Cold Spring Harbor, N.Y.
55. Tyler, G. V., Summers, J., and Snyder, R. L. (1981): Woodchuck hepatitis virus in natural woodchuck populations. *J. Wildlife Dis.*, 17:297–301.
56. Vierucci, A., DeMartino, M., Graziani, E., Rossi, M. E., London, W. T., and Blumberg, B. S. (1982): A mechanism for liver cell injury in viral hepatitis: Effects of hepatitis B virus on neutrophil function in children with chronic active hepatitis. *Pediatr. Res.*, *(in press)*.
57. Werner, B. G., Smolec, J. M., Snyder, R., and Summers, J. (1979): Serological relationship of woodchuck hepatitis virus to human hepatitis B virus. *J. Virol.*, 32:314–322.
58. Williams, G. (1980): The pathogenesis of rat liver cancer caused by chemical carcinogens. *Biocim. Biophys. Acta*, 605:167–189.

Subject Index

A gene mutants, SV40, 44
A31 cells, 275–277
Abortive infections, EBV, 162–169, 171
Actinomycin D, EBV induction block, 164
Acycloguanosine, EBV DNA replication inhibition, 151–152
Ad-SVR6 hybrid virus, 41–42
Ad2, transforming region, comparison, 105–107
Ad2 + D2 hybrid virus, 37–38
Ad2 + ND$_2$ hybrid virus, 38
Ad2 + ND$_4$ hybrid virus, 38
Ad2ts 206 mutant, 98
Ad5, transforming region, comparison, 105–107
Ad7, transforming region, comparison, 105–107
Ad12
  DNA integration pattern, 112–113
  transforming region, comparison, 105–107
ADCC (antibody-dependent cellular cytotoxicity), 229
Adenosine, EBV DNA, 145–146
Adenovirus; see also Human adenovirus
  DNA integration, transformed cells, 111–113
    methylation, 113–114
  DNA replication, 91–95
  early gene expression, 95–97
    proteins, 98–99
    switch to late, 97–98
  genome, functional organization, 86–90
  morphology, 85–86
  serotypes, 84–86
  T antigens, 107–110

transformation, molecular biology, 83–116
  adenovirus comparison, 14
  genetics, 114–116
  region comparison, oncogenicity, 105–107
  virus-associated RNAs, 90–91
Adsorption, EBV, 185–187
African Burkitt tumors, see Burkitt's lymphoma
Ag-4, mtr-III region product, 285–286
AG876, DNA studies, 141
α class, HSV-1, see Immediate early HSV-1 mRNA
Antibodies; see also Monoclonal antibodies
  EBV infection, 229, 231
  hepatitis B virus, 326–327, 329
Antibody-dependent cellular cytotoxicity, EBV, 229
Antigens
  Epstein-Barr virus, 139–141, 151
  hepatitis B virus, 326–327, 330, 336
  HSV-induced, transformation, 298–299
  target cells and T cells, EBV, 223
Ataxia-telangiectasia, 190–191
11att variant, 313–314
Autoregulation, viral, SV40 large T antigen, 31–32

B lymphocytes, EBV, 133–135
  activation, 213–215
  latency, 152–157
  transformation, 151–160, 186, 229
B95-8 culture, EBV
  and P3H-1 strain binding, 185
  polypeptides, 137–139

B95-8 culture, EBV *(contd.)*
  viral DNA studies, 141–145
    sequence deletion, 142
    strain variation, 146, 150
    transformation, 154
BALB/c
  HSV transformation studies, 273–280
  SV40 cell line, immunology, 33–35
BamHI site
  Epstein Barr virus DNA, 143–145
    HpaII resistance, Raji cells, 153–154
    polypeptides, infection, 167
    primates, colinearity, 150
    RNA encoding, sequences, 165
  HSV-1 DNA, 241
    encoding, 248, 251
    RNA expression, 280
    tk gene, 254
  human papillomavirus, 69–70
BamHI-Y, HSV-2 genome, 285–286
β class, HSV-1 mRNA, 240, 242, 255–263
β₂-microglobulin, 198, 224
βγ mRNA expression, HSC-1, 243, 251, 255–263
BglII site, HSV
  DNA sequence integration, F4A1A1 cells, 289–290
  focus formation, 273–275
  mRNA family generation, 259–260
BglII-C
  HSV focus formation, 274
  HSV-2, transformation, 253
BglII-I; *see also* Mtr-1 region
  HSV focus formation, 273, 275, 293
  physical and functional map, 280–283
  primary focus, HSV, 275–276
  transformed cell lines, HSV DNA sequences, 288–289
BglII-N; *see also* Mtr-II region
  and cell lines, 277
  HSV focus formation, 273–277
  HSV-1 and HSV-2 homology, 282–283

HSV-1 mRNA species, 244–245
late mRNA, promoters, HSV, 255–256
Mtr-2 region, HSV-2, 252
pGR136 position, tk experiments, 292–295
physical map and coding capacity, 283–285
transformed cell lines, DNA sequences, 288–290
Biological markers, HSV, 240, 251–255
BJAB cells
  early antigen induction, EBV, 194, 199
  T cell effect, versus EBV, 223
Bovine papillomaviruses
  genome, 61–63
  malignant transformation, 59–60
  physical map, 64–65
  sequences, PPV-1 comparison, 71–73
  transcription, 67–68
  vector use, 73–74
  viral DNA, 66–67
BPVT69, vector use, 73–75
Br322, *see* pBR322
Burkitt's lymphoma
  cytogenetics, 188–191
  Epstein-Barr virus relationship, 135–137, 183
    DNA, 154
    viral RNA, 159–160
  hybrids, 197–198
  versus lymphoblastoid cells, 188
  strain variant, viral DNA, 141
  tumor cell, electron photomicrograph, 138

C-terminal, *see* Carboxy-terminal
C2D cell line, 275, 277
C3, EBV binding antagonism, 185
Ca²⁺-dependent transfection techniques, 196
Cadmium toxicity, 73
Capsid; *see also* Viral capsid antigen
  adenovirus, 85–86

Epstein-Barr virus polypeptides, 138–141

papillomaviruses, 61

Carboxy-terminal

papillomavirus genomes, 73

polyoma virus middle T antigen, 18–22

SV40 large T antigen, 34–35

DNA effects, 50–51

CG dinucleotide, methylation, 316–318

China, Epstein-Barr lymphomas, 136

Chromatin, EBNA stimulation, 192

Chromosome 8, translocation, 134, 189–190

Chromosome 14, translocation, 134, 189–191

Chromosomes, EBV cell lines, 189–191

ClaI site, "deletable" region, HSV genome, 280–281

Class 1 antigens, SV40 cytotoxic T cells, 34

Colcemid treatment, 199

Complement, EBV binding antagonism, 185

Complementary strand synthesis, 91–92

Complementation class I, 112

Complementation group N, *see* Group N mutants

Conserved nucleotide sequences, 65

Control regions, *see* Promoters

COP cells, transformation genetics, 12

Core protein, adenovirus location, 85

COS cells, 39

Coselection, transposition plasmid pGR136, 293

Cyclic AMP, virus activation, 198–199

Cyclosporin A lysing

Epstein-Barr virus malignancies, 135

T cell EBV regression inhibition, 225

Cytogenetics, Burkitt's lymphoma cells, 188–191

Cytomegalovirus, expression, and HSV-1, 241

Cytosine, EBV DNA, 145–146

Cytoskeleton disruption, DNA synthesis, 10

Cytotoxic T cells

EBV transformation, late suppression, 225–227

EBV transformation regression, 217–225, 231

specificity, 223

infectious mononucleosis, 184–185, 230–232

LYDMA specificity, 232

SV40, antitumor response, 33–37

D antigen, 184

D2T

DNA replication, 50

DNA transcription stimulation, 52

SV40 large T antigen study, 37–40

D98/P3HR-1, 198

D98/Raji, 198

Daudi cell line, 197–200

"Delay," EBV B cell transformation, 226–228

Delayed transformation

interferon, EBV, 215–216

T cell override, 219

Deletion mutants, *see* dl mutants

Differentiation, hybrid Burkitt's cells, 197–198

Dihydrofolate reductase gene, 49

Direct repeats, EBV DNA, 142–147, 149–150

dl mutants

adenovirus transformation genetics, 114

transformation effect, polyoma virus, 21–22

viability, and polypeptide IX, 105

dl 313, viability, and polypeptide IX, 105

DNA; *see also specific aspects*

adenovirus, integration, 111–113

Epstein-Barr virus, 141–151

abortive and productive infections, 163

DNA sequences *(contd.)*
  Epstein-Barr virus *(contd.)*
    function, 193–195
    latently infected cells, 152–156
    structure, 141–151, 193–195
    synthesis, 187, 193–197
  Herpesvirus saimiri, transformation, 314–321
  morphological transforming regions, HSV, 280–286
  papillomavirus, 61–63, 66–67
  polyoma virus, large T effect, 24
  polyoma virus, physical map, 4
  SV40 large T effect, 31–32, 39–40
  transfection experiments, HSV, 272–280
  woodchuck hepatitis virus, 334–335
DNA binding protein 128K, 293–297
DNA methylation, *see* Methylation
DNA polymerase
  adenovirus DNA replication, 94–95
  EBV DNA replication, 151–152, 186–187
  hepatitis B virus, 327
  HSV, mapping, 253
DNA replication
  adenovirus, 91–95
  Epstein-Barr virus, origin, 144–145, 151–152
  HSV-1, and gene expression, 240, 242–243
  papillomavirus, 73
  SV40 large T antigen role, 39–40, 50–52
DNA sequences
  adenovirus genomic integration, 113
  adenovirus transforming regions, comparison, 105–107
  Epstein-Barr virus, 144–145
  herpesvirus saimiri, transformation, 315–316
  papillomavirus, 69–73
  polyoma virus, 18–19
  retention in transformed cells, HSV, 287–293

SV40 large T antigen interaction, 37–45
woodchuck hepatitis virus, 334–335
DPB, *see* 72K DNA binding protein
Duck hepatitis B virus, 327, 335–336, 338

E1 region, adenovirus
  kinase activity, 111
  T antigens, 108–110
  transformation role, 101
E1 region, papillomavirus, 72, 74
E1A region, adenovirus
  expression, 95–97
  mutant mapping, 94
  mRNAs, subgroup C, 103
  T antigens, 108–109
  transformation role, 101
    genetics, 114–116
    and polyoma virus, 14
    region comparison, 105–106
    T antigens, 110
E1B region, adenovirus
  expression, 95–96
  kinase activity, 111
  T antigen encoding, 109–110
  transforming regions, comparison, 105–106
  transformation role, 101–105, 110
    and polyoma virus, 14
    polypeptide IX, 101–105
    T antigens, 110
E2 region, adenovirus, 87–89
  gene expression, 95–96
  HE1 cells, methylation, 114
  protein products, 98
E2B region, adenovirus, 87–89
E3 region, adenovirus
  gene expression, 95–96
  protein products, 98–99
E4 region, adenovirus, 95–96, 99
Early antigen, EBV
  EcoRI B fragment, expression, 196
  hybrid activation, 198–200
  identification, 184
  infection, 162–164, 169, 194

Early class, HSV-1 mRNA, 240, 242
 complexity effects, 245–246
 promoters, 255–259
 properties, 257–258
Early events, EBV infection, 166–168,
 187
Early region, papillomavirus, 69–71
EB4, T cell effect, versus EBV, 223
EBNA
 antigenic activity, 151
 antigenic reactivity, EBV encoding,
 160–162
 B lymphocytes, 186
 Burkitt's lymphoma cells, 134, 183
 cytotoxic T cells, 219–225
 EBV transformation effect, 191–193
 hybrids, expression, 199–200
Ecogpt, SV40 genome cotransfection, 49
EcoRI sites
 EBV DNA, 143
 function, 195–197
 homology, 150
 polypeptides, infection, 167
 RNA encoding, sequences, 157–158,
 165
 HSV focus formation, 274
 HSV-1 DNA, 241
EcoRI B fragment, 196
EcoRI J fragment, function, 195–196
EcoRI-L fragment, RNA activation,
 HSV, 280
EcoRI M fragment, HSV DNA poly-
 merase encoding, 253
Elongation, DNA binding protein, ade-
 novirus, 94
Envelope polypeptides, EBV, 138–141,
 185–187
Episomal state, papillomaviruses, 65–67,
 73
Epitheliallike carcinoma cells, 200
Epstein-Barr virus
 abortive and productive infections,
 162–169
 antigenic determinants, 139–141, 185–
 187

cytogenetics, 188–191
 DNA, structure and function, 141–
 151, 193–195
 immunology, transformation, 213–233
 antibody role, 229
 cytotoxic T cells, 217–225
 polypeptides, 137–139
 structural components, 137–151
 transformation and replication, 133–
 172, 185–187
 and EBNA, 191–193
 latency, 151–162
 transformation, biology and function,
 183–200
Equine abortion virus, 295
Eukaryotic vectors, papillomavirus, 73–
 75

F4A1A1, HSV DNA sequences, 288–
 290
F5A3B cell line
 growth in methylcellulose, 278
 HSV DNA sequences, 288
 summary and origins, 275–277
F11A1A, integrated HSV DNA se-
 quences, 289–290
F11A2B cells, 275–277
F11B2A cells, 275, 277
F11B2B cells, transfection, 279
F12A2B cells, integrated HSV DNA se-
 quences, 289–290
Fetal-calf-serum-related cytotoxicity,
 221
Fibers, adenovirus location, 85–86
Fibroblast feeder layers, 216–217
FnuDII, H. saimiri DNA methylation,
 318–319
Focus formation, HSV DNA fragments,
 272–275
Fragments, HSV DNA, 288–289; *see
 also specific fragments*

γ Gene expression, HSV-1, 240, 242–
 243, 255–263

Gastrin, tyrosine modification, 21
Gene expression
  adenovirus, 95–98
  EBV hybrids, 198–200
  HSV, basic patterns, 239–243
    mechanism, 260–263
    RNA activation, 279–280
    "typical" gene, 255–263
  papillomavirus, 68
Genetic heterogeneity, papillomaviruses,
  63–64
Genomic organization
  adenovirus, and function, 86–90
  adenovirus DNA integration, transfor-
    mation, 111–113
  H. saimiri, 311–314
  hepatitis B virus, 327
  HSV, 239–241
  papillomaviruses, 61–63
  polyoma virus, 4–8
  retention in transformed cells, HSV,
    287–293
Glucosamine labeling, polypeptides,
  EBV, 138
Glycoprotein A/B
  HSV-1 genome mapping, 252
  morphological transforming regions,
    295
Glycoprotein C, HSV-1 genome map-
  ping, 252
Glycoprotein complex, EBV, 140
Glycoprotein D, HSV-1 genome map-
  ping, 252
gpt gene, papillomavirus vector, 75
Ground squirrel hepatitis B virus, 335
Group N mutants
  adenovirus transformation, 116
  DNA negative mutants, adenovirus,
    94
Growth conditions, transformation in-
  fluence, 9
Guanine phosphoribosyl transferase
  gene, 75
Guanosine, EPV DNA, 145–146

H genomes
  structure, 311–313
  transformed cells, 314–319
H1591 cell line, 315–316
H-2 system, SV40 antitumor T cells,
  33–34
HaeII sites
  Epstein-Barr virus, 147
  H. saimiri DNA CG methylation, 317
Hamster embryo cells
  HSV DNA study, 274–278
  versus BALB/c cells, 278
HAT selection, 290
HBcAg, 330–331
HBsAg, 330–332
HE1, HE2 and HE3 cells lines, methyl-
  ation, 114
Helper T cells, EBV response, 225, 230
Hepatitis B hyperimmune globulin, 329
Hepatitis B virus, 325–339
  animal occurrence, 333–336
  characteristics, 326–329
  molecular biology, 331–333
  and primary hepacellular carcinoma,
    325–329
Hepatocytes, pathogenesis in PHC, 337–
  338
Herpes simplex virus; see also HSV-1;
  HSV-2
  biochemical aspects, transformation,
    271–300
    DNA sequence retention, 287–293
    morphological transforming regions,
      280–286
  and EBV polypeptides, 137–138
  gene expression, 239–243, 260–263
  host cell function effects, 243
  SV40 relationship, transformation,
    300
  transcription patterns, 239–263
Herpesvirus ateles, lymphocyte transformation, 311
Herpesvirus pan
  antigens, 160

DNA, colinearity with EBV, 148–151
polypeptides, and EBV, 141
Herpesvirus papio
   antigens, 160
   DNA, colinearity with EBV, 150
   DNA, comparison, 148–151
   polypeptides and EBV, 141
Herpesvirus saimiri
   advantages, 307–308
   background, 308–311
   DNA, transformed cells, 314–321
   nononcogenic variants, 313–314
   oncogenic transformation, 307–321
   tumor induction, selected species, 309
   virion DNA structure, 311–314
Hexon, adenovirus, 85–86, 90
HF3 cells, 277–278
HG-52 infection, 297
High-resolution mapping, HSV-1, 248–251
HindIII fragments
   HSV, focus formation, 274
   HSV-1 DNA, 241
      encoding, 248, 251, 259–260, 262
   HSV-2, mtr correspondence, 252–253
   HVPapio DNA, EBV colinearity, 150
   pBR322 cloning, HSV-1, 244
HindIII-G, adenovirus transformation, 101, 110
HindIII-J, 254
HindIII-K
   early mRNA mapping, promoters, 255–256
   HSV-1 mRNA species, 244–246, 248, 251, 262
   mRNA family generation, HSV, 259–260
HindIII-L
   mRNA families, HSV, 259
   transcription initiation, HSV, 262
HL-60, Burkitt's lymphoma hybrid, 197
HLA antigens, EBV, 186, 198, 223–224
Host-range mutants, *see* hr-t mutants

Hpa I cleavage, HSV-1 DNA, 241
HpaI-E transformed cells, 100–101
HpaII
   EBV DNA cleavage, Raji cells, 153–154
   H. saimiri cleavage pattern, 317–318
hr-I genome, 13S mRNA encoding, adenovirus, 115
hr-t mutants
   adenovirus, transformation, 114–115
   polyoma virus, 6–8, 11, 21–22
HSB2 cells, T cell effect, versus EBV, 223
HSV-1
   DNA transforming origins, 280–286
   focus formation, DNA fragments, 272–275
   gene expression, 239–243
   HSV-2 genome homology, transformation, 282–285
   morphological transformation, 252–255
   transcription patterns, 239–263
   "typical" gene, 255–263
HSV-2
   BglII-N fragment, coding, 283–286
   ClaI site, BglII-I fragment, 280–281
   focus formation, DNA fragments, 272–275
   HSV-1 genome homology, transformation, 282–285
   integrated DNA sequences, 293–295
   mammalian cell genome homology, 286
   morphological transformation, 252–255
   mtr identification, 299
   mtr-I equivalent, transformation, 281–283
   polypeptides, transformation, 293–299
Human adenovirus
   subdivisions, 84–86
   transforming region comparison, 105–107

Human embryonic cells, adenovirus, 114

Human papillomavirus
  capsid, 61–63
  genome, 61–63, 71
  malignant transformation, 59
  physical map, 64–65
  sequences, BPV-1 comparison, 71–73
  structure, 69–71
  subtypes, 60
  viral DNA, 66

HVPapio, *see* Herpesvirus papio

Hybrid arrested translation techniques, 254

Hybrid cells
  Burkitt's lymphoma, 197–198
  Herpesvirus saimiri, 316
  HSV DNA retention, tumors, 287–293
  viral expression, EBV, 198–200

i leader, adenovirus mRNA, 89, 98

Ia antigens, Burkitt's lymphoma, 197

IB4 cells, EBV studies, 155–156, 159

ICP4 protein, HSV-1 mRNA coding, 251–252, 262

ICP-7 protein, mtr-III region, 286

ICP-8 protein, 128K protein relationship, 295

ICP-10, mtr-II region, 285–286

"Icron," 333

ICSP-11/12 polypeptide, 295, 297

IgM
  B lymphocytes, EBV, 186
  Burkitt's lymphoma cells, 188, 197

Immediate-early HSV-1 mRNA, 240, 242
  BglII-I fragment relationship, 281
  biological marker correlation, 251–253
  control regions, 255–259
  properties, 257–258

Immortalization
  adenovirus genes, 101
  polyoma virus, T antigens, 24

"Immune inhibition," EBV B cells, 226–228

Immunoglobulins
  B lymphocytes, EBV, 186
  EBV infection effects, 187

Immunology
  Epstein-Barr virus transformation, 213–233
  SV40 large T antigen, 32–37

Immunosuppression, EBV manifestations, 133–135

Infectious mononucleosis; *see also* Epstein-Barr virus
  EBV relationship, 184–185
  immune response, 221
  T cells, 229–230

Initiation
  adenovirus DNA, 93–94
  HSV mRNA, 258, 262
  large T antigen, polyoma virus, 12–14

Interferon, EBV delayed transformation, 215–216

5-Iodo-2-deoxyuridine, 164, 198–200

IR1, Epstein-Barr virus
  DNA sequence, 142–146
  HpaII resistance, Raji cells, 153–157
  RNA encoding, 157–158

IR2, Epstein-Barr virus, 147, 157–158

IR3, Epstein-Barr virus, 147, 155–156

Isolation, HSV-1 mRNA, 243–248

Jijoye cell line, 146–148, 185

19K protein, adenovirus product, 99

21K protein, adenovirus oncogenesis, 110, 115

35/38 protein, HSV mtr, 297–298

45K protein, EBV-infected B cells, LYDMA, 224

48K protein, transformation role, EBNA, 192

53K protein, 191–193

54K protein, 111

55K protein
  adenovirus transformation role, 110
  mutant encoding, 115

56K protein, polyoma virus transformation, 192–193
72K DNA binding protein
adenovirus replication, 93–94
mRNA regulation, 96
as T antigen, 107
128K DNA binding protein, HSV mtr relationship, 293–295
140K protein, 298
K562 hybrid
characterization, 197–198
T cell effect, versus EBV, 223
Kappa chains, Burkitt's lymphoma hybrids, 197
Kinase, *see* Protein kinase
KOS strain, HSV, 240

L-DNA, herpes saimiri, 311–314
L segment, HSV genome
equine abortion virus genome, 295
transformation regions, 274–275
tumor RNA, 288
L th+ cell line, 291–294, 299
L1 protein
coding sequences, 72, 74
papillomavirus, 69
L2 protein, papillomavirus, 69
Lactoperoxidase iodination, 36
Lambda chains, Burkitt's lymphoma hybrids, 197
Large T antigen, polyoma virus
analysis, 5–8
biochemical basis, action, 23–24
dihydrofolate reductase gene amplification, 49
kinase activity, 16
SV40 comparison, 8
transformation, genetics, 10–11
initiation role, 12–14
Large T antigen, SV40
biochemical reactions, 32
cell surface, immunology, 33–37
DNA replication and transcription, 50–52, 191

DNA sequence interaction, 37–45
mutation binding, affinities, 44–45
origin binding, 39–43
EBNA similarity, 191–192, 224
novel derivatives, transformed cells, 47–50
polyoma virus comparison, 8
structure and function, 31–52
subsets and forms, 45–47
Late polypeptides, EBV infection, 168
Late region
adenovirus, 89–90, 97–98
papillomavirus, structure, 69–70
Late DNA expression
EBV infection, 166–167
HSV-1, 240, 242–243, 246
control regions, 255–258
Late suppression, 225–228
Latency phase
EBV expression, 151–162, 171
HSV infection, biological marker, 253
LCL lines, EBV
cytogenetics, 188–191
infection, 187–188
T cell response, 184
"Leaky late" mRNA, HSV-1, 243, 251, 255–263
Leukocytes, lymphokine release, EBV, 217
LH$_1$X$_2$ cell line, 291–292
LH$_2$p136 cell lines, 293–295, 297–299
"Light" form, SV40 large T antigen, 45
Localization, HSV-1 mRNA, 243–248
Long unique region
HSV genome, 240–241
HSV morphological transformation, 252–253
LTR promoter, 272
LYDMA antigen
cytotoxic T cell precursors, 232
EBV, 171, 184, 187
T cell response, EBV regression, 221, 224

Lymphoblastoid cell lines, *see* LCL line, EBV

Lymphocyte-derived membrane antigen, 151

Lymphocytes
EcoRI J fragment, 195–197
H. saimiri transformation, 311

Lymphoid cell lines, EBV infection, 187–188

Lymphokines, EBV transformation inhibition, 217

Lymphomas, *see* Burkitt's lymphoma

M genomes, 311–319

"Major late promoter," adenovirus, 90

Malic enzyme, Burkitt's lymphoma cells, 198

"Manley" polymerase system, 262

Mapping
HSV focus formation regions, 274–275
HSV-1 mRNAs, 240, 248–251
polyoma virus middle T, 20–22

Mastomys natalensis papillomavirus, 59

Membrane antigen complex, EBV, 162–164, 184, 229

Methylation
adenovirus integrated viral sequences, 113–114
EBV DNA, Raji cells, 153–154
herpes virus saimiri DNA, 316–320
papillomavirus, DNA, CpG sites, 67

Methylcellulose, cell line growth, 278

5-Methylcytosine, 316–317

Methylmercury agarose gel electrophoresis, 248–249

β_2-microglobulin, 198, 224

Microinjections
EBNA, DNA synthesis, 192
HSV-1 mRNA translation, 246–248
SV40 genome, nuclei, 50–51

Middle T antigen, polyoma virus
analysis, 5–8
biochemical properties, 14–23
minor forms, 23

and SV40, 8
transformation, 3–25, 192–193

Middle T mutants, polyoma virus, 21–22

Minichromosomal structure, papillomavirus, 62–63

Mitomycin C, T cell effect, EBV, 219, 222

mKSA, immunology, BALB/c mice, 33–34

ml-t mutants, polyoma virus, 7–8, 11, 16, 21–22

Moderate resolution map, HSV-1 mRNAs, 240, 248

Molecular cloning, papillomavirus genomes, 63–65

Molt-4 T cell, EBV adsorption, 186

Monoclonal antibodies
Burkitt's lymphoma cells, 188
EBV antigen recognition, 140
HSV transformation antigens, 298–299
38K protein, HSV-2, 298
LYDMA, 224
middle T, 15, 23
SV40 large T antigen, cell surface, 35
SV40 large T antigen, subset definition, 46–47

MOP 1033, 22

Morphological transformation regions, *see* Mtr-1; Mtr-2; Mtr-3

MspI
EBV DNA cleavage, Raji cells, 153–154
H. saimiri cleavage pattern, 317–318

Mtr-1 region; *see also* BglII-I
cell line variation, 275–277
characterization, 280–286
HSV mapping, 252–253
location, 274–275
HSV-1 role, 299
retention in L tk + cell lines, 291–292
transfection, NIH 3T3 cells, 279–280
transformation role, 293–297
tumor RNA, HSV, 288

Mtr-2 region; *see also* BglII-N
  HSV mapping, 252–253
    location, 274–275
  HSV-2 role, 299–298
  integration in F4A1A1 cells, 290
  LH₂ p136 L th+ cells, 294–295
  physical map and coding, 283–285
  transfection, NIH 3T3 cells, 279
  tumor RNA, HSV, 288
Mtr-III region
  coding and cell DNA homology, 285
  location, 274–275
  transfection, 280
Mutants, viral; *see also specific mutants*
  polyoma virus, 6–8
  SV40 large T antigen, 44, 48, 50–52
Myeloma cells, 188

N mutants, *see* Group N mutants
N-terminal, SV40 large T antigen, 34,
  49–50
Namalwa cells, viral DNA, EBV, 153,
  155
Nasopharyngeal cancer
  and Burkitt's lymphoma hybrids, 200
  epidemiology, EBV relationship, 136
  Epstein-Barr virus DNA, 153
Natural killer cells, EBV, 216, 229–230
New Zealand white rabbit, 309
NG-59 mutant, 21–22
NIH 3T3 cells
  characterization, 277–278
  transfection, HSV, 279
NK cells, EBV, 216, 299–230
Northern blots, HSV mRNA, 246–247
Nucleocapsids, EBV polypeptides, 138–
  140

Oligo(dt)-primed cDNA, 157–160
"Oncogenes," 272
"One-hit" kinetics, EBV, 186
Origins, DNA
  EBV DNA replication, 145
  SV40 large T antigen, 39–43, 50–52
Oropharynx, EBV, 231

Owl monkey kidney cells, 309–310,
  312–313

P3HR-1 clone
  DNA, comparative study, 146–148
  DNA, transformation, 154–155
  polypeptides, 137–139
  Raji cell line infection, 137, 163–169
  receptors, EBV, 185
  viral DNA sequence deletion, 142
p53 protein, SV40, 36, 46–47
Papillomavirus, 59–76
  bovine, *see* Bovine papillomavirus
  characterization, 63–65
  eukaryotic vector use, 73–75
  human, *see* Human papillomavirus
  molecular cloning, 63–65
  sequence studies and organization, 69–
    73
  state and expression, host cell, 65–68
  structural properties, 61–63
Papovavirus, EBV sequence homology,
  145
PBASCOMP program, 72
Penton base, adenovirus location, 85–86
Periodic-acid-Schiff staining, 138
Permissive phase, EBV expression, 171
"Persistent" polypeptides, 168
pBR322
  EBV DNA cloning, pkH47, 159
  HSV transformed lines, 293
  HSV-1 HindIII fragment cloning, 244
  as shuttle vector, papillomavirus, 73–
    75
pDG401
  BglII-N, map, 284
  focus formation, HSV-2, 274, 278
pGR62 DNA, 284, 293
pGR136 plasmid, 292–294
pGR236 plasmid, 292–293
Philadelphia chromosome, 190
Phosphonoacetic acid
  EBV DNA inhibition, 140, 151–152
  transformation block, 186

Phosphonoformic acid, EBV DNA replication inhibition, 151–152
Phosphorylation regulation
  adenovirus E1B polypeptides, 110–111
  EBV polypeptides, 168
  hepatitis B virus, 328
  middle T, polyoma virus, 15–25
Phosphotyrosine, 16–17, 20–21
pkH47, EBV RNA study, 159
Plasma membrane
  EBV antigenic polypeptide, 139–141
  polyoma virus middle T, 18–25
Plasmids, *see specific plasmids*
"Poison" sequences, 293
Polyadenylation sites, HSV, 259–260
Polyoma virus
  versus EBV, transformation, 192–193
  gene associations, transformation, 10–14
  genomic organization, 4–8
  versus papillomavirus, genome, 69
  SV40 comparison, 8
  transformation properties, biochemistry, 3–25
Polypeptide IX, adenovirus, 101–105
Polypeptide synthesis; *see also specific polypeptides*
  adenovirus, 87–89
  EBV, 137–141, 161–162
pp60src, *see* Rous sarcoma virus
Preproinsulin, papillomavirus, 73, 75
Primary hepatocellular carcinoma, 325–339
  clinical and pathological features, 326
  hepatitis B virus biology, 331–333
  prevalence and distribution, 325
Primates
  EBV DNA comparison, 148–150
  H. saimiri tumor induction, 309–310
Productive infections, EBV, 162–169
Promoters
  adenovirus, 87–90, 100
  hepatitis B virus, hypothesis, 336
  HSV-1 genes, 255–259
  polypeptide IX, 105

Protein kinase activity
  adenovirus transformed cells, 110–111
  EBNA, 192
  hepatitis B virus, 328
  middle T, polyoma virus, 15–20
  SV40 large T antigen, 45
Proteins; *see also* K proteins
  Epstein-Barr virus transformed cells, 160–162
  polyoma virus, 5–6
  productive and abortive infections, EBV, 166–169
Pseudorabies virus, 241
Pulse-chase experiments, SV40 large T antigen, 46
PvuII fragment, 294–295

R antigen, 184
R cells, primary hepatocellular carcinoma, 337–338
R6T, SV40 DNA interactions, 41–42
Raji cell line
  EBV DNA, 153–155
  EBV RNA, 159
  hybrids, viral expression, 198–200
  P3HR-1 infection, 137, 148, 163–169, 194
ras gene, papillomavirus vector, 73
Rat preproinsulin, 73–75
Rat-1 cells, middle-T antigen transformation, 13
Rat-3T3 cells, *see* 3T3 cells
Receptors, EBV, 185–187
Reciprocal translocation, 189–190
Recognition, EBV, 185–187
Regression of transformation, 217–228
Restriction endonuclease; *see also specific endonucleases*
  EBV, DNA, 146, 149, 154
  HSV-1 DNA, 241
"Restringent," EBV infection, B lymphocytes, 152
Revertants, ad12-transformed cells, 113
Rheumatoid-arthritis-associated nuclear antigen, 161–162

RNA; *see also* mRNA
  abortive and productive infections, EBV, 163–168
  detection by hybridization, HSV, 287–288
  EBV, transformation, 156–160
  H. saimiri, 319
  hepatitis B virus, 327–328
cRNA derivatives, SV40, 42–43
RNA-protein complexes, adenovirus, 91
RNA polymerase II, HSV DNA, 262–263
RNA polymerase III, adenovirus, 90
mRNA
  adenovirus, early gene expression, 95–97
  adenovirus, genome relationship, 86–90
  adenovirus transforming regions, 101–107
    mutant encoding, 115–116
    structures, 102
  EBV, transformation, 156–160
  HSV genome location, 282–283
  HSV-1 infection, 239-243, 262
    isolation and translation, 243–248
    promoters, 255–259
  papillomavirus, transcription, 67–68
  polyoma virus, 5–6
  SV40 large T antigen, 40–41
9SmRNA, T antigen encoding, 109
12SmRNA, adenovirus, 108, 112, 115–116
13SmRNA, adenovirus
  E1 region coding, 103–104
  hr-I genome encoding, 115–116
  T antigen encoding, 107–110
22SmRNA, adenovirus, 103–104, 107, 109
snRNPs (RNA-protein complexes), 91
Rous sarcoma virus
  phosphotyrosine levels, transformation, 17
  plasma membrane, transforming protein, 20
  tyrosine modification, amino acids, 21

S cells, primary hepatocellular carcinoma, 337–338
S1 digests, HSV 1, mRNA location, 248–251
S295C strain, H. saimiri, 310, 312–313
Sa/I, linkage map, EBV homology, 150
Saguinus species, H. saimiri tumor induction, 309
SD-15 mutant, 21–22
Serotype 12, adenovirus genome integration, 112
Shared promoters, HSV, 259–260
Shope cottontail rabbit papillomavirus, 59, 61–63, 66–67
Short unique region, HSV-1 genome, 240–241
Simian virus 40, 31–52
  A gene, 94
  Epstein-Barr virus similarities, 192
  functional map, 38
  and human papillomavirus, genome, 69
  large T antigen, structure and function, 31–52
    cell surface, immunology, 33–37
    DNA interactions, 37–45
  polyoma virus comparison, 8
  subsets, 45–47
SmaI, H. saimiri DNA methylation, 317
Small T antigen, polyoma virus
  analysis, 5–8
  biochemical basis, action, 23–24
  kinase activity, 16
  SV40 comparison, 8, 14
  transformation, 14
SMHI strain, 312–313
SMHIatt, 313–314
Sodium butyrate, EBV infection, 162–163
Squirrel monkey, H. saimiri, 308
SSt1 enzyme, recognition site, 147
Strain-variation hypothesis
  African Burkitt-lymphoma, 135–136
  viral DNA, Burkitt's lymphoma, 141, 146, 150

Strand-displacement synthesis, 91–92
Subgroup C adenoviruses, 103–104
Super T antigens, SV40, 47–48
Suppressor T cells, EBV infection, 229–232
"Surface T," SV40, 36
SV40, *see* Simian virus 40
SVRE9, 38, 48
SV3T3-20-G
  function, SV40 large T antigen, 38
  truncated SV40 T-antigen template, 49–50
SV3T3-20-K, function, SV40 large T antigen, 38
SV3T3-38-D, 38, 48
SV80, mutant large T antigens, 48
SVE 5Kb, 38
"Switch on," 128K protein, 295

T-antigen-origin binding, 39–40
T antigens
  adenovirus, 107–110
  EBNA resemblance, 183
  polyoma virus, 5–8
T(R6T), 38
T cell growth factor cells
  cyclospin A effect override, 225
  EBV transformed cell effect, 219
T cells; *see also* Cytotoxic T cells
  EBV delayed transformation, 215, 229–232
  EBV transformation late suppression, 225–228
  EBV transformation regression, 217–225
  H. saimiri infection, 311
3T3 cells, 13; *see also* NIH 3T3 cells
TATA box, HSV mRNA, 260
Terminal protein, adenovirus DNA, 91–93
Terminal repeats, EBV, 142–143, 149–150, 154
5′ termini shift, mRNAs, SV40, 40–41
12-O-tetra-decanoylphorbol-12-acetate, *see* TPA

Tg cells, 219–221
333-8-9 cells, 287
Thymidine, EBV DNA, 145–146
Thymidine kinase gene
  BglII-I fragment relationship, 280–281
  EBV coding, 196
  HSV mtr involvement, 290–295, 299
  HSV-1 marker use, 253–254
  nucleotide sequences, HSV-1, 257–258
  retention in transformed cells, HSV, 287
  SV40, large T antigen, 51
  transcription, HSV, 262
TPA (12-O-tetra-decanoylphorbol-12-acetate)
  EBV infection, 162–163, 166
  H. saimiri DNA methylation, 318–319
Transcription, *see* Viral transcription
Transfection, HSV DNA fragments, 272–280
Translation, HSV-1 mRNA species, 243–248, 251–255
Translocation, Burkitt's lymphoma, 189–190
Transposition plasmid pGR136, 293
Transposon Th5, 75
Trisomy, EBV cell lines, 189
13 trisomy, 112–113
"True-late" mRNAs, HSV-1, 255–263
Truncated T antigens, SV40, 49–50
ts7 mutation, mtr-III, HSV genome, 286
ts125 mutation, adenovirus, 94
H5ts125 mutation, adenovirus genome integration, 112
ts mutation ad2ts206, 98
ts mutations, SV40, 38
ts-a mutations, polyoma virus, 6–8
  kinase activity, 16–17
  transformation genetics, 11, 13
TSTA, LYDMA similarity, 224
Tumor-specific transplantation antigen
  and 19K protein, 99
  SV40, 34, 36

293 cell line, adenovirus transformation, 114
Tyrosine, middle T phosphorylation, 16–17, 20–21
Tyrosine 315, 20–22

U1 region, structure, 142–143
U2 region
  P3HR-1 virus DNA, transformation, 148
  RNA encoding, 157–158
  structure, 142–143
U3. . .U5 regions
  linkage, IB4 and Namalwa cells, 155–156
  RNA encoding, 157–158
  structure, 142
U698 cell, receptor defect, 185
UL region, structure, 142–143
Ultraviolet irradiation, HSV DNA, 287
Unique regions; see also specific regions
  EBV DNA, 142–143, 155–156
  linkage, Namalwa and IB4 cells, 155–156
  RNA encoding, 157–158
US region, structure, 142–143

Vectors, eukaryotic, papillomavirus, 73–75
Viral capsid antigen; see also Capsid
  EBV infection, 162–163
  hybrid activation, EBV, 198–200
  identification, 184
  polypeptides, EBV, 140–141
Viral envelope, EBV, polypeptides, 138–141

Viral gene expression, see Gene expression
Viral transcription
  adenovirus, 86–90
    expression, 95–98
    transformation, 101–103
  Epstein-Barr virus, 156–160
  papillomavirus genomes, 67–68
  SV40 large T antigen, 40
Viral transformation, see under specific viruses
Virion
  adenovirus, 86
  hepatitis B virus, 326–327
  H. saimiri, 311–314
VP22 HSV-1 gene product, 252

W91 clone, DNA studies, 141
Woodchuck hepatitis virus, 333–334, 338

XbaI cleavage
  HVPapio DNA, EBV colinearity, 150
  HSV-1, 241
  HSV-1(F)DNA, focus formation, 273–274
XhoI fragment W, 244–245

y leader, adenovirus mRNA, 89

z leader, adenovirus mRNA, 89
Zinkernagel-Doherty phenomenon, 19K protein, 99
Zonal sedimentation, SV40 large T antigen, 45–46